Guide to Antimicrobial Use in Animals

Guide to Antimicrobial Use in Animals

Edited by

Luca Guardabassi

Department of Veterinary Pathobiology
Faculty of Life Sciences
University of Copenhagen
Denmark

Lars B. Jensen

National Food Institute
Technical University of Denmark
Denmark

Hilde Kruse

Department for Health Surveillance
National Veterinary Institute
Norway

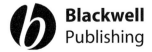
Blackwell
Publishing

Blackwell Publishing editorial offices:
Blackwell Publishing Ltd, 9600 Garsington Road, Oxford OX4 2DQ, UK
Tel: +44 (0)1865 776868
Blackwell Publishing Professional, 2121 State Avenue, Ames, Iowa 50014-8300, USA
Tel: +1 515 292 0140
Blackwell Publishing Asia Pty Ltd, 550 Swanston Street, Carlton, Victoria 3053, Australia
Tel: +61 (0)3 8359 1011

First published 2008 by Blackwell Publishing Ltd

ISBN: 9781405150798

Library of Congress Cataloging-in-Publication Data

Guide to antimicrobial use in animals/edited by Luca Guardabassi,
Lars Bogø Jensen, Hilde Kruse.
    p. ; cm.
Includes bibliographical references and index.
ISBN-13: 978-1-4051-5079-8 (hardback : alk. paper)
ISBN-10: 1-4051-5079-3 (hardback : alk. paper)
1. Anti-infective agents in veterinary medicine. 2. Drug resistance
in microorganisms. I. Guardabassi, Luca. II. Jensen, Lars Bogø.
III. Kruse, Hilde.
[DNLM: 1. Anti-Infective Agents–therapeutic use. 2. Drug
Therapy–veterinary. 3. Animals, Domestic. 4. Anti-Infective
Agents–adverse effects. 5. Anti-Infective Agents–standards. 6. Drug
Resistance, Microbial. SF 918.A48 G946 2008]
SF918.A48G85 2008
636.089′69041–dc22

2007036834

A catalogue record for this title is available from the British Library

Set in 9.5/11.5 Minion by Newgen Imaging Systems Pvt. Ltd., Chennai, India
Printed and bound in Singapore by Fabulous Printers Pte Ltd

The publisher's policy is to use permanent paper from mills that operate a sustainable forestry policy, and which has been manufactured from pulp processed using acid-free and elementary chlorine-free practices. Furthermore, the publisher ensures that the text paper and cover board used have met acceptable environmental accreditation standards.

For further information on Blackwell Publishing, visit our website:
www.BlackwellVet.com

CONTENTS

FOREWORD

It is a pleasure to be invited to write a foreword for a book which will provide vital information for one of the commonest activities in veterinary practice, the prescription of antimicrobial agents. This is a process which easily becomes routine, but can often lead to suboptimal use and enhanced risk of generation of antimicrobial resistance, not only amongst the pathogens causing the current disease, but also in non-pathogenic microbes which may then act as reservoirs of resistance genes.

One of my heroes in the field of medicine is Ignac Semmelweis who recognised, in 1847, the value of washing and disinfection in the control of puerperal fever, a cause of much death at that time in women admitted to obstetrical wards with dystochia. He was not aware of how his methods worked and his disinfection methods were resented by busy clinicians; despite evidence that they were very effective in reducing mortality, it was some time before they were widely adopted. Indeed it was only after the existence of bacteria had been demonstrated by Louis Pasteur that surgeons began to recognise how infection occurred and started to develop efficient methods to combat sepsis. Joseph Lister was at the forefront of this technology and his paper in *The Lancet* in 1867 (1) on 'Illustration of the antiseptic system of treatment in surgery' was a landmark in the use of antimicrobial agents in the battle against infection.

By the early years of the 20th Century Lister's disinfection methods were rather discredited in surgery where the focus was now on asepsis. However, increasing numbers of substances were now being investigated and developed for the treatment of established infections. Most significant amongst these studies was the work of Paul Ehrlich and his development, in 1909, of Salvarsan as an effective treatment for syphilis. He coined the term 'chemotherapy' and his work stimulated a search for other effective antimicrobial

substances for the treatment of infectious disease. The breakthrough occurred in the 1930s when Gerhard Domagk developed Prontosil and showed that it was effective in human streptococcal septicaemia. Although Prontosil was protected by patents, it was soon recognised that it was broken down in the body to release sulfanilamide, which was not patented, and this opened the way for the development of the sulfonamides and their application in a wide variety of bacterial infections.

Although Lister is best known for his advocacy of phenol (carbolic acid), he also recognised that fungal extracts could inactivate infections and used them to irrigate wounds. Thus Lister began to use what we subsequently came to know as antibiotic some 60 years prior to Alexander Flemming's description in the *British Journal of Experimental Pathology* in 1929 (2) of the antibacterial action of extracts of the mould, *Penicillium notatum*. Although Flemming showed that his extract could be used to treat infection, he failed to obtain support enabling him to exploit his discovery. It was a decade later that the combined talents of the biochemist, Ernest Chain and pharmacologist, Howard Florey, led to the development in the 1940s of methods that could be used for the production of amounts useful in the treatment of human infection.

Alexander Flemming reviewed the development and use of antimicrobials in a lecture entitled 'Chemotherapy: yesterday, today and tomorrow', which he delivered in 1946 (3). He commented on the huge advances that had been made in the chemotherapy of bacterial infection during the past 10 years. These advances continued apace and resulted in the wide range of antimicrobial agents which we now have available. Flemming commented on the problem of bacterial resistance and the promotion of such resistance by the misuse of antimicrobials. He expressed the hope that, as it became more widely available, penicillin would not be abused as the sulfonamides had been. Interestingly, he looked forward to the use of penicillin in veterinary medicine.

Veterinary use of antimicrobials is now very substantial in all fields of animal industry, in pets and in animal conservation. Veterinarians face the dual problems of developing antimicrobial resistance and concerns from human medicine about the potential for animal use to drive this process and make human products less effective. This is of course a two-way process, but veterinary treatment is already prejudiced by the appearance of organisms such as multi-resistant *Staphylococcus aureus*, *Escherichia coli* and *Pseudomonas aeruginosa*. The appearance of multi-resistant *S. intermedius* and its recognition now in both North America and in Europe is a particular concern. With a lack of new and potent antimicrobials in the pipeline we are facing a crisis which can only be faced by much wiser use of the drugs that we have.

The *Guide to Antimicrobial Use in Animals*, therefore, arrives at a very opportune time, providing a comprehensive analysis of the problems and solutions relating to the veterinary use of antimicrobials. The very approachable format allowing easy reference will make it convenient for use in veterinary practice.

The ample supporting material explaining and justifying the recommendations will also enable clinicians and others using antimicrobial agents to make well-informed decisions. It is to be hoped that this book will become an essential reference in both small and large animal practice, helping veterinarians to optimise their antimicrobial treatment practices and protocols. Were they still with us, I am sure that Semmelweis, Lister and Flemming would join me in applauding its publication.

David Lloyd
December 2007

References

1. Lister, J. (1867). Illustration of the antiseptic system of treatment in surgery. *The Lancet*, Sept. 21st, 1867, p. 354.
2. Fleming, A. (1929). On the antibacterial action of cultures of a penicillium with special reference to their use in the isolation of *B. influenzae*. *British Journal of Experimental Pathology* **10**: 226–36.
3. Flemming, A. (1946). Chemotherapy: yesterday today and tomorrow. Reprinted in *Fifty Years of Antimicrobials: Past Perspectives and Future Trends* (eds. Hunter, P.A., Darby, G.K., Russell, N.J.) Cambridge University Press, Cambridge, 1995, pp. 1–18.

PREFACE

In 1968, the government of the UK appointed a Joint Committee led by Professor Michael Swann to obtain information about the use of antimicrobial agents in animal husbandry and veterinary medicine, to consider the implications for human and animal health, and to make recommendations based on evidence sought from published work, from public and private organizations, professional bodies, trade associations, research workers and other interested parties. This was the first historical attempt to provide guidelines for antimicrobial use in animals, with particular focus on the use of growth promoters in animal production. In the report presented to parliament, the Joint Committee emphasized the importance of independent information being available to the veterinary profession. They wrote: 'We were often conscious of the relative paucity of independent sources of advice, particularly of advice based on critical observation, on the proper use of antibiotics and the dangers of misusing them. The availability of such independent advice, and of vigorous professional discussion and continuing postgraduate education, can do nothing but good and is an important factor in the maintenance of responsible professional attitudes'. Forty years after the publication of the Swann report, there is still a need for unbiased scientific advice on antimicrobial use in animals. This topic is controversial due to the complexity of antimicrobial drug resistance as a biological phenomenon, the paucity of scientific data on how to minimize the negative consequences of antimicrobial therapy on resistance development, and the difficulty in assessing the actual impact of antimicrobial use in animals to resistance problems in human medicine. The topic is also particularly subject to multiple opinions and divergence as it involves ethical issues on animal welfare and human health as well as economic interests by the pharmaceutical industry, the food industry and various professional categories, including farmers, veterinarians, pharmacists and researchers. As a consequence of all these factors, the debate on antimicrobial use in animals is often vigorous and not always scientific and unbiased.

The present book was conceived to provide independent advice and to promote continuing postgraduate education on antimicrobial use in animals. Prudent and rational antimicrobial use is a part of good veterinary practice and recognizing the human and animal health importance of antimicrobial agents and the need to preserve their efficacy has become an important aspect of the veterinary profession. The book represents an attempt to convert theoretical notions of prudent and rational antimicrobial use into a set of animal- and disease-specific guidelines for antimicrobial use covering both companion animals and food-producing animals, including aquaculture. In order to ensure the necessary multidisciplinary expertise and the required independence and impartiality for this difficult task, the contributors were selected from international experts from different backgrounds, including academics and researchers in the areas of veterinary clinical medicine, pharmacology, microbiology and epidemiology, members of national or international public health organizations, and farm consultants. In case of any controversies, the contributors made efforts to reach consensus or to compromise between divergent positions.

The book is composed of six general chapters and six specific chapters on antimicrobial use in swine, poultry, cattle, horses, small animals and aquaculture. The general principles of prudent and rational antimicrobial use in animals introduced in Chapter 1 form the basis of the guidelines presented in the book. Chapter 2 provides a thorough description and presents evidence of the risks to human health associated with antimicrobial use in animals. Chapter 3 emphasizes the importance of antimicrobial resistance risk assessment in developing policies and implementing guidelines on antimicrobial use in animals.

Chapter 4 summarizes the most serious resistance problems in human medicine and provides up-to-date classification of antimicrobial drugs based on their clinical importance in human medicine. Chapter 5 is an overview of the present legislation on antimicrobial use in animals in Australia, the USA, the EU and Japan. Treatment strategies aimed at minimizing resistance development in animals are delineated in Chapter 6. The following six chapters are dedicated to specific animal groups and contain tables indicating the drugs of choice for treating common bacterial diseases. Each of these chapters were given authority by a multidisciplinary team of experts in complementary disciplines. The antimicrobial choices proposed in the tables are inspired by the need for preserving the efficacy of clinically important antimicrobials and do not necessarily reflect the current trends in antimicrobial prescription and usage.

The final product is a practically oriented reference on the use of antimicrobial agents in animals.

As such, the book targets veterinary practitioners, lecturers and students at veterinary universities and other interested readers. We hope that the book is readable and enjoyable for such a broad audience and can serve as a reference on this important topic. A number of references are listed at the end of each chapter for those interested in additional information and greater depth in a particular topic. The use of tables has been maximized and the layout of the chapters has been designed to ensure easy and rapid consultation in veterinary practice. The editors trust that the guidelines presented in the book will be useful in supporting decisions on antimicrobial use by veterinarians. Obviously, the guidelines should not be considered a limitation of clinical freedom or a substitute for veterinary judgment, but rather a valuable source of scientific advice that veterinarians can consult when taking decisions on antimicrobial use.

The book 'can do nothing but good', Professor Michael Swann would say.

ACKNOWLEDGEMENTS

This book would have never been realized without the contributions by 38 authors representing 14 countries and 5 continents. We are indebted to all of them for their excellent work. Their names and affiliations are listed in the List of Contributors. A special acknowledgement is due to Professor Ove Svendsen, who passed away during the production of the book. We will all miss him.

The editors also wish to acknowledge the constructive comments by many international experts who kindly agreed to review the individual manuscripts: Rohana Subasinghe, Food and Agriculture Organization of the UN; Morten Sichlau Bruun and Inger Dalsgaard, Danish Institute for Fisheries Research; Paula Fedorka-Cray, USDAARS-Antimicrobial Resistance Research Unit; Bruno Gonzalez-Zorn, Universidad Complutense de Madrid, Spain; Erik Jacobsen and Henrik Casper Wegener, Danish Technical University; David Lloyd, Royal Veterinary College, UK; Henrik Christian Lundegaard, Ansager Veterinary Hospital, Denmark; Jens Peter Nielsen and Karl Pedersen, University of Copenhagen, Denmark; Mark Papich, North Carolina University, USA; Satu Pyörälä, University of Helsinki, Finland; Stefan Schwarz, Bundesforschungsanstalt für Landwirtschaft, Germany; Arnfinn Sundsfjord, University of Tromsø, Norway; Linda Tollefson, US Food and Drug Administration; Pier Louis Toutain, Ecole Nationale Vétérinaire, Toulouse, France; Neil Woodford, Health Protection Agency, UK; Olav Østerås and Henning Sørum, The Norwegian School of Veterinary Science.

The staff at Blackwell assisted us with their expertise in the publication of this book. Special thanks to the Commissioning Editors Samantha Jackson and Justinia Wood, their assistants Adam Burbage and Sophie Gillanders, and the Senior Production Editor Emma Lonie. Thanks also to the team at Newgen Imaging Systems for the editing and production of the book.

CONTRIBUTORS

Frank M. Aarestrup
National Food Institute
Technical University of Denmark
Copenhagen
Denmark
Email: faa@food.dtu.dk

Awa Aidara-Kane
Department of Food Safety, Zoonoses & Foodborne
    Diseases
World Health Organization
Geneve
Switzerland
Email: aidarakanea@who.int

Frederick J. Angulo
Division of Foodborne, Bacterial and Mycotic
    Diseases
National Center for Zoonotic, Vectorborne, and
    Enteric Diseases
Centers for Disease Control and Prevention
Atlanta, GA
USA
Email: fja0@cdc.gov

Keith Edward Baptiste
Department of Large Animal Sciences
Faculty of Life Sciences
University of Copenhagen
Denmark
Email: keb@kvl.dk

Viveca Baverud
Department of Bacteriology
National Veterinary Institute
Uppsala, Sweden
Email: viveca.baverud@telia.com

David G. S. Burch
Octagon Services Ltd
Old Windsor, Berkshire
UK
Email: D.Burch@Octagon-Services.Demon.Co.Uk

Peter Collignon
Canberra Clinical School
Australian National University
Canberra
Australia
Email: Peter.Collignon@act.gov.au

Peter D. Constable
Department of Veterinary Clinical Sciences
School of Veterinary Medicine
Purdue University
West Lafayette, IN
USA
Email: constabl@purdue.edu

Flavio Corsin
Network in Aquaculture Centres in Asia-Pacific
    (NACA)
c/o NAFIQAVED
Ministry of Fisheries
Ba Dinh District, Ha Noi
Vietnam
Email: flavio.corsin@gmail.com

Patrice Courvalin
Unité des Agents Antibactériens
Institut Pasteur, Paris
France
Email: pcourval@pasteur.fr

Timothy S. Cummings
College of Veterinary Medicine
Mississippi State University
Mississipipi State, MS
USA
Email: Cummings@cvm.msstate.edu

C. Oliver Duran
Moss Veterinary Partners
Naas, Co. Kildare
Ireland
Email: oliver.duran@mossvet.ie

Yuuko S. Endoh
National Veterinary Assay Laboratory
Ministry of Agriculture, Forestry and Fisheries (MAFF)
Tokyo
Japan
Email: endoyuk@nval.go.jp

Linda A. Frank
Department of Small Animal Clinical Sciences
College of Veterinary Medicine
University of Tennessee
Knoxville, TN
USA
Email: lfrank@utk.edu

Kornelia Grein
European Medicines Agency (EMEA)
Canary Wharf, London
UK
Email: Kornelia.Grein@emea.europa.eu

Luca Guardabassi
Department of Veterinary Pathobiology
Faculty of Life Sciences
University of Copenhagen
Frederiksberg C
Denmark
Email: lg@life.ku.dk

Tor Einar Horsberg
Department of Food Safety and Infection Biology
Norwegian School of Veterinary Science
Oslo
Norway
Email: TorEinar.Horsberg@veths.no

Geoffrey A. Houser
Department of Small Animal Clinical Sciences
Faculty of Life Sciences
University of Copenhagen
Denmark
Email: geh@life.ku.dk

Lars B. Jensen
National Food Institute
Technical University of Denmark
Copenhagen
Denmark
Email: lje@food.dtu.dk

Hilde Kruse*
Department for Health Surveillance
National Veterinary Institute
Oslo
Norway
Email: hik@ecr.euro.who.int

Alain Le Breton
Fish Consultant
Grenade sur Garonne
France
Email: le-breton.alain@wanadoo.fr

Peter Lees
Department of Veterinary Basic Sciences
Royal Veterinary College
North Mymms
UK
Email: PLees@RVC.AC.UK

Ulrich Löhren
PHW-Group
Lohmann & Co. AG
Central Diagnostic Laboratory
Rechterfeld
Germany
Email: Ulrich.Loehren@wiesenhof.de

Scott McEwen
Department of Population Medicine
University of Guelph
Guelph, Ontario
Canada
Email: smcewen@uoguelph.ca

Kåre Mølbak
Department of Epidemiology
Statens Serum Institut
Copenhagen
Denmark
Email: KRM@ssi.dk

Mark G. Papich
Department of Molecular Biomedical Sciences
College of Veterinary Medicine
Raliegh, NC
USA
Email: mark_papich@ncsu.edu

* Regional Adviser for Food Safety, WHO European Centre for Environment and Health, Rome, WHO Regional Office for Europe.

Satu Pyörälä
Department of Production Animal Medicine
Faculty of Veterinary Medicine
University of Helsinki
Saarentaus
Finland
Email: spyorala@mappi.helsinki.fi

Antonia Ricci
OIE Reference Laboratory for Salmonellosis
Istituto Zooprofilattico Sperimentale
    delle Venezie
Legnano, Padova
Italy
Email: aricci@izsvenezie.it

Geoffrey W. Smith
Department of Population Health and
    Pathobiology
College of Veterinary Medicine
North Carolina State University
USA
Email: Geoffrey_Smith@ncsu.edu

Peter R. Smith
Department of Microbiology
National University of Ireland
Galway
Ireland
Email: peterrsmith@eircom.net

Emma Snary
Centre for Epidemiology & Risk Analysis
Veterinary Laboratories Agency – Weybridge
Addlestone, Surrey
UK
Email: e.l.snary@vla.defra.gsi.gov.uk

Ove Svendsen
Department of Veterinary Pathobiology
Faculty of Life Sciences
University of Copenhagen
Denmark

Linda Tollefson
US Food and Drug Administration
Rockville, MD
USA
Email: linda.tollefson@fda.hhs.gov

Pierre-Louis Toutain
Ecole Nationale Vétérinaire
Toulouse
France
Email: pl.toutain@envt.fr

Angelo A. Valois
Australian Government Department of
    Agriculture, Fisheries and Forestry
Canberra, ACT
Australia
Email: Angelo.Valois@daff.gov.au

J. Scott Weese
Department of Clinical Studies
Ontario Veterinary College
University of Guelph
Guelph, Ontario
Canada
Email: jsweese@uoguelph.ca

Henrik C. Wegener
National Food Institute
Technical University of Denmark
Søborg
Denmark
Email: HCW@food.dtu.dk

Camilla Wiuff
Section for HAI & IC
Health Protection Scotland
Glasgow
UK
Email: Camilla.Wiuff@hps.scot.nhs.uk

Chapter 1

PRINCIPLES OF PRUDENT AND RATIONAL USE OF ANTIMICROBIALS IN ANIMALS

Luca Guardabassi and Hilde Kruse

1.1 Introduction

Throughout history, infectious diseases have been a major threat to human and animal health and a prominent cause of morbidity and mortality. The introduction of antimicrobial agents (Box 1.1) in the 1930s (sulfonamides) and 1940s (penicillin) revolutionized human medicine by substantially reducing morbidity and mortality rates from bacterial diseases. However, it was soon observed that bacteria could become resistant to antimicrobials, and resistant strains emerged shortly after the introduction of every new antimicrobial drug. Resistance is a natural and unavoidable consequence of antimicrobial use. Exposure to antimicrobials selects for resistant bacteria and results in an ecological disadvantage for susceptible bacteria. This phenomenon can be easily reproduced in the laboratory by cultivating a mixed bacterial population in the presence of an antimicrobial drug: in accordance with the Darwinian principle 'survival of the fittest', resistant strains overgrow their susceptible counterparts, which are either killed or inhibited depending on the type and concentration of the drug. Because of their intrinsic selective properties, antimicrobials have been progressively loosing their efficacy in the therapy of various bacterial infections. The emergence and spread of antimicrobial resistance associated with the difficulties encountered in the discovery of novel antimicrobial agents has resulted in a major medical challenge and a serious public health problem.

Antimicrobial use in animals originated over 50 years ago when chlortetracycline fermentation waste was found to enhance animal growth and health. Since then, major changes have taken place in food animal production as well as in companion animal medicine. Intensification of food animal production has led to radical changes in the size, structure and management

---

Box 1.1 Antimicrobial agents, antibiotics, disinfectants and antiseptics.

Antimicrobial agents, or more simply *antimicrobials*, are chemical compounds that kill or inhibit the growth of microorganisms. They are naturally produced by microorganisms such as fungi (e.g. penicillin) and bacteria (e.g. tetracycline and erythromycin), or can be synthetically (e.g. sulfonamides and fluoroquinolones) or semi-synthetically produced (e.g. amoxicillin, clarithromycin and doxycycline). According to the original definition by the Nobel laureate S. A. Waksman, the term *antibiotic* only refers to natural compounds of microbial origin. However, the term is often used as a synonym for any antimicrobial agent by both professionals and lay-persons alike. Antimicrobials targeting bacteria are generally referred to as *antibacterial agents*; although some of them (e.g. sulfonamides and tetracyclines) are also active against protozoa. Some antimicrobial agents affect bacterial and human or animal cells equally due to lack of selective toxicity, and can therefore only be used on inanimate objects (*disinfectants*) or on external surfaces of the body (*antiseptics*).

of farms. Modern production systems have enabled better disease control by improving hygiene barriers and measures, but have made animals more vulnerable to disease because of high animal densities and stressful conditions. At the same time, the number of companion animals has substantially increased in modern society, with such animals being increasingly regarded as family members, resulting in increased expenditure on veterinary care and antimicrobial therapy. Partly as a result of these changes, the use of antimicrobials has become widespread in both animal production and veterinary medicine. Today it is estimated that more than half of all antimicrobials produced worldwide are used in animals.

Resistance to antimicrobials developed a long time before the introduction of antimicrobial agents in human and veterinary medicine. It most likely originated millions of years ago from antibiotic-producing bacteria living in soil, and was subsequently transferred to bacterial species of medical interest (1). Bacteria have developed various mechanisms to neutralize the action of antimicrobial agents. The most common are enzymatic drug inactivation, modification or replacement of the drug target, active drug efflux and reduced drug uptake (2). Resistance can be either intrinsic or acquired by conjugation, transformation or

transduction (Box 1.2). Since distinct resistance genes are frequently clustered together, horizontal transfer of a single genetic element can result in the acquisition by recipient bacteria of resistance to multiple unrelated antimicrobials (*multi-resistance*).

Independent of the modality by which resistance is acquired, the use of antimicrobial agents creates optimal conditions for the emergence and dissemination of resistant bacteria. It should be noted that resistance to a certain antimicrobial agent can even be selected by the use of another agent (Box 1.3). The spread of antimicrobial resistance does not respect phylogenetic or ecological borders. Animal-to-human transmission may occur by various means including food and

---

Box 1.2 Intrinsic and acquired resistance.

Intrinsic or *natural resistance* is due to a structural or functional trait inherently associated with a bacterial species, a genus or even a larger group. For example, Gram-negative bacteria are intrinsically resistant to glycopeptides because their outer membrane is impermeable to such antibiotics. *Acquired resistance* is due to genetic changes in the bacterial genome, which can be a consequence of either random mutation in housekeeping genes or horizontal acquisition of foreign genes. Bacteria can acquire antimicrobial resistance genes by uptake of free DNA (*transformation*), via bacteriophages (*transduction*) or by cell-to-cell transfer (*conjugation*). Conjugation is the most important mechanism for the transfer of resistance genes due to its broad-host range and the frequent location of resistance genes on conjugative elements such as plasmids or transposons. In some cases, resistance can also result from a combination of mutation and gene transfer events (e.g. resistance to cephalosporins due extended-spectrum β-lactamases).

Box 1.3 Cross- and co-selection.

Resistance to one antimicrobial agent can be selected for by another agent following two mechanisms: *cross-selection* and *co-selection*. Cross-selection refers to the presence of a single resistance gene or mutation conferring resistance to two or more antimicrobial agents (*cross-resistance*), usually belonging to the same antimicrobial class. Co-selection is due to the co-existence of distinct genes or mutations in the same bacterial strain, each conferring resistance to a different class of drug (*co-resistance*). An example of cross-selection is provided by certain antimicrobial drugs licensed for animal use, such as tylosin, avoparcin and enrofloxacin, which have the ability to cross-select for resistance to structurally related drugs used in human medicine, such as erythromycin (macrolides), vancomycin (glycopeptides) and ciprofloxacin (fluoroquinolones), respectively. Tylosin and tetracycline, two antibiotics commonly used in swine production, are likely to co-select for glycopeptide resistance in porcine enterococci since genes conferring resistance (*ermB* and *tetM*, respectively) are often located on plasmids carrying the *vanA* glycopeptide resistance gene. Similarly, some heavy metals also have the potential to select for resistance to antimicrobial agents due to the fact that the genes encoding resistance to the various groups of molecules often co-exist on the same genetic structure. For example, the *tcrB* gene that confers resistance to copper sulfate, a heavy metal used as a feed supplement in swine and as a foot antiseptic in cattle, has recently been found to be closely located upstream of *vanA* on enterococcal plasmids of porcine origin. High levels of copper in the feed have been shown to co-select macrolide- and glycopeptide-resistant enterococci in pigs (4).

water supply as well as direct contact with animals or manure. Resistance genes can be transferred between bacteria that belong to unrelated species and originate from distinct ecological niches. Mobile genetic elements harbouring resistance genes can be easily transferred horizontally between bacteria from terrestrial animals, fish and humans (3). Furthermore, resistance genes and resistant bacteria can spread across geographical boundaries through movement of people, animals, feed and food. This implies that antimicrobial use in animals may have consequences for the resistance situation in humans, and that resistance problems in one country can spread to another country. Antimicrobial resistance in human and 'non-human' environments are interdependent on a global scale. Consequently, when addressing the problems of antimicrobial resistance, one has to take a global and holistic approach that embraces different sectors and ecological niches.

Antimicrobial resistance is a global public health problem, and growing scientific evidence indicates that it is negatively impacted by both human and animal antimicrobial usage (Chapter 2). The objective of this book is to transform the general principles of prudent antimicrobial use into a set of species- and disease-specific guidelines for antimicrobial use in animals, including food animal production, large animal and small animal medicine and aquaculture. The intention of the editors was to provide veterinary practitioners and students with a practical and user-friendly guide to antimicrobial prescription. The book should orient veterinary practitioners towards prudent and rational antimicrobial use and inform them about the importance of preserving the efficacy of critically important antimicrobials in human medicine. This first chapter introduces the modalities by which antimicrobial agents are administered to animals (Section 1.2) and describes the history and the general principles of prudent and rational antimicrobial use (Box 1.4) (Sections 1.3 and 1.4). Above all, it provides the reader with the information necessary to understand and interpret the guidelines presented in the following chapters (Section 1.5).

1.2 Antimicrobial use in animals

Antimicrobial agents can be individually administered to animals to treat (*therapy*) or prevent (*prophylaxis*) disease. In animal production, antimicrobials can also

---

> **Box 1.4**   Prudent and rational use of antimicrobials.
>
> There are no finite definitions of 'prudent' and 'rational' in relation to antimicrobial use. Both terms are frequently used to suggest a responsible attitude to antimicrobial use, aimed at minimizing the development and spread of antimicrobial resistance while maximizing therapeutic efficacy. This attitude, and its objectives, apply both to human and veterinary medicine. Sometimes the terms 'prudent' and 'rational' are used more or less synonymously. However, they refer to slightly different aspects. *Prudent use* has the overall goal of reducing antimicrobial usage, with particular emphasis on the relative use of broad-spectrum and critically important drugs. *Rational use* refers to rational administration of antimicrobials to the individual with the purpose of optimizing clinical efficacy while minimizing development of resistance.

---

be administered to clinically healthy animals belonging to the same flock or pen as animals with clinical signs (a form of prophylaxis called *metaphylaxis*), or for improving animal growth (*growth promotion*). Metaphylaxis is typically used during disease outbreaks in aquaculture and in poultry, but is also used in swine and cattle. Infections are treated before their clinical appearance and the treatment period is usually shorter than for therapeutic treatment. The use of the term 'methaphylaxis' is controversial, as this word does not exist in the English dictionary and refers to situations where antimicrobials are used for both therapeutic and prophylactic purposes. However, the editors have decided to keep this term in the book as it is well understood by people working in the animal sector and refers to a particular form of prophylaxis in the presence of disease.

For the purpose of growth promotion, antimicrobial drugs are used as a feed supplement and are continuously administered at sub-therapeutic doses. The mechanisms by which antimicrobial growth promoters exert their effects on feed efficiency and weight gain are still not fully understood. Data show that the claimed benefits derived from the use of growth promoters may not be realized in modern production systems and tend to be greater in situations where hygienic conditions are poor (5). Most authors agree that the benefits of growth promoters can be minimized, if not annulled, by improving hygiene, management conditions, and other measures aiming at disease control, such as biosecurity and vaccination.

Among food animals, flock medication is the only feasible means of treatment in poultry, whereas treatment can be given to either the individual or group in swine and cattle. Systemic antimicrobial treatment can be administered orally, through medicated feed or water, or by injections – usually as an initiation of antimicrobial treatment typically followed by systemic or local treatment. Local antimicrobial treatment includes intramammary infusion for mastitis treatment, intrauterine treatment and topical skin, ear and eye treatment. With regard to farmed fish, antimicrobial treatment is almost always administered by medicated feed, although some brood stock may be treated individually by injection or immersion. Antimicrobial treatment is usually administered on an individual basis to pets. Systemic treatment is conducted orally, by the administration of tablets or mixtures, or by injections. Local antimicrobial treatment includes topical skin, ear and eye treatment.

Antimicrobials used in animals are generally the same as, or closely related to, antimicrobials used in humans. Tetracyclines constitute the antimicrobial class quantitatively most used in animals, followed by macrolides, pleuromutilins, lincosamides, penicillins, sulfonamides, aminoglycosides, fluoroquinolones, cephalosporins and phenicols (6). The types of agents used in humans and animals vary between countries. In Denmark, penicillins accounts for approximately 70% of all dosages given to humans, whereas the most commonly used antimicrobials in swine production are macrolides (70%) and tetracyclines (21%) (7). In Norway in 2004, pure penicillin preparations represented 43% and 42% of the total antimicrobial usage in humans and terrestrial animals respectively, tetracyclines only 17% and 3% respectively (8). Qualitative and quantitative differences can be observed between distinct animal species or groups, even within the same country. For example, data from Denmark shows that a large proportion of the preparations containing aminopenicillins with clavulanic acid, cephalosporins and fluoroquinolones used in veterinary practice are administered to pet animals (9). Worldwide, there are marked differences in relation to regulation, market availability, dispensation and usage of veterinary antimicrobial products (Chapter 5). In many countries, drugs licensed for human use are administered to animals, and veterinary products are used in animal species that are not indicated as appropriate on the label (*off-label use*).

The most common antimicrobial drugs used presently or in the past as growth promoters include macrolides (tylosin and spiramycin), polypeptides (bacitracin), glycolipids (bambermycin), streptogramins (virginiamycin), glycopeptides (avoparcin), quinoxalines (carbadox and olaquindox), everninomycins (avilamycin) and ionophores (monensin and salinomycin). The distinction between growth promotion and prophylactic use is not always clear since growth promoters also contribute to the prevention of certain diseases and can be administered for this purpose. Some countries allow antimicrobials that are used therapeutically to also be used as growth promoters in sub-therapeutic doses. In the USA, antimicrobial agents such as penicillin, erythromycin, tylosin and tetracycline are approved for both growth promotion and therapeutic use. In Europe, the legislation for use of growth promoters originates from the Swann report (10), and antimicrobials for therapeutic use were not authorized for growth promotion here.

Due to the international scientific attention and documentation regarding the public health risks associated with the use of growth promoters in animal husbandry, some countries, including the EU, have banned or are in the process of phasing out such use. This policy is in accordance with the recommendations proposed by WHO in 2000 (11) and endorsed by FAO and OIE in 2003 (12) (Section 1.3). The effects on total antimicrobial consumption that resulted from the ban of growth promoters in 1995 were investigated in Denmark (7). The total consumption of antimicrobial agents in food animals was reduced by approximately half in the period between 1994 (206 tonnes) and 2004 (101 tonnes). While a marked increase in the consumption of antimicrobial agents used for therapy was also observed, with 48 tonnes used in 1996 and 101 tonnes used in 2003, the increase observed since 2000 was most likely due to an epidemic of PMWS (Post-weaning Multisystemic Wasting Syndrome) in pigs. In Norway and Sweden, the ban of growth promoters was not followed by an increase in therapeutic use of antimicrobial agents (13).

In most countries, it is very difficult to collect good information on the consumption of antimicrobial agents for veterinary and growth promoting purposes in animals. Quantitative figures are very rare and estimates are available for only a few countries. In the USA, antimicrobial consumption in animals showed an evident increase from 1951 to 1978 (14). The total production of feed additives grew from 110 tonnes in 1951 to 5580 tonnes in 1978, and an even more pronounced increase was observed for medical use in humans and animals, which increased from 580 to 6080 tonnes during the same period. The European Agency for the Evaluation of Medical Products (EMEA) estimated the amount of antimicrobial agents used to produce the same amount of meat in different EU countries in 1997 (15). Although such data should be interpreted with caution, substantial differences were observed between the various countries, suggesting that there is room for reduction of antimicrobial usage.

1.3 History of prudent antimicrobial use

During the past 40 years, there has been controversy over the impact of antimicrobial use in animals upon antimicrobial resistance in human medicine. The use of antimicrobial growth promoters in animals particularly has created a heated debate. The major obstacle in determining whether resistant bacteria arising from animal sources present an important threat to human health is the difficulty in tracing all the postulated steps from animal to human disease. This issue is complicated by the fact that animals and humans receive the same kind of antimicrobials, are colonized with common or closely related bacterial species and their environments are not separate. Although the controversy still continues to a certain degree today, it is generally acknowledged and well documented that the use of antimicrobials in animals can have an impact on public health (Chapter 2). The following sections describe the historical process leading to recognition of the human health risks and the consequent formulation of principles of prudent antimicrobial use.

1.3.1 The Swann report

Concern about possible influence of antimicrobial use in animals upon human health led to the appointment of the Joint Committee on the use of Antibiotics in Animal Husbandry and Veterinary Medicine in Great Britain in 1968. The task of this committee, chaired by M. M. Swann, was to obtain information about the present and prospective use of antimicrobials in animal husbandry and veterinary medicine with particular reference to antimicrobial resistance; to consider the implications for animal husbandry and for human and animal health; and to make recommendations for the use of antimicrobials. The Swann

report (10) recommended that antimicrobial agents be excluded from animal feed (unless specifically prescribed for such use) if they were used as therapeutic agents in human or animal medicine or if they were associated with the development of cross-resistance to drugs that were used in humans. The Swann report was the foundation for the development of policy on prudent use of antimicrobials and regulation on antimicrobial use in many countries.

The British Government implemented the recommendations given by the Swann committee in 1971. Antimicrobials were officially classified into two groups. The first group consisted of agents approved for use in animal feeds as growth promoters, and included bacitracin, virginiamycin and bambermycins. The second group consisted of agents for therapeutic purposes, whose use was restricted to specific prescription by a medical or veterinary practitioner. Hence, therapeutic antimicrobials were removed from sub-therapeutic use. Other western European countries and Japan also followed the recommendations given in the Swann report but, in contrast, no new legislation was enacted in the USA or Canada. The use of antimicrobials as feed additives remains liberal in North America because it is considered good practice in animal health management. In 2005 the US Food and Drug Administration (FDA) withdrew the approval of enrofloxacin in poultry due to the assessed public health risk relating to development of quinolone resistance in *Campylobacter*. This action represents the first time an antimicrobial was withdrawn in the USA because of resistance concerns.

1.3.2 Relevant activities by FAO, OIE and WHO

In recent years it has become clear that containment of antimicrobial resistance, as a consequence of the complexity and multi-dimensionality of the antimicrobial resistance problem, relies on a holistic, cross-sectional and international approach. The human, animal and plant sectors all have a shared responsibility and role in efforts to prevent and minimize antimicrobial resistance selection by both human and non-human use of antimicrobials. Managing human health risks from non-human usage of antimicrobials and the resulting antimicrobial resistant bacteria requires national and international interdisciplinary cooperation. Therefore, since 1997, the World Health Organization (WHO) has, in collaboration with the

Food and Agriculture Organization (FAO) or FAO and the World Organisation for Animal Health (OIE), convened a number of consultations to address non-human antimicrobial usage and associated antimicrobial resistance and possible public health problems.

In 1997, WHO convened a meeting in Berlin addressing the medical impact of the use of antimicrobials in food animals (16). At this meeting, it was concluded that 'there is direct evidence that antimicrobial use in animals selects for antimicrobial-resistant non-typhoid *Salmonella* serotypes. These bacteria have been transmitted to humans in food or through direct contact with animals'. Notably, the experts recommended managing risk at the producer level through the prudent use of antimicrobials. Because of the human health importance of fluoroquinolones and the public health concern of increasing resistance to them, particularly in *Salmonella* and *Campylobacter*, WHO convened a meeting in Geneva in 1998 addressing the use of quinolones in food-producing animals and the potential impact on human health (17). The participants agreed that the use of antimicrobials selects for resistance, and that resistant *Salmonella*, *Escherichia coli* and *Campylobacter* in the food supply pose a public health risk. It was concluded that 'the use of fluoroquinolones in food animals has led to the emergence of fluoroquinolone-resistant *Campylobacter* and of *Salmonella* with reduced susceptibility to fluoroquinolones'.

Acknowledging that antimicrobial resistance is a multi-factorial problem and thus requires a multidisciplinary approach, WHO, with the participation of FAO and OIE, convened in 2000 an expert consultation that developed 'WHO global principles for the containment of antimicrobial resistance in animals intended for food' (11). The purpose of these 'global principles' is to minimize the negative public health impact of the use of antimicrobial agents in food-producing animals, whilst at the same time providing for their safe and effective use in veterinary medicine. The principles provide a framework of recommendations to reduce the overuse and misuse of antimicrobials in food animals for the protection of human health and are part of a comprehensive WHO Global Strategy for the containment of antimicrobial resistance. Amongst others, the 'global principles' underlined that antimicrobial growth promoters that belong to classes of antimicrobial agents used (or submitted for approval) in humans and animals

should be terminated or rapidly phased-out in the absence of risk-based evaluations, and that risk-based evaluations of all antimicrobial growth promoters should be continued. The importance of establishing national monitoring programmes for antimicrobial resistance in bacteria from animals, food of animal origin and humans and for antimicrobial usage in food animals was highlighted. In November 2002, WHO convened an independent multidisciplinary international expert panel in Foulum, Denmark, to review the potential consequences to human health, animal health and welfare, environmental impact, animal production, and national economy resulting from Denmark's programme for termination of the use of antimicrobial growth promoters in food animal production, particularly swine and broiler chicken (18). The review showed that it is possible, at least for some animal production systems, to abandon the use of antimicrobial growth promoters in animal production without any significant increase in therapeutic use or any considerable loss of productivity.

The Codex Alimentarius is a body under the auspices of FAO and WHO that develops food standards, guidelines and related texts such as codes of practice under the Joint FAO/WHO Food Standards Programme. Its main purposes are to protect the health of consumers and to ensure fair trade practices in the international food trade. The Executive Committee of the Codex Alimentarius Commission, in 2001, recommended that FAO, WHO and OIE give consideration to convening a multidisciplinary expert consultation to advise the Commission on the human health risks associated with antimicrobial use in agriculture, including aquaculture and veterinary medicine. As a response, FAO, WHO and OIE jointly convened a two-step approach consisting of two expert workshops. The first workshop, which was held in December 2003 in Geneva, conducted a scientific assessment of antimicrobial resistance risks arising from all non-human uses of antimicrobials in animals, and formulated recommendations and options for future risk management actions (19). The second workshop, held in March 2004 in Oslo, Norway, considered the broad range of possible risk management options for antimicrobial resistance from non-human usage of antimicrobials (12).

The first expert workshop in Geneva concluded that there is clear evidence of adverse human health consequences due to resistant organisms resulting from non-human usage of antimicrobials (see also Chapter 2). The food-borne route was recognized as the major transmission pathway for resistant bacteria and resistance genes from food animals to humans. However, it was acknowledged that other routes of transmission exist. Available scientific evidence shows that antimicrobial usage in horticulture, aquaculture and companion animals can also result in the spread of resistant bacteria and resistance genes to humans. The workshop concluded that residues of antimicrobials in foods, under present regulatory regimes, represent a significantly less important human health risk than the risk related to antimicrobial resistance. The workshop recommended implementation of WHO global principles for the containment of antimicrobial resistance in animals intended for foods. They also recommended to follow OIE Guidelines on responsible and prudent antimicrobial use to establish national surveillance programmes on animal usage of antimicrobials and on antimicrobial resistance in bacteria from food and animals, and to implement strategies to prevent the transmission of resistant bacteria from animals to humans through the food chain and the dissemination of bacteria resistant to critically important antimicrobial agents in human medicine (19).

The second expert workshop in Oslo underlined that it is possible to reduce the necessity for antimicrobials in agriculture and aquaculture through stringent implementation of good agricultural practices, including good animal husbandry and good veterinary practices (12). The need for rapid implementation by governments and all stakeholders of the principles laid down in WHO and OIE guidelines was stressed. It was recommended that a Codex/OIE Task Force be established to develop risk management options for antimicrobial resistance related to non-human use of antimicrobials. The workshop emphasized that the risks associated with non-human antimicrobial use should be part of the human safety assessment for regulatory decisions in relation to veterinary antimicrobials and that 'critically important' classes of antimicrobials for humans and animals should be identified. As a follow-up to this, the WHO convened in 2005 and 2007 two expert workshops to specifically address identification of critically important antimicrobials for humans (Chapter 4). The OIE has identified those antimicrobials that are considered critical for animal health. The two lists are currently being discussed by international experts.

1.4 Prudent and rational antimicrobial use: global approach and basic principles

In order to minimize the possible impact of animal antimicrobial usage on public and animal health, various international organizations such as the WHO, OIE, FAO and the EU Commission have in recent years emphasized the importance of prudent and rational antimicrobial use in animals. This has been recognized by professional associations such as the World Veterinary Association (WVA), the International Federation of Agricultural Producers (IFAP), the World Federation of the Animal Health Industry (COMISA), the Federation of Veterinarians of Europe (FVE), the American College of Veterinary Internal Medicine (ACVIM) and the American Veterinary Medical Associations (AVMA), as well as by national and international authorities. All these entities have emphasized to a lesser or greater degree that prudent antimicrobial use is important, not only to safeguard the efficacy of antimicrobial drugs in veterinary medicine but, even more so, to prevent the emergence and spread of undesirable resistance phenotypes in zoonotic pathogens as well as in commensal bacteria that can be transmitted between animals and humans. In the following sections, a set of basic principles identified as important for executing prudent and rational antimicrobial use are listed and discussed. These principles focus on the use of antimicrobials in veterinary practice and do not take into consideration governmental measures such as licensing and control, which are under the responsibility of the national competent regulatory agencies. In the formulation of this set of principles, particular attention was devoted to addressing both benefits to animal health and consequences to public health.

1.4.1 Disease prevention as a tool for reducing antimicrobial use

It is of utmost importance that antimicrobial use is not seen in isolation from infection control. The best way of minimizing the need for, and use of, antimicrobials and thereby aiding the containment of antimicrobial resistance, is by preventing disease. Prevention is better than cure, not only in relation to antimicrobial resistance, but also from an animal welfare perspective and, in the long run, from an economic viewpoint. Successful disease control relies on an holistic approach encompassing animal husbandry and management, nutrition, animal welfare and vaccination. Infection control plans should be implemented in all animal facilities and veterinary practices, including those working with companion animals. Routine prophylactic use of antimicrobials should never be used as a substitute for health management. In relation to veterinary surgery, it is generally unnecessary to administer antimicrobials in routine surgical procedures since aseptic techniques and hygiene measures can replace the need for antimicrobials in most cases.

An excellent example of how antimicrobial use in animals may be drastically reduced by the introduction of adequate measures for disease prevention is provided by Norway. In this country, the annual usage of veterinary antimicrobial agents in terrestrial animals decreased gradually by 40% from 1995 to 2001. Since then, the annual usage has remained on a relatively constant level. This significant reduction is due to a campaign by professional organizations within animal husbandry implemented in the mid-1990s. The campaign focused on preventive veterinary medicine and prudent use of antimicrobials. With respect to aquaculture, which represents one of the main industries in this country, the annual usage of antimicrobial agents in farmed fish declined by 98% from 1987 to 2004. During the same period, the total production of farmed fish increased massively, indicating that animal and public health can be safeguarded without affecting economical profit for stakeholders. This significant decrease in the usage of antimicrobial agents in Norwegian aquaculture was mainly attributed to the introduction of effective vaccines, as well as to improved health management (8).

1.4.2 Accurate diagnosis and antimicrobial susceptibility testing

Empirical use of antimicrobials should be avoided whenever possible and antimicrobials should be preferably prescribed on the basis of laboratory diagnosis and antimicrobial susceptibility testing. The use of antimicrobials should always be based upon examination of the clinical case, diagnosis of a bacterial infection and selection of a clinically efficacious antimicrobial agent. Antimicrobials should only be used when it is known or strongly suspected that the disease is caused by bacteria, since viruses are not susceptible to antibacterial therapy. Ideally, the

causal infectious agent should be identified at the species level and its antimicrobial susceptibility be ascertained before initiating antimicrobial therapy. However, in certain situations, such as when the animal is seriously ill or there is an outbreak with high mortality or rapid spread, therapy may be initiated on the basis of clinical diagnosis (empirical treatment). The resistance patterns of certain animal pathogens such as Pasteurellaceae, *Bordetella bronchiseptica*, *Actinobacillus*, beta-haemolytic streptococci and *Erysipelothrix rhusiopathiae* can be predicted with relatively high certainty, and generally the use of penicillin G is sufficient to cure infections caused by these microorganisms. On the other hand, the susceptibility patterns of other bacteria, such as staphylococci, *E. coli* and *Salmonella* can hardly be predicted. For these bacteria, susceptibility testing is strongly recommended, if possible before initiation of antimicrobial treatment.

Collection of local data on antimicrobial susceptibility is the first step to rational antimicrobial use. Antimicrobial resistance should be monitored over time at the herd or hospital level and data should be kept in apposite records. If available, data generated at the national level are also important for guiding choice of antimicrobials. Monitoring reveals the emergence of new antimicrobial resistance trends and is essential in guiding the choice of appropriate drugs for empirical treatment. Antimicrobial susceptibility testing should be done according to internationally recognized standards. A wide range of standardized methods are currently available, such as those of the Clinical Laboratory and Standards Institute (CLSI) in the USA, the British Society for Antimicrobial Chemotherapy (BSAC), the Comité de l'Antibiogramme de la Société Française de Microbiologie (CA-SFM), the Swedish Reference Group for Antibiotics (SRGA) and the Deutsches Institut für Normung (DIN). If the veterinary practice does not have the human and economical resources necessary to run a diagnostic service with standardized antimicrobial susceptibility testing methods, clinical specimens should be sent to an accredited diagnostic laboratory.

1.4.3 Justification of antimicrobial use

Before initiating antimicrobial therapy, even in the case of a correct diagnosis, the practitioner should ascertain that such therapy is justified. No treatment is a possible alternative, for instance, in a situation where the disease can be controlled by other means such as stamping out in the case of a serious infectious animal disease, or the slaughter of an old cow with recurrent mastitis. Ideally, only diseased animals should be treated, and the treatment should be as individual as possible. However, in the case of poultry and farmed fish this is not practical, and mass-treatment is accepted following a relevant diagnosis. Metaphylaxis, where clinically healthy animals are treated along with their diseased 'neighbours', should be avoided. Prophylaxis should be kept to a minimum. While some prophylactic use can be medically justified, for example in relation to elected or prolonged surgery, quite often prophylaxis is used to counteract unhygienic routines or bad management. This practice is imprudent and in some countries even illegal.

1.4.4 Choice of an appropriate antimicrobial product and administration route

From a strictly clinical point of view, four factors have to be considered when selecting an antimicrobial agent: clinical efficacy, toxicity to the host, risk for development of resistance and adverse effects on the commensal flora. Clinical efficacy requires not only that the pathogen is susceptible to the selected drug, but also that the drug is able to penetrate and be active at the site of infection. Attention should also be paid to the immune status of the animal and the type of infection since bacteriostatic drugs have a slower effect and rely on an active immune system to control the infection, and are therefore not appropriate for the treatment of acute life-threatening infections or for immunosuppressed animals. Other host-related factors such as pregnancy, age and allergies should also be considered in order to avoid undesirable effects on the health of the animal.

The spectrum of activity of the drug, its importance in human medicine and route of administration are the most important factors in accomplishing prudent and rational antimicrobial use. Consideration should be given to the potential public health consequences of resistance to the antimicrobial in question. In general, narrow-spectrum and older antimicrobials, if appropriate and available, should be preferred to broad-spectrum drugs. Broad-spectrum antimicrobials exert a selective pressure on a larger number of microorganisms than narrow-spectrum antimicrobials and are therefore more prone to selecting for resistance

development and spread. Antimicrobials identified as critically important in human medicine (see Chapter 4) should only be used if justified. In the editors' opinion, certain aminoglycosides (gentamicin and amikacin), cephalosporins (cefadroxil, cefalexin, cefazolin, ceftiofur and cefquinome) and fluoroquinolones (enrofloxacin, danofloxacin, difloxacin, ibafloxacin, orbifloxacin, marbofloxacin and sarafloxacin) should, as far as possible, be avoided in the veterinary sector due to their critical importance in human medicine. In view of the recent emergence of methicillin-resistant *Staphylococcus aureus* (MRSA) in animals, antistaphylococcal penicillins (cloxacillin, dicloxacillin and nafcillin) should only be considered for treating infections caused by penicillase-producing staphylococci. Broad-spectrum drugs or antimicrobial combinations should in general only be used if justified by the resistance profile of the pathogen, the nature of the disease (e.g. acute course and high mortality), and the economic or affective value of the animal. As a general rule, the use of antimicrobial combinations should be avoided due to their broadened spectrum of activity, increased potential for resistance development and possible pharmacological antagonism. The only exception is that of sulfonamides, which are usually combined with diaminopyrimidines (trimethoprim, baquiloprim and ormethoprim) because of the synergistic effect between these two antimicrobial classes. The use of other synergistic combinations of antimicrobials, such as that between penicillins and aminoglycosides, should be avoided in animals because of their importance in the treatment of acute hospital infections in humans caused by enterococci and streptococci. It is a well-established fact that combined or sequential treatment with bacteriostatic and bactericidal drugs produces an antagonistic effect.

The route of administration should also be considered in order to minimize the impact of antimicrobial treatment on development of resistance. Local treatment should be preferred to systemic treatment when the infection is localized and accessible by topical products (e.g. eye, ear, udder and wound infections). When systemic treatment is necessary in animal production, intramuscular and intravenous injections are preferable to oral administration to avoid disturbance of the normal gut flora. Furthermore, medication by feed and, to a lesser degree, water, may result in insufficient uptake by diseased animals due to loss of appetite, thus reducing the effects of medication and increasing the risks of resistance development.

Additional risks associated with oral administration include heterogeneous distribution of the drug in the feed, interference of feed ingredients on drug activity, and irrational handling or dosing of the drug by the farmer. In aquaculture facilities, where antimicrobial drugs are introduced directly into aquatic environments, pharmacological factors such as drug bioavailability, stability and toxicity to aquatic organisms in the neighbouring environment should also be considered in order to minimize environmental impact. In all circumstances, veterinary practitioners should only prescribe antimicrobial formulations that are approved for the species and the indication concerned. Off-label use of antimicrobials should be exceptional and always under the professional responsibility of the veterinarian. In particular, this practice should be limited to cases where no other suitable product is available.

1.4.5 Appropriate dosage regimen

Appropriate dosage regimen (dose level, dose interval and treatment duration) is of fundamental importance to ensure rational antimicrobial use. It is essential to administer antimicrobials in accordance with the recommended dosage regimen to minimize therapy failures, exploit the efficacy potential of the drug and comply with the regulated withdrawal times. Each antimicrobial class has its own pharmacodynamic and pharmacokinetic properties that are expressed when the recommended dosage regimen is applied. Low doses, increased dose intervals and reduced treatment duration can lead to recrudescence of the infection and may increase the risk of selecting resistant organisms. On the other hand, the treatment period should never be prolonged unnecessarily as this will affect withdrawal times and amplify the adverse effects on the commensal flora. It should be noted that the dose regimens indicated on the label instructions of veterinary antimicrobial formulations are determined on the basis of the antimicrobial concentrations achieved in the serum of healthy animals. However, as previously mentioned, drug intake can be significantly reduced in diseased animals due to loss of appetite. Based on these considerations, the higher dose levels reported on label instructions can be chosen with the purpose of minimizing the risk of resistance development (Chapter 6). Toxic effects must be taken into consideration, and label instructions should always be strictly followed with regard to withdrawal periods and storage instructions.

An important aspect of antimicrobial misuse is patients' non-compliance. Questionnaire surveys among human patients have shown that, contrary to doctors' expectations, non-compliance seems to be common worldwide. Patients frequently miss one or more doses of an antimicrobial treatment, or stop treatment before the end of the course (20). This phenomenon is likely to enhance the emergence of resistant strains during treatment because of the low antimicrobial concentration or short antimicrobial exposure attained in body tissues. Non-compliance in prescribed antimicrobial treatment regimes is also likely to occur in veterinary medicine, where antimicrobials are usually administered to animal patients by a third party. Accordingly, veterinarians have the important role of informing farmers and animal owners or managers about the importance of complying with the prescribed dosage regimens.

1.4.6 Ethical aspects related to prescription and dispensation of antimicrobial drugs

Prudent and rational antimicrobial use should be regarded as an important ethical issue in the veterinary profession. Veterinarians have the ethical obligation to use and prescribe, when indicated appropriate antimicrobials to cure infections in their patients, thus contributing to the health and well-being of animals. However, for the sake of public health, veterinarians also have the responsibility of the adoption of prudent and rational use of antimicrobials. In addition, they have the important function of informing farmers and animal owners or managers about the potential public health consequences associated with imprudent or irrational use of antimicrobial agents in animals, and instructing them in correct handling and administration of antimicrobial products. It has been recently indicated that profit from the sale of antimicrobial agents negatively impacts on prescribing practices (21). This assumption is based on the observation that antimicrobial use is higher in countries where antimicrobials are dispensed by veterinarians and the direct sale of drugs generates a significant part of their income. The amount of prescribed antimicrobials can be significantly reduced by eliminating the economic advantages associated with drug dispensation by veterinarians. The discussion on whether dispensation of antimicrobials in animals should be assigned to other professional figures or entities is not within the scope of this book. However, over-prescription or prescription of unnecessary expensive antimicrobial products is clearly an unethical practice in the veterinary profession.

1.5 The need to shift from general principles to practice guidelines

The basic principles indicated in the previous section and the general guidelines for antimicrobial use currently available in official documents and on websites of national and international organizations are of great value as part of the overall strategy for limiting the emergence and spread of antimicrobial resistance in animals. However, prior to the publication of this book, with the exclusion of sporadic initiatives at the national level, a concrete guide for veterinarians on the choice of antimicrobial agents for treatment of specific animal infections was not available at the international level. The book takes advantage of the recent international initiatives on prudent use of antimicrobial agents in animals (Section 1.3). The antimicrobials that are necessary to preserve for use in human medical therapy and those that are needed to treat diseases in animals are now being delineated and commented on by the global health community.

In this book, internationally recognized experts in microbiology, pharmacology and veterinary medicine were asked to draft species-and disease-specific guidelines for antimicrobial use in animals (Chapters 7–12). The selection of expert authors for the various chapters took into account multi-disciplinarity and geographical spread. The practice guidelines presented in this book do not necessarily reflect the current trends in antimicrobial prescription and usage. Where appropriate and feasible, improvements are aimed at preserving the efficacy of important drugs in human medicine. When interpreting the guidelines, local patterns of antimicrobial usage in both humans and animals should be borne in mind. In fact, the frequency of usage and the clinical importance of an antimicrobial agent in human medicine may vary considerably depending on the country. Furthermore, significant geographical differences also exist in relation to the resistance patterns of both human and veterinary pathogens.

The authors of this chapter believe that prudent and rational antimicrobial use is a part of good veterinary practice. Recognizing the human and animal health importance of antimicrobial agents and the need to preserve their efficacy is an important aspect in the veterinary profession. However, prudent and rational antimicrobial use should not be considered a limitation of clinical freedom in the veterinary profession, and the guidelines presented in this book should not be regarded as a substitute for veterinary judgement. Veterinarians should adopt the principles of evidence-based medicine when taking decisions on animal care, including prescription of antimicrobial drugs. This book was conceived to promote veterinary education and provide veterinary practitioners with a useful guide where such evidence is conflicting or lacking. Hopefully, the book will contribute to increased awareness of the resistance problem among veterinarians and help to balance their ethical obligations regarding animal and public health.

References

1. Aarestrup, F.M. (2006). The origin, evolution and global dissemination of antimicrobial resistance. In *Antimicrobial Resistance in Bacteria of Animal Origin* (ed. Aarestrup, F.M.). ASM Press, American Society for Microbiology, Washington DC, pp. 339–60.
2. Guardabassi, L. and Courvalin, P. (2006). Modes of antimicrobial action and mechanisms of bacterial resistance. In *Antimicrobial Resistance in Bacteria of Animal Origin* (ed. Aarestrup, F.M.). ASM Press, American Society for Microbiology, Washington DC, pp. 1–18.
3. Kruse, H. and Sorum, H. (1994). Transfer of multiple drug resistance plasmids between bacteria of diverse origins in natural microenvironments. *Appl. Environ. Microbiol.* 60: 4015–21.
4. Hasman, H., Kempf, I., Chidaine, B. *et al.* (2007). Copper resistance in *Enterococcus faecium*, mediated by the tcrB gene, is selected by supplementation of pig feed with copper sulphate. *Appl. Environ. Microbiol.* 72: 5784–9.
5. Barug, D., de Jong J., Kies, A.K. and Verstegen, M.W.A. (eds.) (2006). *Antimicrobial Growth Promoters: Where Do We Go From Here?* Wageningen Academic Publishers, The Netherlands.
6. Schwarz, S. and Chaslus-Dancla, E. (2001). Use of antimicrobials in veterinary medicine and mechanisms of resistance. *Vet. Res.* 32: 201–25.
7. Anonymous (2005). *DANMAP 2004 – Use of antimicrobial agents and occurrence of antimicrobial resistance in bacteria from food animals, foods and humans in Denmark.* Statens Serum Institut, Danish Veterinary and Food Administration, Danish Medicines Agency and Danish Institute for Food and Veterinary Research; Copenhagen. Available at http://www.danmap.org/pdfFiles/Danmap_2004.pdf

8. NORM/NORM-VET (2005). *Usage of antimicrobial agents and occurrence of antimicrobial resistance in Norway*. Tromsø/Oslo 2006. ISSN:1502-2307. Available at http://www.ventist.no/nor/tjenester/publikasjoner/norm_norm_vet_rapporten

9. Guardabassi, L., Schwarz, S. and Lloyd, D.H. (2004). Pet animals as reservoirs of antimicrobial resistant bacteria. *J. Antimicrob. Chemother.* 54: 321–32.

10. Swann Report (1969). Joint Committee on the Use of Antibiotics in Animal Husbandry and Veterinary Medicine. Report. HMSO, London. Presented to Parliament in November 1969.

11. World Health Organization (2000). *WHO Global principles for the containment of antimicrobial resistance in animals intended for food*. Report of a WHO Consultation with the participation of the Food and Agriculture Organization of the United Nations and the Office International des Epizooties, Geneva, Switzerland, 5–9 June 2000. Geneva, WHO. Available at http://whqlibdoc.who.int/hq/2000/WHO_CDS_CSR_APH_2000.4.pdf

12. World Organisation for Animal Health, World Health Organization, and Food and Agriculture Organization of the United Nations (2004). *Joint FAO/OIE/WHO 2nd Workshop on Non-human Antimicrobial Usage and Antimicrobial Resistance: Management Options*, 15–18 March 2004, Oslo, Norway. Available at http://www.who.int/foodsafety/publications/micro/en/exec.pdf

13. Grave, K., Jensen, V.F., Odensvik, K. *et al.* (2006). Usage of veterinary therapeutic antimicrobials in Denmark, Norway and Sweden following termination of antimicrobial growth promoter use. *Prev. Vet. Med.* 75: 123–32.

14. Black, W.D. (1984). The use of antimicrobial drugs in agriculture. *Can. J. Physiol. Pharmacol.* 62: 1044–8.

15. European Agency for the Evaluation of Medical Products (1999). *Antibiotic resistance in the European nion associated with therapeutic use of veterinary medicines*. Report and qualitative risk assessment by the committee for veterinary medicinal products. 14 July. Available at http://www.emea.europa.eu/htms/vet/swp/srantimicrobial.htm

16. World Health Organization (1997). *The medical impact of the use of antimicrobials in food animals*. Report of a WHO, Meeting, Berlin, Germany, 13–17 October 1997. Geneva, WHO. http://www.who.int/emc/diseases/zoo/oct97.pdf

17. World Health Organization (1998). *Use of quinolones in food animals and potential impact on human health: report and proceedings of a WHO meeting, Geneva, Switzerland, 2–5 June 1998*. Geneva, Available at http://whqlibdoc.who.int/hq/1998/WHO_EMC_ZDI_98.12_(p1-p130).pdf

18. World Health Organization (2003). *Impact of antimicrobial growth promoter termination in Denmark*. The WHO international review panel's evaluation of the termination of the use of antimicrobial growth promoters in Denmark. 6–7 November 2002, Foulum, Denmark. Available at http://www.who.int/salmsurv/links/gssamrgrowthreportstory/en

19. World Organisation for Animal Health World, Health Organization, and Food and Agriculture Organization of the United Nations (2004). *Joint First FAO/OIE/WHO expert workshop on non-human antimicrobial asage and antimicrobial resistance: scientific assessment*, Geneva, 1–5 December 2003. Available at http://www.who.int/foodsafety/publications/micro/en/report.pdf

20. Pechère, J.C., Cenedese, C., Muller, O. *et al.* (2002). Attitudinal classification of patients receiving antibiotic treatment for mild respiratory tract infections. *Int. J. Antimicrob. Ag.* 20: 399–406.

21. Grave, K. and Wegener, H. C. (2006). Comment on: Veterinarians profit on drug dispensing. *Prev. Vet. Med.* 77: 306–8.

Chapter 2

HUMAN HEALTH RISKS ASSOCIATED WITH ANTIMICROBIAL USE IN ANIMALS

Lars B. Jensen, Frederick J. Angulo, Kåre Mølbak
and Henrik C. Wegener

Antimicrobials select for resistant bacteria irrespective of the reservoir where they are used. A number of bacteria that are pathogenic to humans have animal reservoirs and can be transmitted to humans by either contaminated food (*food-borne transmission*), exposure to animal carriers (*direct transmission*) or contaminated environments (*environmental transmission*). Furthermore, animal bacteria that are not pathogenic to humans can serve as donors of resistance genes to human pathogens. Most antimicrobial resistance genes are situated on mobile genetic elements (MGE) such as plasmids, transposons and integrons that can be transferred more or less frequently between bacterial species and genera. MGE and the resistance genes they carry originated a long time before antimicrobials were discovered by humans, as indicated by the recovery of antimicrobial resistance plasmids in bacterial isolates from the pre-antimicrobial era (1). Most likely, the genes conferring antimicrobial resistance in pathogenic bacteria originated millions of years ago from ancestor genes in antibiotic-producing bacteria and other soil bacteria (2, 3). It should be noted that our knowledge of resistance genes is largely based on studies of pathogenic bacteria. However, commensal and environmental bacteria represent a vast reservoir of resistance genes. This natural reservoir could include novel resistance genes and mechanisms that might be picked up by pathogenic bacteria in the presence of favourable conditions, for example following the use of novel antimicrobial agents.

Although the use of antimicrobial agents in human medicine, animal production and veterinary medicine is not responsible for the origin of antimicrobial resistance, it has certainly contributed to the spread of resistant bacteria. As a matter of fact, when bacteria are exposed to antimicrobials, resistant strains overgrow their susceptible counterparts and become prevalent in the bacterial population, thereby facilitating the spread of resistance across bacterial, host and geographical borders. Antimicrobial usage also influences the evolution of resistance genes and their clustering on MGE. An example of how resistance genes adapt to the introduction of novel antimicrobial agents is provided by the evolution of β-lactamases. Shortly after the introduction of new β-lactams resistant to β-lactamases, enzymes able to degrade the novel compounds rapidly emerged as a result of mutations in previously existing β-lactamase genes. Today, more than 200 β-lactamases have been identified, each characterised by a well-defined spectrum of activity (4). Clustering of resistance genes on MGE can be selected by the use of chemically unrelated antimicrobials. As a result, bacteria harbouring MGE typically display co-resistance to multiple antimicrobial classes.

While selection of resistant bacteria by antimicrobial usage in animals, zoonotic transmission and horizontal transfer of resistance genes between animal and human bacteria have been documented by various types of scientific evidence, quantification of the occurrence of these events *in vivo* is extremely difficult. Consequently, the public health significance of the use of antimicrobials in animals remains the subject of intense debate. This chapter highlights the available scientific evidence regarding (i) the association between antimicrobial use and occurrence of antimicrobial resistance in animals (Section 2.1); (ii) the occurrence of food-borne, direct and environmental transmission of antimicrobial resistance from animals to humans (Sections 2.2–2.4); and (iii) the consequences of antimicrobial resistance in human infections with zoonotic bacteria (Section 2.5).

2.1 Association between antimicrobial use and occurrence of antimicrobial resistance in animals

Usually, a correlation exists between the patterns and amount of antimicrobial usage and the occurrence of antimicrobial resistance (Figure 2.1). Various

monitoring programs in Europe have determined associations between data on antimicrobial usage and the prevalence of antimicrobial resistant bacteria in animals and food products (5–7). Among these, the Danish surveillance programme (DANMAP) was initiated at the time when the use of growth promoters was terminated in this country. This has provided a unique opportunity to study the effects of the ban on the prevalence of resistant bacteria in food animals. After the ban of avoparcin (a growth promoter chemically related to the glycopeptide vancomycin) in Denmark in 1995, the prevalence of vancomycin-resistant enterococci (VRE) in poultry diminished drastically. Three years after the ban, the prevalence of VRE in poultry fell from more than 72% in 1995 to 2% in 2005 (Figure 2.2). However, VRE has persisted in poultry and can still be detected a decade after the

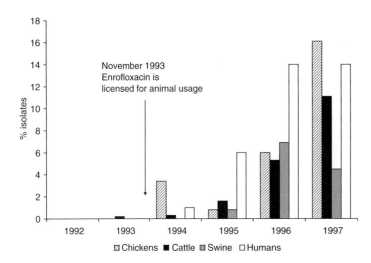

Figure 2.1 Prevalence (%) of fluoroquinolone-resistant *Salmonella* DT104 in chickens, cattle, swine and humans in the UK before and after the introduction of enrofloxacin in animal production in 1993. Reproduced with permission from reference 13.

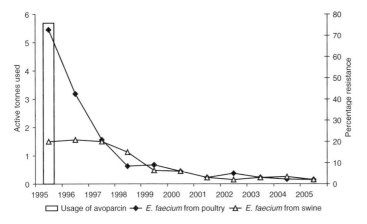

Figure 2.2 Prevalence of vancomycin-resistant *Enterococcus faecium* in Danish poultry and swine following the ban of the growth promoter avoparcin in 1995. Reproduced with permission from reference 5.

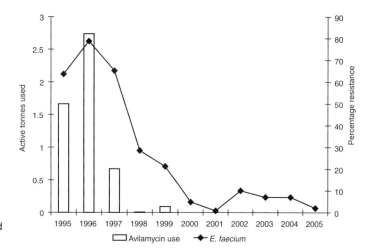

Figure 2.3 Association between avilamycin use and prevalence (%) of avilamycin-resistant *Enterococcus faecium* in poultry, poultry meat and healthy humans in Denmark. Reproduced with permission from reference 5.

ban when using selective methods for isolation of VRE (5). An equivalent reduction in avilamycin resistance was detected in *E. faecium* isolates from poultry following the ban of this growth promoter in Denmark (Figure 2.3). The prevalence of VRE in Danish swine remained stable three years after the avoparcin ban, until 1998, when the growth promoter tylosin (a macrolide) was banned (Figure 2.2). The ban of tylosin as a growth promoter was found to reduce the prevalence of VRE in swine. Genetic characterisation of porcine VRE revealed the presence of large plasmids encoding resistance to glycopeptides, macrolides and copper in the majority of the strains, suggesting that vancomycin resistance could have been co-selected by the use of tylosin in the three first years after the avoparcin ban (8).

The introduction of fluoroquinolones in animal production has been followed by the appearance of fluoroquinolone resistance in bacteria isolated from food animals and, subsequently, in zoonotic bacteria isolated from human infections. This is another example of the effects of antimicrobial usage on antimicrobial resistance in the animal reservoir. Fluoroquinolones are, in several countries, the drugs of choice for treatment of severe zoonotic infections caused by *Salmonella* and *Campylobacter*, and the emergence of fluoroquinolone resistance in these bacterial species is a matter of increasing concern. The selective effects associated with the use of fluoroquinolones in animals were first observed in The Netherlands, where the practice of medicating water with enrofloxacin in poultry production was

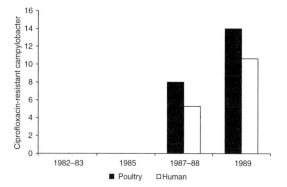

Figure 2.4 Prevalence of ciprofloxacin-resistant *Campylobacter* in poultry and humans following the introduction of enrofloxacin in poultry production in the Netherlands. Reproduced with permission from (9).

followed by the emergence of fluoroquinolone-resistant *Campylobacter* in both poultry and humans (see Figure 2.4) (9). Since then, several studies have documented an increase in the occurrence of fluoroquinolone-resistant *Campylobacter* in food animals and humans following the introduction of fluoroquinolones in animal production (10). Similar associations have been observed in *Salmonella*. In Germany, an increase in the occurrence of fluoroquinolone-resistant *Salmonella* Typhimurium DT204c was observed after the introduction of enrofloxacin in veterinary medicine in 1989 (11). In the UK, fluoroquinolone resistance in *Salmonella* Hadar, *S.* Virchow and *S.* Typhimurium DT104 substantially increased following the licensing of enrofloxacin and danofloxacin for veterinary use in 1993 and 1996 respectively (12) (Figure 2.1).

In the former East Germany, the antimicrobial nourseothricin, a streptothricin, was introduced in the mid-1980s as a growth promoter in swine production. Since streptothricins had never been used in either human or veterinary medicine, the study of nourseothricin resistance provided useful information on the effects of growth promoters in animal production, dissemination of resistant bacteria to humans, and horizontal transfer of the resistance genes to human bacteria, including pathogens. Shortly after nourseothricin was introduced as a growth promoter in swine, *Escherichia coli* containing plasmids conferring nourseothricin resistance were frequently found in faeces from swine and farm workers. Within 2 years, similar nourseothricin-resistant *E. coli* were isolated from family members of swine farm workers and from cases of urinary tract infections in adjacent communities, but not from people and animals in control areas without nourseothricin use (13). Nourseothricin resistance was subsequently detected in human *Salmonella* and *Shigella* isolates (14). Since *Shigella* is a pathogen of primates and does not occur in the intestinal tract of swine, this finding provided indirect evidence that horizontal transfer of nourseothricin resistance had occurred in the intestinal tract of humans.

2.2 Food-borne transmission of antimicrobial resistance from animals to humans

Most infections with antimicrobial-resistant *Salmonella* in industrialised countries are acquired by consumption of food products from swine, poultry and cattle (15). For antimicrobial-resistant *Campylobacter*, poultry is the principal reservoir. Resistant *E. coli* and enterococci can also be acquired from swine, poultry and cattle, but the relative importance of the major food animal reservoirs compared with human and environmental reservoirs is difficult to disentangle and quantify based on current knowledge. Several lines of evidence have demonstrated food-borne transmission of antimicrobial resistance from animals to humans, including outbreak investigations, epidemiological investigations of sporadic infections, field studies,

case reports, geographical and temporal associations, and molecular typing comparing isolates from human and animal sources. Numerous studies have indicated an association between antimicrobial use in food animals and antimicrobial resistance in humans by one or more of these lines of evidence (16).

2.2.1 Outbreak investigations

Although outbreaks only represent a fraction of the cases of infections caused by food-borne pathogens, including *Salmonella*, much insight into the epidemiology of food-borne diseases has been provided by investigation of outbreaks. Several outbreak investigations of antimicrobial-resistant *Salmonella* infections in humans have combined epidemiological fieldwork and laboratory subtyping techniques to trace antimicrobial-resistant *Salmonella* through the food distribution system to farms, and use of antimicrobial agents on the farms was found to be associated with the resistance patterns of *Salmonella* isolates from humans. A review of outbreaks of *Salmonella* infection indicated that outbreaks caused by antimicrobial-resistant strains were more likely to have a food animal source than outbreaks caused by antimicrobial-susceptible *Salmonella* (17). Among the most notable outbreak investigations have been the tracing of human tetracycline-resistant *Salmonella* infections to the addition of tetracycline to cattle feed (18) and the tracing of human chloramphenicol-resistant *Salmonella* infections to the illegal use of chloramphenicol on dairy farms (19). An outbreak of human nalidixic-acid-resistant *S.* Typhimurium DT104 infections in the UK was traced to a dairy farm where fluoroquinolones were used in the dairy cattle in the month prior to the outbreak (20). In Denmark, the first outbreak of nalidixic acid-resistant *S.* Typhimurium DT104 was traced back through the food chain to a local farm by use of typing methods (21). Another Danish outbreak of multi-resistant *Salmonella* DT104 was traced to import of Italian meat (22).

2.2.2 Epidemiological investigations

Several recent epidemiological investigations of sporadic cases of human *Salmonella* infections have demonstrated that persons with antimicrobial-resistant infections are more likely to have visited or lived on a farm before the onset of illness than persons infected with antimicrobial-susceptible infections. These findings have been demonstrated in a case–control study of antimicrobial-resistant *S.* Typhimurium DT104 infections (23), and multidrug resistant *Salmonella* Newport infections (24). A case–control study in the USA of persons infected with fluoroquinolone-resistant *Campylobacter* also found that these persons were more likely to have eaten chicken or turkey outside the home than controls. Since chicken and turkey are not imported into the USA, this finding provides evidence that poultry is an important source of domestically acquired fluoroquinolone-resistant *Campylobacter* infections in the country (25).

2.2.3 Field studies

Levy and colleagues (26) conducted prospective field experiments to demonstrate how antimicrobial use in food animals selects for the emergence and dissemination of resistance determinants. They found that the tetracycline resistance among *E. coli* in faecal samples from chickens increased within one week of introduction of animal feed containing tetracycline. Importantly, as long as the chickens were fed animal feed containing tetracycline, the proportion of tetracycline-resistant intestinal coliforms was also greater among members of the immediate farm family, and remained higher than intestinal coliforms from neighbourhood control families (26).

2.2.4 Case reports

There are several individual case reports of farmers, members of their families or other persons who have been directly exposed to antimicrobial-resistant bacteria from food animals. For example, the first reported case of domestically acquired ceftriaxone-resistant *Salmonella* in the USA involved the child of a veterinarian. Before the child's illness, the father was treating several herds of cattle for *Salmonella*. Ceftriaxone-resistant and ceftriaxone-susceptible *Salmonella* were isolated from ill cattle treated by the veterinarian. These isolates and the child's ceftriaxone-resistant isolate were shown to be very similar by pulsed-field gel electrophoresis (PFGE). It appears likely that the *Salmonella* strain developed ceftriaxone resistance in the cattle and then was transmitted to the child (27).

Multi-resistant *E. coli, Salmonella, Shigella flexneri* and staphylococci have been detected in aquatic products like *ready to eat* shrimps, thus indicating another potential source of food-borne transmission of antimicrobial resistance (28). Not only may resistant bacteria from aquacultures be transferred to humans, but also MGE containing resistance genes can be transferred to pathogenic bacteria, as suggested by the recovery of identical antimicrobial resistance plasmids in aquaculture and human clinical isolates (29, 30). Transfer of transposon-mediated tetracycline resistance from aquatic *Aeromonas* to human commensal *E. coli* has been reproduced under laboratory conditions (30).

2.2.5 Geographical and temporal associations

In countries such as Denmark, where quantitative data on antimicrobial use in food animals are available, correlations have been shown between the amount of antimicrobials used in food animals and the occurrence of antimicrobial resistance in selected bacteria (5). Even in countries without surveillance on antimicrobial use in food animals, temporal associations have been demonstrated between the first approved use of an antimicrobial agent in food animals and an increase in antimicrobial resistance. The effects of the approval of fluoroquinolones for animal use have been documented in various European countries (see Section 2.1). In the USA, a marked increase in the proportion of domestically acquired *Campylobacter* infections that were fluoroquinolone-resistant was observed following the first approved use of fluoroquinolones in food animals in 1995 (31). Geographical comparisons between countries with distinct patterns of antimicrobial usage in food animals have led to similar conclusions on zoonotic transmission of fluoroquinolone-resistant *Campylobacter*. For example, domestically acquired *Campylobacter* infections are commonly fluoroquinolone-resistant in European and North American countries that allow use of fluoroquinolones in food animals. However, domestically acquired *Campylobacter* infections are susceptible to fluoroquinolones in Australia, where fluoroquinolones are not used in food animals (32). In Norway, fluoroquinolone resistance among *Campylobacter jejuni* of human origin have remained very low, most likely reflecting the low prevalence of fluoroquinolone resistance among *Campylobacter* of broiler origin (33).

2.2.6 Molecular typing

Molecular typing has provided evidence for the association between avoparcin use in food animals and VRE occurrence in humans. Before the EU ban of avoparcin as a growth promoter in 1997, various studies detected VRE in the intestinal tract of healthy individuals (34–36). Molecular subtyping of VRE isolates from swine, chickens, healthy humans and hospitalised patients indicated genetic similarity between some isolates from animals and healthy humans (37). Although recent studies on the population structure of VRE have clearly shown that hospital strains generally differ from those occurring in food animals (38), typing of the MGE associated with glycopeptide resistance (Tn*1546*) has suggested horizontal gene transfer between animal and human enterococci. In particular, one of the three essential glycopeptide resistance genes in Tn*1546* (*vanX*) is characterised by single nucleotide (T or G) variants that are associated with strain origin. Among food animals, the G variants are only found in poultry isolates and the T variants in swine isolates. Among human isolates, the G and T variants are evenly distributed. Furthermore, human isolates from Muslim countries, where swine are not raised or consumed, only carry the G mutation (39).

After the introduction of the aminoglycoside apramycin for veterinary usage at the beginning of the 1980s, apramycin resistance emerged among *E. coli* isolates from cattle and swine in France and in the UK (40, 41). Apramycin has never been used for treatment of infections in humans. The resistance gene (*aac*(3)IV) encoding apramycin resistance confers cross-resistance to other aminoglycosides used in human medicine (tobramycin, gentamicin, kanamycin and neomycin) but the presence of this gene was first observed after the introduction of apramycin in veterinary practice (42). The apramycin resistance gene and similar resistance plasmids were subsequently found in *Salmonella* from animals and in human clinical *E. coli*, *Salmonella* and *Klebsiella pneumoniae* (43–45). These observations strongly indicated that apramycin resistance was primarily selected by the use of this antibiotic in food animals and was subsequently transferred to human pathogenic bacteria.

Molecular evidence also suggests an association between the use of gentamicin in food animals, particularly in chickens and turkeys in the USA, and the occurrence of high-level gentamicin-resistant enterococci in humans. The gentamicin resistance genes occurring in resistant enterococci isolated from animals corresponded to those found in enterococcal isolates from food products of the same animal species. Furthermore, although much diversity was evident among high-level gentamicin-resistant enterococci, indistinguishable strains were found in human and pork isolates, and human and grocery store chicken isolates (46). Similarly, genetic associations between *Salmonella* isolates from animals and humans have been demonstrated by molecular typing. For example, in a study on human fluoroquinolone-resistant *Salmonella* Choleraesuis infections in Taiwan (47), molecular typing allowed the authors to conclude that swine were the source of the human infections.

Molecular characterisation of MGE in bacteria isolated from fish has suggested an aquatic origin for the antimicrobial resistance determinants characteristic of the pandemic clone *S.* Typhimurium DT104, that have caused numerous outbreaks of salmonellosis in humans worldwide (6). Furthermore, spread of a *Salmonella* Agona found in imported fish meat from Peru was identified as the cause of an international outbreak (48).

2.3 Direct transmission of antimicrobial resistance from animals to humans

While food-borne transmission has been extensively described in the scientific literature, other routes have been less studied. However, there is increasing evidence to show that direct contact with animals can, under certain circumstances, play an important role in the transmission of resistance. This represents an occupational hazard for workers handling animals or animal products, such as farmers, veterinarians and meat producers. Also, people attending animal exhibitions or visiting farms may be exposed to this route of transmission (49, 50).

2.3.1 Transmission by contact with food animals

There are several case reports of farmers, veterinarians, members of their families or other persons who have become directly infected with antimicrobial-resistant bacteria by contact with food animals.

As mentioned in section 2.2.4 the first case reported was between a child of a veterinarian and cattle (27). In the Netherlands, indistinguishable PFGE patterns were displayed by *S.* Typhimurium DT104 isolated from a child, a swine and a calf living in the same farm (51). In the USA, transmission of multidrug-resistant *S.* Typhimurium has been documented in veterinary facilities and animal shelters. Transmission was likely to have occurred from animals to humans since humans became infected after animal illness (52).

Transmission of methicillin-resistant *Staphylococcus aureus* (MRSA) has recently been reported between swine and swine-farmers in the Netherlands (53) (see Chapter 7). In the same country, indistinguishable clones of *E. coli* and VRE were previously reported in farmers and their animals (35). A recent study conducted in Canada (54) has shown that use of antimicrobials and other management factors in swine farming may lead to increased antimicrobial resistance among faecal *E. coli* in farm residents. Altogether these data indicate that this route of transmission may have been overlooked in the past.

2.3.2 Transmission by contact with companion animals

The role of companion animals in the dissemination of antimicrobial resistance has been given little attention when compared with that of food animals. Cases of transmission of antimicrobial resistance by contact with companion animals are usually sporadic and more difficult to recognise. However, companion animals such as horses, dogs, cats and exotic pet animals have shown to be reservoirs of resistant bacteria, including species with a potential for zoonotic transmission and resistance phenotypes of clinical interest, like multidrug-resistant *S.* Typhimurium DT104 and MRSA (55). Even though the total amount of antimicrobials used in companion animals is lower than in food animals, broad-spectrum drugs of critical importance in human medicine are frequently used in companion animal medicine. In Denmark, 65% and 33% of the total veterinary use of cephalosporins and fluoroquinolones respectively, are used for companion animals (5). Despite their importance in human medicine, the use of fluoroquinolones or cephalosporins in dogs is comparatively higher than in humans (see Chapter 11).

Although *Salmonella* is generally regarded a food-borne pathogen, it has been estimated that up to 6% of salmonellosis cases are attributable to contact with exotic pets (56, 57). A direct correlation has been documented between the number of *Salmonella* Marina cases reported to the *Salmonella* surveillance programme in the USA and the number of iguanas imported annually in this country between 1982 and 1994 (58). Outbreak investigations have associated multi-drug-resistant *S.* Typhimurium with purchase of rodents (59) or reptiles (60). Similarly, household pets, especially cats, are a recognised source of human infection with multidrug-resistant *S.* Typhimurium. In 1999, various outbreaks of multidrug-resistant *S.* Typhimurium were reported at small animal facilities in the USA (61). Pet ownership is a recognised risk factor for sporadic campylobacteriosis among young children (62, 63). In a Danish study in 2001 (64), over 20% of healthy puppies were found to be healthy carriers of *C. jejuni*. Direct evidence of *C. jejuni* transmission between household dogs and young patients has been documented by DNA fingerprinting techniques (65, 66), including transmission of a fluroquinolone-resistant strain (65).

MRSA is increasingly reported in companion animals (66). The first indication that companion animals could be a source of human MRSA infection was provided in 2003 by a study in which recurrent infection in a human patient was associated with carriage by the family dog (67). Subsequently, MRSA carriage in pet animals has been associated with cases of infection in pet owners (68) and veterinarians (69). Transmission of MRSA between companion animals and veterinary staff has been reported in Canada (70), in the UK and in Ireland (71). Animal-to-human transmission is suggested by the fact that the MRSA clones found in equine and small animal practitioners generally correspond to those occurring in horses and small animals respectively (70, 71). Furthermore, the proportion of nasal MRSA carriage in veterinary personnel appears to be significantly higher when compared to the estimated prevalence in the community (72).

Direct transmission of bacteria, including antimicrobial-resistant bacteria, from pets to people working or living in contact with these animals is further supported by the common isolation of *Staphylococcus intermedius* from the nasal cavity of veterinarians (73) and owners of dog affected by atopic dermatitis (74). *S. intermedius intermedius* is a commensal staphylococcal species in domestic pets that is frequently associated with opportunistic skin, ear and urinary tract infections in dogs. The fact that *S. intermedius* is normally rare in the nasal cavity of humans suggests dog-to-human transmission. Strains carried by dog owners generally correlate with strains recovered from their dogs and display resistance to multiple antimicrobial agents, including penicillins, fusidic acid, macrolides, lincosamides, tetracyclines and chloramphenicol (74).

2.4 Environmental transmission of antimicrobial resistance from animals to humans

Environmental exposure of humans to antimicrobial-resistant bacteria of animal origin can occur under many different circumstances, including various occupational and leisure activities. For example, the spread of manure on farm land can be a significant source of resistant bacteria in agricultural environments. Resistant bacteria of animal faecal origin cannot usually adapt to live outside the host but may be able to survive in the environment for a limited period of time, during which they can transfer resistance genes to soil bacteria (75). Various investigations have shown that the use of swine manure results in the transfer of resistant bacteria from the farm to the surrounding environment, including aquatic environments (76, 77). In Asia, manure originating from food animal production facilities is placed in aquaculture pounds, where the organic compounds are utilised to support growth of photosynthetic organisms. Via this direct link, resistant bacteria selected by the intensive use of antimicrobials in swine and poultry production are directly released into the aquatic environment, together with antimicrobial residues in animal faeces and medicated feed. As a consequence of this practice, high numbers of resistant bacteria have been detected in the sediment from integrated fish farms (78, 79).

Environmental transmission of antimicrobial resistance from animals to humans may also take place by air pollution. High numbers of antimicrobial-resistant staphylococci (80) and enterococci (81) have been detected in the air inside swine facilities. Dust particles from animal facilities have also been shown to contain measurable concentrations of antimicrobials (82). Therefore, it appears that farm workers are exposed daily to resistant bacteria as well as to antimicrobial residues that can potentially select for the resistant bacteria once they have been inhaled. Transmission by air pollution also represents a risk for

people living in the vicinity of farms as indicated by the recovery of resistant bacteria in an air plume collected downwind from a confined and concentrated animal feeding operation (83).

2.5 Consequences of antimicrobial resistance in human infections with zoonotic bacteria

Evidence is accumulating that antimicrobial resistance in zoonotic bacteria has human health consequences (15, 84) (Table 2.1). Such consequences include infections that would not otherwise have occurred if the pathogens were not resistant, increased frequency of treatment failures and increased severity of infection. The latter includes prolonged duration of illness, increased frequency of bloodstream infections, increased hospitalisation and increased mortality.

2.5.1 Infections that would not have otherwise occurred

Antimicrobial usage disturbs the microbiota of the intestinal tract, placing treated individuals at increased risk of clinical salmonellosis if they are also colonised with a *Salmonella* strain that is resistant to that agent (84). Individuals taking an antimicrobial are therefore at increased risk of developing illness with pathogens resistant to the used antimicrobial. Furthermore, exposure to contaminated foodstuff can result in asymptomatic colonisation with food-borne bacteria that can be selected for by therapeutic treatment and result in colonisation progression to clinical disease. Some of these effects have been demonstrated in case–control studies of persons infected with antimicrobial resistant *Salmonella*. Persons exposed to antimicrobials for unrelated reasons, such as treatment of an upper respiratory tract infection, were at increased risk of infection with the antimicrobial-resistant *Salmonella* (18). As an example, in a milk-borne outbreak of a multidrug-resistant strain of *S.* Typhimurium in 1985 with 116 000 cases, patients who were undergoing antimicrobial therapy with an antimicrobial drug to which the outbreak strain was resistant had been drinking significantly less milk than patients who had not been taking antimicrobial drugs. This suggested that the infectious dose is lower for persons receiving antimicrobial therapy than it is for persons who do not receive treatment (85). This

Table 2.1 Potential effects of the emergence of antimicrobial drug resistance in food-borne bacteria on human health. Adapted from (15)

Reduced efficacy of early empirical treatment	Antimicrobial drug treatment is not advocated for most cases of gastroenteritis. However, for patients with severe underlying illness or with suspected extraintestinal spread, treatment should be initiated prior to microbiological diagnosis. In these cases, resistance to clinically important drugs will increase the risk of treatment failure
Limited choice of treatment after the diagnosis	Drug resistance to clinically important classes of antimicrobial drugs will limit the choices of drugs, and may lead to increasing costs of treatment
Increased transmission	Drug-resistant bacteria have a selective advantage in patients treated with antimicrobial drugs for other reasons Resistant strains may easily gain foothold in settings where antimicrobials are used, such as hospitals. Hence, increased transmission may often occur among individuals with underlying illness
Horizontal transmission of resistance genes	Genes encoding for antimicrobial drug resistance are often located on mobile genetic elements, such as plasmids, transposons and integrons. These may be transferred to other bacteria
Increased virulence	There is evidence that resistant bacteria cause more invasive infections and increased mortality, perhaps due to co-selection of virulence traits or improved fitness of drug-resistant bacterial pathogens

effect has also been demonstrated in the laboratory when the use of the antibiotic streptomycin in mice dramatically lowers the dose needed to infect the mouse with a streptomycin-resistant strain (86).

The increased risk of *Salmonella* transmission among persons exposed to antimicrobial agents for unrelated reasons has been estimated. Cohen and Tauxe (87) looked at the attributable fraction of cases in relation to antimicrobial treatment in selected outbreaks involving antimicrobial resistant *Salmonella* strains. Overall between 16 and 64% of cases would not have occured if the exposed person had not had antimicrobial treatment or the infectious strain had been sensitive to antimicrobials. Because taking antimicrobial agents for a variety of reasons is common in different parts of the world, antimicrobial resistance in *Salmonella* results in infections, hospitalisations and deaths that would not have occurred in the absence of resistance. Barza and Travers reviewed the literature on attributable fraction of cases and concluded that antimicrobial resistance in *Salmonella* and *Campylobacter* results in 29 379 *Salmonella* infections that would not otherwise have occurred – leading to 342 hospitalisation cases and 12 deaths – and 17 688 *C. jejuni* infections that would not otherwise have occurred – leading to 95 hospitalisations each year in the USA (84).

Keeping in mind that the prevalence of drug resistance in S. Typhimurium, the most common *Salmonella*

serotype in the USA, is 40%, increased transmission as a result of drug resistance is of real public health significance. Also, persons who have an underlying illness or are being treated for other disorders may face more severe clinical consequences of the infection. This interaction may, in some situations, explain why infections with antimicrobial drug-resistant bacteria may appear to be more virulent than those with drug-susceptible bacteria. It may also explain why outbreaks with drug-resistant food-borne bacteria so commonly occur in hospital settings where antimicrobial drugs are used for a variety of indications. A similar effect may occur in food animals, which are also frequently exposed to antimicrobial agents, though the extent that antimicrobial resistance in *Salmonella*, *Campylobacter*, and perhaps other bacteria results in increased transmission of these bacteria between food animals that are exposed to antimicrobial agents has not been described. If such use does promote the spread of resistant strains among food animals, it seems likely that this may result in increased transmission of those strains to humans.

2.5.2 Increased frequency of treatment failures and increased severity of infection

Increased frequency of treatment failures and increased severity of infection may be manifested by prolonged duration of illness, increased frequency of bloodstream infections, increased hospitalisation or increased mortality. The association between an increased frequency of antimicrobial resistance *Salmonella* and an increased frequency of hospitalisation has been demonstrated in several studies. A study of 28 *Salmonella* outbreaks investigated by the Centers for Disease Control and Prevention (CDC) between 1971 and 1983 found that outbreaks caused by antimicrobial-resistant *Salmonella* resulted in a greater hospitalisation rate and greater case-fatality rate than outbreaks caused by susceptible infections (7). Recently, this analysis has been repeated on *Salmonella* outbreaks investigated by CDC between 1984 and 2002. Again, outbreaks caused by antimicrobial-resistant *Salmonella* resulted in a greater hospitalisation rate than outbreaks caused by susceptible infections (88).

A study of 758 persons with sporadic *Salmonella* infections in 1989–1990 found that persons infected with antimicrobial-resistant isolates were more likely to be hospitalised and hospitalised longer (89). A more comprehensive study of sporadic *Salmonella* infections has been completed for the Foodborne Diseases Active Surveillance Network (FoodNet) and National Antimicrobial Resistance Monitoring System (NARMS) in the USA (90). Unlike the study by Lee (89), this analysis controlled for the serotype of *Salmonella*. Among *Salmonella* isolates tested in NARMS from 1996 to 2001, *Salmonella* isolates resistant to antimicrobial agents were more frequently isolated from blood than susceptible isolates. A particularly high frequency of isolation from blood was observed among isolates resistant to five or more antimicrobial agents. Among patients interviewed, persons with *Salmonella* isolates resistant to antimicrobial agents were more frequently hospitalised with bloodstream infection than susceptible infections. Again, there was a particularly high frequency of hospitalisation with bloodstream infection among persons infected with isolates resistant to five or more antimicrobial agents.

In a comprehensive study of sporadic *S.* Typhimurium and *Campylobacter* infections in Denmark among patients with culture-confirmed infections, of 1323 patients infected with quinolone-resistant *S.* Typhimurium, 46 (3.5%) were hospitalised with invasive illness within 90 days of acquiring the infection and 16 (1.2%) died within 90 days of being infected. After adjusting for age, sex and co-morbidity, the infection with quinolone-resistant *S.* Typhimurium was associated with a 3.15 fold higher risk of invasive illness or death within 90 days from infection when compared to infections with (pan) susceptible strains (91). Furthermore, if infected with fluoroquinolone-resistant *Campylobacter,* a greater risk of death or invasive illness exists when compared to susceptible strains. Of 3471 patients infected with *C. jejuni* or *C. coli*, 22 (0.63%) had an adverse event within 90 days. When comparing macrolide (erythromycin) and quinolone-resistant *Campylobacter* infections, to infections with susceptible *Campylobacter,* a five to six fold increase, respectively, of having an adverse event after 90 days was detected (92).

Treatment failures resulting in death have been rare among *Salmonella* cases, but may be expected to increase as the prevalence of resistance to clinically important antimicrobial agents increases among *Salmonella*. In the best described study of such treatment failures, an outbreak of nalidixic acid-resistant *S.* Typhimurium DT104 in Denmark resulted in hospitalisation of 23 patients and 2 deaths (21). Both patients who died had been treated with a fluoroquinolone for their *Salmonella* infections; in both instances, it was concluded that the fluoroquinolone resistance contributed to the deaths (21).

A comprehensive study of mortality associated with antimicrobial resistance among *S.* Typhimurium was conducted in Denmark among patients with culture-confirmed infections from 1995 to 1999 (92). To determine the increase in mortality compared to the general population, cases were matched to 10 persons from the registry by age, sex, county and co-morbidity. Overall, persons with *Salmonella* infections had a 2.3 times higher mortality than the general population, while persons with ampicillin-resistant *Salmonella* infections had a 4.8 times higher mortality than the general population. Furthermore, persons with quinolone-resistant infections (10.3 times higher) and with multidrug-resistant infections (13.1 times higher) had a remarkably higher chance of dying in the 2 years following specimen collection than the general population.

Although antimicrobial resistance among *Salmonella* Typhi is not related to use of antimicrobial agents in animals, prolonged duration of illness has also been demonstrated among persons infected with nalidixic acid-resistant *Salmonella* Typhi treated with fluoroquinolones. Such apparent treatment failures have been sufficiently common among persons infected with strains having borderline MIC (Minimal Inhibitory Concentration) to fluoroquinolones that several groups have suggested that the breakpoints used to define fluoroquinolone resistance in *Salmonella* and other enteric bacteria be lowered (93, 94).

An association between resistance and longer duration of illness has been demonstrated in four recent case–control studies of fluoroquinolone-resistant *Campylobacter* infections (31, 93–96). In these studies, among persons treated with fluoroquinolones, the median duration of diarrhoea in persons infected with fluoroquinolone-resistant *Campylobacter* was several days longer than the median duration of diarrhoea in persons with susceptible infections.

Taken together, these data provide evidence of the clinical and public health consequences of drug resistance in zoonotic agents. Mitigation of drug resistance in bacteria that are transmitted from animals to man is likely to be of benefit for human health.

References

1. Hughes, V. M. and Datta, N. (1983). Conjugative plasmids in bacteria of the pre-antibiotic era. *Nature* 302: 725–726.
2. Weisblum, B. (1995). Erythromycin resistance by ribosome modification. *Antimicrob. Agents Chemother.* 39(3): 577–585.
3. Guardabassi, L., Christensen, H., Hasman, H. and Dalsgaard, A. (2004). Members of the genera *Paenibacillus* and *Rhodococcus* harbor genes homologous to enterococcal glycopeptide resistance genes VanA and VanB. *Antimicrob. Agents Chemother.* 48(12): 4915–4918.
4. Bush, K. (2001). New beta-lactamases in Gram negative bacteria: diversity and impact on the selection of antimicrobial therapy. *Clin. Infect. Dis.* 32: 1085–1089.
5. Anonymous. (2006). *DANMAP, 2005: Use of antimicrobial agents and occurrence of antimicrobial resistance in bacteria from food animals, foods and humans in Denmark.* Available at http://www.dfvf.dk/Files/Filer/Zoonosecentret/Publikationer/Danmap/Danmap_2005.pdf
6. MARAN 2003 (2004). *Monitoring of antimicrobial resistance and antibiotic usage in animals in The Netherlands.* Available at http://www.cidc-lelystad.wur.nl/NR/rdonlyres/7F79ACE60–FD241–AB-81B2-BB17FA89603C/11381/MARAN2003web1.pdf
7. NORM/NORM-VET 2005 (2006). *Consumption of antimicrobial agents and occurrence of resistance in Norway.* Available at http://www.vetinst.no/zoo/index.asp?startID=&topExpand=&subExpand=&strUrl=1000586i
8. Hasman, H. and Aarestrup, F.M. (2003) Relationship between copper, glycopeptide, and macrolide resistance among *Enterococcus faecium* strains isolated from pigs in Denmark between 1997 and 2003. *Antimicrob. Agents Chemother.* 49(1): 454–456.
9. Endtz, H.P., Ruijs, G.J., van Klingeren, B., Jansen, W.H., van der Reyden, T. and Mouton, R. P. (1991). Quinolone resistance in campylobacter isolated from man and poultry following the introduction of fluoroquinolones in veterinary medicine. *J. Antimicrob. Chemother.* 27: 199–208.
10. Engberg, J., Aarestrup, F.M., Smidt, P.G., Nachamkin, I. and Taylor, D.E. (2001). Quinolone and macrolide resistance in *Campylobacter jejuni* and *coli*: a review of mechanisms and trends over time of resistance profiles in human isolates. *Emerg. Infect. Dis.* 7: 24–34.
11. Helmuth, R. (2000). Antibiotic resistance in *Salmonella*. In Wray, C. and Wray, A. (eds.), *Salmonella in domestic animals.* CAB International, Wallingford pp. 89–106.
12. Threlfall, E.J., Ward, L.R., Skinner, J.A. and Rowe, B. (1997). Increase in multiple antibiotic resistance in nontyphoidal salmonellas from humans in England and Wales: a comparison of data for 1994 and 1996. *Microb. Drug Resist.* 3: 263–266.
13. Hummel, R., Tschäpe, H. and Witte, W. (1986). Spread of plasmid-mediated nourseothricin resistance due to antibiotic use in animal husbandry. *J. Basic Microbiol.* 26: 461–466.
14. Witte, W., Tschäpe, H., Klare, I. and Werner, W. (2000). Antibiotics in animal feed. *Acta Vet. Scand.* 93(Suppl): 37–45.
15. Mølbak, K. (2005). Human health consequences of antimicrobial drug-resistant *Salmonella* and other foodborne pathogens. *Clin. Infect. Dis.* 4: 1613–1620.
16. Angulo, F.J., Nargund, V.N. and Chiller, T.C. (2004). Evidence of an association between use of antimicrobial agents in food animals and antimicrobial resistance among bacteria isolated from humans and the human health consequence of such resistance. *J. Vet. Med.* 51: 374–379.
17. Holmberg, S.D. Solomon, S.L. and Blake, A. (1987). Health and economic impacts of antimicrobial resistance. *Rev. Infect. Dis.* 9(6): 1065–1078.
18. Holmberg, S.D., Osterholm, M.T., Senger, K.A. and Cohen, M.L. (1984). Drug-resistant *Salmonella* from animals fed antimicrobials. *N. Engl. J. Med.* 311: 617–622.
19. Spika, J., Waterman, S., Hoo, G. *et al.* (1987). Chloramphenicol-resistant *Salmonella* Newport traced through hamburger to dairy farms: a major persisting source of human salmonellosis in California. *N. Engl. J. Med.* 316: 565–570.
20. Walker, R.A., Lawson, A.J., Lindsay, E.A. *et al.* (2000). Decreased susceptibility to ciprofloxacin in outbreak-associated multiresistant *Salmonella* Typhimurium DT104. *Vet. Rec.* 147(14): 395–396.
21. Mølbak, K., Baggesen, D.L., Aarestrup, F.M. *et al.* (1999). An outbreak of multi-drug resistant, quinolone-resistant *Salmonella enterica* serotype Typhimurium DT104. *N. Engl. J. Med.* 341: 1420–1425.
22. Ethelberg, S., Sørensen, G., Kristensen, B. *et al.* (2007). Outbreak with multi-resistant *Salmonella* Typhimurium

DT104 linked to Carpaccio, Denmark, 2005. *Epidemiol. Infect.* 5: 1–8.

23. Glynn, M.K., Reddy, V. Hutwagner, L. *et al.* (2004). Prior antimicrobial agent use increases the risk of sporadic infections with multidrug-resistant *Salmonella enterica* serotype Typhimurium a FoodNet case–control study. *Clin. Infect. Dis.* 38(Suppl 3): S227–S236.

24. Varma, J.K., Marcus, R., Stenzel, S.A. *et al.* (2006). Highly resistant Salmonella Newport-MDRAmpC transmitted through the domestic US food supply: a FoodNet case–control study of sporadic *Salmonella* Newport infections, 2002–2003. *J. Infect. Dis.* 194(2): 222–230.

25. Kassenborg, H.D., Smith, K.E., Vugia, D.J. *et al.* (2004). Emerging Infections Program FoodNet Working Group, 2004: Fluoroquinolone-resistant *Campylobacter* infections: eating poultry outside the home and foreign travel are risk factors. *Clin. Infect. Dis.* 38 (Suppl 3): S279–S284.

26. Levy, S., Fitzerald, G. and Macone, A. (1976). Changes in intestinal flora of farm personell after introduction of a tetracycline-supplemented feed on a farm. *N. Engl. J. Med.* 295: 583–588.

27. Fey, P.D., Safranek, T.J., Rupp, M.E., *et al.* (2000). Ceftriaxone-resistant salmonella infection acquired by a child from cattle. *N. Engl. J. Med.* 342: 1242–1249.

28. Duran, G.M. and Marshall, D.L. (2005). Ready to eat shrimps as an international vehicle of antibiotic resistant bacteria. *J. Food Prot.* 68: 2395–2401.

29. Adams, C.A., Austin, B., Meaden, P.G. and McIntosh, D. (1998). Molecular characterization of plasmid mediated oxytetracycline resistance in *Aeromonas salmonicida*. *Appl. Environ. Microbiol.* 64: 4194–4201.

30. Rhodes, G., Huys, G., Swings, J. *et al.* (2000). Distribution of oxytetracycline resistance plasmids between *Aeromonas* in hospitals and aquaculture environments: implication of Tn*1721* in dissemination of the tetracycline resistant determinant TetA. *Appl. Environ. Microbiol.* 66: 2883–3890.

31. Smith, K.E., Besser, J.M., Hedberg, C.W. *et al.* (1999). Quinolone-resistant *Campylobacter jejuni* infections in Minnesota, 1992–1998. *N. Engl. J. Med.* 340(20): 1525–1532.

32. Unicomb, L., Ferguson, J., Riley, T.V. and Collignon, P. (2003). Fluoroquinolone resistance in *Campylobacter* absent from isolates, Australia. *Emerg. Infect. Dis.* 9(11): 1482–1483.

33. Norström, M., Hofshagen, M., Stavnes, T., Schau, J., Lassen, J. and Kruuse, H. (2006). Antimicrobial resistance in *Campylobacter jejuni* from humans and broilers in Norway. *Epidemiol. Infect.* 134(1): 127–130.

34. Klare, I., Badstubner, D., Konstabel, C., Bohme, G., Claus, H. and Witte, W. (1999). Decreased incidence of VanA-type vancomycin-resistant enterococci isolated from poultry meat and from fecal samples of humans in the community after discontinuation of avoparcin usage in animal husbandry. *Microb. Drug Resist.* 5(1): 45–53.

35. van den Bogaard, A.E., Mertens, P., London, N.H. and Stobberingh, E.E. (1997). High prevalence of colonization with vancomycin- and pristinamycin-resistant enterococci in healthy humans and pigs in The Netherlands: is addition of antibiotics to animal feed to blame? *J. Antimicrob. Chemother.* 40: 454–456.

36. van den Bogaard, A.E., Bruinsma, N. and Stobberingh, E.E. (2000). The effect of banning avoparcin on VRE carriage in The Netherlands. *J. Antimicrob. Chemother.* 46: 146–148.

37. Bruinsma, N., Willems, R.J., van den Bogaard, A.E. *et al.* (2002). Different levels of genetic homogeneity in vancomycin-resistant and susceptible *Enterococcus faecium* isolates from different human and animal sources analysed by amplified-fragment length polymorphism. *Antimicrob. Agents Chemother.* 46: 2779–2783.

38. Willems, R. and Boten, M. (2007). Glycopeptide-resistant enterococci: deciphering virulence, resistance and epidemicity. *Curr. Opin. Infect. Dis.* 20(4): 384–390.

39. Jensen, L.B. (1998). Differences in the occurrence of two base-pair variants of Tn*1546* from vancomycin resistant enterococci from humans, pigs and poultry. *Antimicrob. Agents Chemother.* 42: 2463–2464.

40. Chaslus-Dancla, E. and Lafont, J.P. (1985). Resistance to gentamicin and apramycin in *Escherichia coli* from calves in France. *Vet. Rec.* 117: 90–91.

41. Wray, C., Hedges, R.W., Shannon, K.P. and Bradley, D.E. (1986). Apramycin and gentamicin resistance in *Escherichia coli* and salmonellas isolated from farm animals. *J. Hyg.* 97(39): 445–456.

42. Hedges, R.W. and Shannon, K.P. (1984). Resistance to apramycin in *Escherichia coli* isolated from animals: detection of a novel aminoglycoside-modifying enzyme. *J. Gen. Microbiol.* 130: 473–482.

43. Chaslus-Dancla, E., Martel, J.L, Carlier, C., Lafont, J.P. and Courvalin, P. (1986). Emergence of aminoglycoside 3-*N*-acetyltransferase IV in *Escherichia coli* and *Salmonella* Typhimurium isolated from animals in France. *Antimicrob. Agents Chemother.* 29: 239–243.

44. Hunter, J.E., Shelley, J.C., Walton, J.R., Hart, C.A. and Bennett, M. (1992). Apramycin resistance plasmids in *Escherichia coli*: possible transfer to *Salmonella* Typhimurium in calves. *Epidemiol. Infect.* 108: 271–278.

45. Johnson, A.P., Burns, L., Woodford, N. *et al.* (1994). Gentamicin resistance in clinical isolates of *Escherichia coli* encoded by genes of veterinary origin. *J. Med. Microbiol.* 40: 221–226.

46. Donabedian, S.M., Thal, L.A, Hershberger, E. *et al.* (2003). Molecular characterization of gentamicin-resistant Enterococci in the United States: evidence of spread from animals to humans through food. *J. Clin. Microbiol.* 41(3): 1109–1113.

47. Chiu, C.H., Wu, T.L., Su, L.H., *et al.* (2002). The emergence in Taiwan of fluoroquinolone resistance in *Salmonella enterica* serotype Choleraesuis. *N. Engl. J. Med.* 346(6): 413–419.

48. Clark, G.M., Kaufmann, A.F. and Gangarosa, E.J. (1973). Epidemiology of an international outbreak of *Salmonella* Agona. *The Lancet* 2: 490–493.

49. Bender, J.B. and Shulman, S.A. (2004). Anomalies in public contact subcommittee and National Association of State Public Health Veterinarians. Reports of zoonotic disease outbreaks associated with animal exhibits and availability of recommendations for preventing zoonotic disease transmission from animals to people in such settings. *J. Am. Vet. Med. Assoc.* 224: 1105–1109.

50. Heuvelink, A.E., van Heerwaarden, C., Zwartkruis-Nahuis, J.T. *et al.* (2002). *Escherichia coli* O157 infection associated with a petting zoo. *Epidemiol. Infect.* 129: 295–302.

51. Hendriksen, S.W.M., Orsel, K., Wagenaar, J.A., Miko, A. and van Duijkeren, E. (2004). Animal to human transmission of *Salmonella* Typhimurium DT104A variant. *Emerg. Infect. Dis.* 12: 2225–2227.

52. Wright, J.G., Tengelsen, L.A., Smith, K.E. *et al.* (2005). Multidrug-resistant *Salmonella* Typhimurium in four animal facilities. *Emerg. Infect. Dis.* 11: 1235–1241.

53. Voss, A., Loeffen, F., Bakker, J., Klaassen, C. and Wulf, M. (2005). Methicillin-resistant *Staphylococcus aureus* in pig farming. *Emerg. Infect. Dis.* 11: 1965–1966.

54. Akwar, T.H., Poppe, C., Wilson, J. *et al.* (2007). Risk factors for antimicrobial resistance among fecal *Escherichia coli* from residents on forty-three swine farms. *Microb. Drug Resist.* 13: 69–76.

55. Guardabassi, L., Schwarz, S. and Lloyd, D. (2004). Pet animals as reservoirs of antimicrobial resistant bacteria. *J. Antimicrob. Chemother.* 54: 321–332.

56. Centers for Disease Control and Prevention (CDC). (2003). Reptile-associated salmonellosis-selected states 1998–2002. *MMWR* 52: 1206–1209.

57. Woodward, D.L., Khakhria, R. and Johnson, W.M. (1997). Human Salmonellosis associated with exotic pets. *J. Clin. Microbiol.* 35: 2786–2790.

58. Mermin, J., Hoar, B. and Angulo, F.J. (1997). Iguanas and *Salmonella* Marina infection in children: a reflection of the increasing incidence of reptile-associated Salmonellosis in the United States. *Pediatrics* 99: 399–402.

59. Centers for Disease Control and Prevention (CDC) (2003). Outbreak of multidrug-resistant *Salmonella* Typhimurium associated with rodents purchase in retail pet stores – United States, December 2003–October 2004. *MMWR* 54: 429–433.

60. Centers for Disease Control and Prevention (CDC) (2005). Salmonellosis associated with pet turtles – Wisconsin and Wyoming 2004. *MMWR* 54: 223–236.

61. Centers for Disease Control and Prevention (2001). Outbreaks of multidrug-resistant *Salmonella* Typhimurium associated with veterinary facilities-Idaho, Minnesota and Washington, 1999. *MMWR* 50: 701–704.

62. Tenkate, T.D. and Stafford, R.J. (2001). Risk factors for campylobacter infection in infants and young children: a matched case–control study. *Epidemiol. Infect.* 127: 399–404.

63. Carrique-Mas, J., Andersson, Y., Hjertqvist, M. *et al.* (2005). Risk factors for domestic sporadic campylobacteriosis among young children in Sweden. *Scand. J. Infect. Dis.* 37: 101–110.

64. Damborg, P., Olsen, K.E., Møller Nielsen, E. and Guardabassi, L. (2004). Occurrence of *Campylobacter jejuni* in pets living with human patients infected with *C. jejuni. J. Clin. Microbiol.* 42: 1363–1364.

65. Wolfs, T.F.W., Duim, B., Geelen, S.P.M. *et al.* (2001). Neonathal septis by *Campylobacter jejuni*: genetically proven transmission from a household puppy. *Clin. Infect. Dis.* 32: 97–99.

66. Leonard, F.C. and Markay, B.K. (2007). Methicillin-resistant *Staphylococcus aureus* in animal: a review. *Vet. J.* (in press). doi: 10.1016/j.tvjl.2006.11.008

67. Manian, F.A. (2003). Asymptomatic nasal carriage of mupirocin-resistant, methicillin-resistant *Staphylococcus aureus* (MRSA) in pet dog associated with MRSA infections in household contact. *Clin. Infect. Dis.* 36: 26–28.

68. van Duijkeren, E., Wolfhagen, M.J., Heck, M.E. and Wannet, W.J. (2005). Transmission of panton-valentine leucocidin-positive methicillin-resistant *Staphylococcus aureus* strain between humans and a dog. *J. Clin. Microbiol.* 43(12): 6209–6211.

69. Weese, J.S., Dick, H., Willey, B.M. *et al.* (2006). Suspected transmission of methicillin-resistant *Staphylococcus aureus* between domestic pets and humans in veterinary clinics and in the household. *Vet. Microbiol.* 115: 148–155.

70. Weese, J.S., Rousseau, J., Traub-Darfatz, J.L., Willey, B.M., McGeer, A.J. and Low, D.E. (2005). Community-associated methicillin-resistant *Staphylococcus aureus* in horses and humans who work with horses. *J. Am. Vet. Med. Assoc.* 226: 580–583.

71. Moodley, A., Stegger, M., Bagcigil, A.F. *et al.* (2006). PFGE and *spa* typing of methicillin-resistant *Staphylococcus aureus* isolated from domestic animals and veterinary staff in the UK and Ireland. *J. Antimicrob. Chemother.* 58: 1118–1123.

72. Hanselman, B.A., Kruth, S.A., Rousseau, J. *et al.* (2006). Methicillin-resistant *Staphylococcus aureus* colonization in veterinary personnel. *Emerg. Infect. Dis.* 12: 1933–1938.

73. Harvey, R.G., Marples, R.R. and Noble, W.C. (1994). Nasal carriage of *Staphylococcus intermedius* in humans in contact with dogs. *Microb. Ecol. Health Dis.* 7: 225–227.

74. Guardabassi, L., Loeber, M.E. and Jacobson, A. (2004). Transmission of multiple antimicrobial resistant *Staphylococcus intermedius* between dogs affected by deep pyoderma and their owners. *Vet. Microbiol.* 98: 23–27.

75. Agersø, Y., Sengeløv, G. and Jensen, L.B. (2004). Development of a rapid method for direct detection of *tet*(M) genes in soil from Danish farmland. *Environ. Int.* 30: 117–122.

76. Sengeløv, G., Agersø, Y., Halling-Sørensen, B., Andersen, J.S. and Jensen, L.B. (2003). Bacterial antibiotic resistance levels in Danish farmland as a result of treatment with pig manure slurry. *Environ. Int.* 28: 587–595.

77. Chee-Sanford, J.C., Aminov, R.I., Krapac, I.J. *et al.* (2001). Occurrence and diversity of tetracycline resistance genes in lagoons and groundwater underlying two swine production facilities. *Appl. Environ. Microbiol.* 67: 1494–1502.

78. Petersen, A., Andersen, J.S., Kaawmak, T. *et al.* (2002). Impact of integrated fish farming on antimicrobial resistance in a pond environment. *Appl. Environ. Microbiol.* 68: 6036–6042.

79. Lee, T.X., Munekage, Y. and Kato, S.-I. (2005). Antibiotic resistance in bacteria from shrimp farming in mangrove areas. *Sci. Total Environ.* 349: 95–105.

80. Chapin, A., Rule, A., Gibson, K., Buckley, T. and Schwab, K. (2005). Airborne multidrug resistant bacteria isolated from a concentrated swine feeding operation. *Environ. Health Perspect.* 113: 137–142.

81. Green, C.F., Gibbs, S.G., Tarwater, P.M. *et al.* (2006). Bacterial plume emanating from the air surrounding swine confinement operations. *J. Occup. Environ. Hyg.* 3: 9–15.

82. Hamscher, G., Pawelzick, H.T., Sczesny, S. *et al.* (2003). Antibiotics in dust originating from a pig-fattening farm: a new source of health hazard for farmers. *Environ. Health Perspect.* 111: 1590–1594.

83. Gibbs, S.G., Green, C.F., Tarwater, P.M. *et al.* (2006). Isolation of antibiotic resistant bacteria from air plume downwind of a swine confined and concentrated animal feeding operation. *Environ. Health Perspect.* 114: 1032–1037.

84. Barza, M. and Travers, K. (2002). Excess infections due to antimicrobial resistance: the 'attributable fraction'. *Clin. Infect. Dis.* 34: 126–130.

85. Ryan, C.A., Nickels, M.K., Hargrett-Bean, N.T. *et al.* (1987). Massive outbreak of antimicrobial-resistant salmonellosis traced to pasteurized milk. *J. Am. Med. Assoc.* 258: 3269–3274.

86. Bohnhoff, M. and Miller, C.P. (1962). Enhanced susceptibility to *Salmonella* infection in streptomycin-treated mice. *J. Infect. Dis.* 111: 117–127.

87. Cohen, M.L. and Tauxe, R.V. (1986). Drug-resistant *Salmonella* in the United States: an epidemiologic perspective. *Science* 234: 964–969.

88. Varma, J.K., Green, K.D., Ovitt, J. *et al.* (2005). Hospitalization and antimicrobial resistance in *Salmonella* outbreaks, 1984–2002. *Emerg. Infect. Dis.* 11: 943–946.

89. Lee L.A., Puhr, N.D., Maloney, E.K. *et al.* (1994). Increase in antimicrobial-resistant *Salmonella* infections in the United States 1989–1990. *J. Infect. Dis.* 170: 128–134.

90. Varma, J.K., Mølbak, K., Barrett, *et al.* (2005). Antimicrobial-resistant nontyphoidal *Salmonella* is associated with excess bloodstream infections and hospitalizations. *J. Infect. Dis.* 191(4): 554–561.

91. Helms M., Simonsen J. and Mølbak K. (2004). Quinolone resistance is associated with increased risk of invasive illness or death during infection with *Salmonella* serotype Typhimurium. *J. Infect. Dis.* 190: 1652–1654.

92. Helms M., Vastrup, P., Gerner-Smidt, P. and Mølbak, K. (2002). Excess mortality associated with antimicrobial drug-resistant *Salmonella* Typhimurium. *Emerg. Infect. Dis.* 8: 490–495.

93. Crump, J.A., Barrett, T.J., Nelson, J.T. and Angulo, F.J. (2003). Reevaluating fluoroquinolone breakpoints for *Salmonella* enterica serotype Typhi and for non-Typhi salmonellae. *Clin. Infect. Dis.* 37: 75–81.

94. Nelson, J.M., Chiller, T.M., Powers, J.H. and Angulo, F.J. (2007). Fluoroquinolone-resistant *Campylobacter* species and the withdrawal of fluoroquinolones from use in poultry: a public health success story. *Clin. Infect. Dis.* 44: 977–980.

95. Neimann, J., Engberg, J., Mølbak, K. and Wegener, H.C. (2003). A case–control study of risk factors for sporadic campylobacter infections in Denmark. *Epidemiol. Infect.* 130: 353–366.

96. Engberg J., Neimann, J., Nielsen, E.M. *et al.* (2004). Quinolone-resistant *Campylobacter* infections: risk factors and clinical consequences. *Emerg. Infect. Dis.* 10: 1056–1063.

Chapter 3

ANTIMICROBIAL RESISTANCE RISK ASSESSMENT

Emma Snary and Scott McEwen

Veterinary drug regulatory agencies and others charged with managing antimicrobial resistance risks must decide which, if any, actions should be taken to reduce them. Although there is much evidence that antimicrobial use provides potent selection pressure for antimicrobial resistance in bacteria, there is considerable debate and uncertainty concerning the mechanisms and magnitude of risks to public health from antimicrobial use in animals. Furthermore, the many stakeholders affected by these decisions (e.g. farmers, veterinarians, pharmaceutical companies, consumers) frequently have varying and sometimes conflicting interests in the decisions. Therefore, risk assessment is often advocated to support these risk management decisions because, if properly conducted and presented, it can help to ensure that the relevant scientific information is brought to bear on the decision in an objective, complete and systematic manner (1, 2). As part of the evidence base for risk management actions (e.g. establish standards, use of technologies, limits on practices), guidelines and other recommendations for food safety, risk assessment is used to enhance consumer protection and facilitate international trade. In addition, it is frequently used as a risk management tool for the identification of data gaps/research needs, thereby enabling future commissioned research/surveillance work to be more focused on generating information that will reduce the uncertainty around the risk estimate. Another of its strengths is identification of stages in the manufacture, distribution, handling and consumption of foods that contribute to an increased risk of infection with an antimicrobial resistant organism. Once identified, such stages within the food chain

are often used as potential targets for risk management strategies. Consequently, resources and effort can be directed to the stage where the risk of antimicrobial-resistant bacteria can be most effectively reduced.

Risk is of course only one consideration in such decision-making; others include possible benefits of antimicrobial use to animal health, the cost of food animal production and animal welfare. The aims of the Antimicrobial Resistance Risk Assessment (ARRA) tend to vary according to the objectives of the sponsor/risk manager, but may include the following: to derive a qualitative or quantitative estimate of the risks to human health due to antimicrobial resistance attributable to the veterinary use of antimicrobials; to identify and incorporate uncertainty in risk estimation and identify gaps in scientific understanding; to investigate the consequences to veterinary medicine and to investigate impacts of control strategies on the risk to public health. This chapter provides an introduction to ARRA, how it can be used to inform governmental policy and guidelines, some methodological considerations, examples of ARRA, and some discussion on its potential future.

3.1 Introduction

3.1.1 The risk analysis and risk assessment frameworks

Risk assessment is a component of risk analysis, which is a formal process used to assess, communicate and manage risk. In the area of veterinary public health, the principal framework used for risk analysis is that set by the Codex Alimentarius Commission (3) under their remit as an international standard-setting organisation for foods in international trade. Under the Codex definition, risk analysis consists of three components; these are: risk management, risk communication and risk assessment, where risk assessment has four components: (i) hazard identification, (ii) hazard characterisation, (iii) exposure assessment, and (iv) risk characterisation. However, in the area of ARRA there are two commonly used risk analysis frameworks and the second framework, as defined by

the World Organisation for Animal Health (OIE) is slightly different to the Codex framework (4, 5). The OIE framework considers hazard identification as a separate component of risk analysis, while the Codex framework considers it to be a part of risk assessment. The Codex and OIE definitions for risk communication and risk management are similar – and are self-explanatory. However, there are also differences in the definitions for risk assessment since under the OIE system this component consists of release assessment, exposure assessment, consequence assessment and risk estimation. Table 3.1 summarises the differences

Table 3.1 Comparison of the Codex (3) and World Organisation for Animal Health, OIE (4, 5) Risk Analysis frameworks

Codex Alimentarius Commission	World Organisation for Animal Health (OIE)
	Hazard Identification: process of identifying the pathogenic agents ('hazards') which could potentially cause adverse effects.
Risk Assessment:	**Risk Assessment:**
Hazard Identification: the identification of biological, chemical, and physical agents capable of causing adverse health effects and which may be present in a particular food or group of foods.	*Release Assessment:* describes the biological pathway(s) necessary for an activity to 'release' (i.e. introduce) pathogenic agents into a particular environment, and estimates the probability of that complete process occurring.
Hazard Characterisation: the evaluation of the nature of the adverse health effects associated with biological, chemical and physical agents which may be present in food. For chemical agents, a dose–response assessment should be performed. For biological or physical agents, a dose–response assessment should be performed if the data are obtainable.	*Exposure Assessment:* describes the biological pathway(s) necessary for exposure of animals and humans to the hazards (in this case the pathogenic agents) released from a given risk source, and estimating the probability of the exposure(s) occurring.
Exposure Assessment: the evaluation of the likely intake of biological, chemical, and physical agents via food as well as exposures from other sources if relevant.	*Consequence Assessment:* describes the potential consequences (direct or indirect) of a given exposure and estimates the probability of them occurring.
Risk Characterisation: the estimation, including attendant uncertainties, of the probability of occurrence and severity of known or potential adverse health effects in a given population based on hazard identification, hazard characterisation and exposure assessment.	*Risk Estimation:* integrates the results from the release assessment, exposure assessment and consequence assessment to produce overall measures of risks associated with the hazards identified at the outset.
Risk Management: the process, distinct from risk assessment, of weighing policy alternatives, in consultation with all interested parties, considering risk assessment and other factors relevant for the health protection of consumers and for the promotion of fair trade practices, and, if needed, selecting appropriate prevention and control options.	**Risk Management:** the process of identifying, selecting and implementing measures that can be applied to reduce the level of risk.
Risk Communication: the interactive exchange of information and opinions throughout the risk analysis process concerning risk, risk-related factors and risk perceptions, among risk assessors, risk managers, consumers, industry, the academic community and other interested parties, including the explanation of risk assessment findings and the basis of risk management decisions.	**Risk Communication:** interactive exchange of information on risk among risk assessors, risk managers and other interested parties.

between the two frameworks. To further complicate matters, some of the ARRA published to date have not strictly followed either the Codex or OIE framework, particularly those employing the so-called 'top–down' approach based on human health surveillance data. An example of this approach is provided later in Section 3.2 as the FDA Fluoroquinolone-resistant *Campylobacter* ARRA (6).

Hazard identification

Antimicrobials are chemicals, and acquired resistance to antimicrobials is an attribute of certain microbes, particularly bacteria. Thus, ARRA has a theoretical basis in both chemical and microbial risk assessment (MRA). Chemical risk assessment has a comparatively longer tradition and is widely used for regulatory purposes in the environmental health field (7, 8). In contrast, MRA, which takes into account the population dynamics of bacteria, is relatively new and its role is still being established in the regulation of microbial hazards (9).

In the area of ARRA the hazards of interest are commonly bacteria, identified to the species or genera level, that express acquired resistance to a particular drug (e.g. vancomycin-resistant *Enterococcus* spp.) or to a class of drugs (e.g. fluoroquinolone-resistant *Campylobacter*). While this designation of the hazard has some clinical relevance and therefore intuitive appeal, in the future there may be advantages to identifying the resistance gene as the identified hazard since genes can be transfered between bacteria and the same resistance phenotype can be associated with distinct genes. Within the hazard identification phase information on the relevant hazard of interest is collected and provides clarification on what hazard the risk assessment will focus.

Hazard characterisation

The hazard characterisation step is used to assess the consequence of exposure to the hazard of interest. In the area of food safety, there are many possible health effects and it is therefore important that the effect of interest is defined by the risk question (see Section 3.1.2). Examples in the area of antimicrobial resistance might include infection, illness, treatment failure or even death. In order to ascertain the risk of infection or illness, given exposure to a certain number of organisms, dose–response relationships are used.

Such relationships are possible to describe to a certain degree due to available data sources such as experimental feeding trials, outbreak investigations or trials involving surrogate hosts or pathogens (10). However, all of the data types have important disadvantages that hinder their ability to describe the inherent variability in human response. For example, the probability of infection will be based on factors such as the host (e.g. age, immunostatus); the food matrix (e.g. fat content) and the hazard itself (e.g. virulence and dose).

Exposure assessment

The exposure assessment step is often the most complex in the risk assessment, particularly if a full farm-to-consumption pathway is developed (see Figure 3.1). As described in Table 3.1, the aim of the exposure assessment is to estimate the frequency and amount of the hazard to which a human is exposed, and these are therefore considered throughout the exposure pathway; further information on this part of the risk assessment is available in Lammerding and Fazil (12). The consideration of the amount of hazard is important because this is used in the hazard characterisation step in the form of a dose–response relationship. In addition, considering both prevalence (e.g. percentage of test-positive animals in the study population; percentage of a specific bacterium resistant to a certain drug) and microbial load (e.g. bacterial concentrations expressed as colony forming units (CFU)/g of faeces or meat) provides more options for control. This can be particularly useful when infection in the animal population is difficult to control and where a reduction in the microbial load in food or other vehicle might prove a more effective risk management option than prevalence reduction in animals.

Risk Characterisation

Finally, the Risk characterisation phase combines the exposure assessment and hazard characterisation, and the final risk estimate is obtained.

3.1.2 The risk assessment process

The risk assessment process is iterative and is illustrated in Figure 3.2. For any risk assessment, the first step is the definition of the risk question. This is a critical step in the process as it will affect the structure of the risk assessment, so it is important that both the

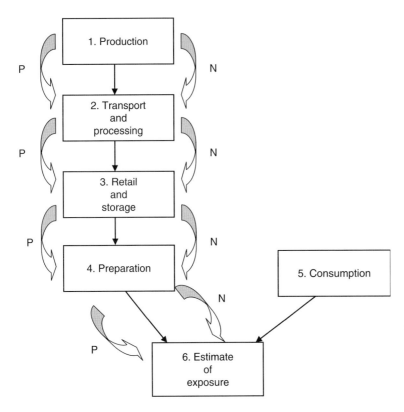

Figure 3.1 Modular pathway to describe the farm-to-consumption pathway. P: changes in prevalence; N: changes in concentration of organisms. Reprinted from WHO/FAO (11) with permission.

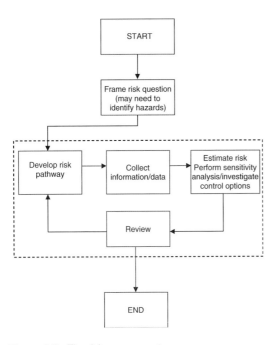

Figure 3.2 The risk assessment process.

risk assessor and risk manager are in agreement at this early stage and that adequate time and thought is given to this task. The risk question might address a specific hazard of interest (e.g. fluoroquinolone-resistant *Campylobacter)* or a number of potential hazards (e.g. antimicrobial-resistant *Campylobacter)* which will mean that the risk assessor and manager will have to identify the hazards of interest. It should also include the consequence of interest (e.g. the risk of human infection per serving of chicken; the risk of human infection per year; the number of human cases; the number of treatment failures due to fluoroquinolone treatment, etc.). Factors such as the time period, country of interest and any control options that the risk manager wishes to be investigated should also be identified at this early stage.

The risk pathway describes all of the steps (or processes) that may impact upon the risk. It requires the consideration of any factor that may increase or decrease the risk, which may mean a change in the prevalence or a change in the concentration of organisms. As the risk pathway is the 'backbone' of any risk assessment it is important that it is developed in consultation with both the risk manager and other scientists within the project team, for example, epidemiologists, veterinarians and microbiologists (medical and veterinary). The risk assessor has the difficult task of balancing the factors that might impact upon the risk, with the practical implications of including them in the risk pathway, that is time, data availability and uncertainty associated with the identified factors. One approach to risk pathways is to use a scenario or probability tree, where probabilities are assigned to each event; these are often used in animal health import risk assessment but not so much in food safety/ARRA risk assessment due to the desire to include considerations of both prevalence and microbial load.

The collection of information and data is an important stage of the risk assessment process and can be very time consuming, especially if there are considerable data gaps or deficiencies. The data requirements are identified by the risk pathway and typical sources of data are investigated, such as the published literature, unpublished literature and industry data. If data cannot be obtained for a particular parameter then expert opinion can be elicited, and this method has been used in ARRA (e.g. Bywater and Casewell (13); Anderson *et al.* (14)).

Once the risk pathway is defined and the data/information gathered the risk can be assessed. Generally there are three types of risk assessment; these are qualitative, semi-quantitative and quantitative, each of which are discussed in Section 3.2. Once the overall risk has been estimated, additional analyses can be undertaken, for example 'what-if' scenarios can be used to investigate the impact of risk management control measures.

It is essential that risk assessments are peer-reviewed, as with all scientific disciplines, but it is perhaps even more important here because of its use to inform risk management decisions. The review is often carried out within the risk assessment team, but it is preferable to also seek external peer review. Multiple reviewers from different disciplines (e.g. microbiology, epidemiology, risk modelling) are frequently used. The risk assessment methods as well as the data and assumptions need to be considered, as all of these factors will affect the quality of the model and hence confidence in the final risk estimate. Due to this extensive review, it is essential that the risk assessment is transparent, in particular that data sources and assumptions are documented and if the model is quantitative that the mathematical methodology is as clear

as possible. Review and revision should be an iterative process; the reviewers should provide feedback and constructive criticism, which the risk assessor can consider when revising the assessment.

3.1.3 Antimicrobial Resistance Risk Assessment

As described in Chapter 1, since the publication of the Swann report in 1969 (15) the veterinary use of antimicrobials has been in the public eye and, in particular, the question of the impact of veterinary antimicrobial use on human health has been, and is still, heavily debated. Because of this, ARRAs are being used to estimate the magnitude of the link between the veterinary use of antimicrobials and the emergence of resistant organisms in humans. Traditionally, ARRAs have only considered veterinary drugs that are already being used (i.e. post-approval); however, more recently, some countries are using ARRA techniques for pre-approval of both new veterinary drugs and veterinary drugs having their licences renewed (e.g. FDA-CVM (16)). Given the role of ARRAs as a means by which governmental policy and guidelines can be informed, it is important that the assessment is scientifically valid, uses the best scientific information available, is transparent and peer-reviewed. Ideally, the ARRA should be carried out independently of the risk management activity, even if the risk assessors and risk managers are within the same government agency. Principles for conducting risk assessments have been provided by both Codex Alimentarius and the OIE, and they both include the attributes listed above.

3.2 Methodological considerations for ARRA

There are three main approaches for the ARRA: qualitative, semi-quantitative and quantitative. It is important to note that whichever method is adopted the risk assessment process described above and depicted in Figure 3.2 remains the same; that is a risk question is selected, a risk pathway developed, data collected and the risk assessed. All 3 types of risk assessment are valid according to Codex and OIE and there is no golden rule of when to develop a qualitative, semi-quantitative or quantitative ARRA. When choosing which method to adopt, the most important criterion is whether the assessment is 'fit for purpose', which, broadly speaking, can be defined as when a risk assessment has answered the risk question given the available resources (time, risk assessor expertise, etc.).

It is important to mention two characteristics associated with data; uncertainty and variability. These are defined as (17):

- *Uncertainty*: lack of knowledge (level of ignorance) about the parameters that characterise the physical system that is being modelled. It can sometimes be reduced through further measurement or study, or through consulting more experts. Example: wide confidence limits on parameter estimates as a result of small sample sizes.
- *Variability*: effect of chance and is a function of the system. It is not reducible through either study or further measurement, but may be reduced through changing the physical system. Example: variation among animals in a given population with respect to the number of antimicrobial resistant bacteria shed per gram of faeces.

Total uncertainty is defined as the combination of uncertainty and variability.

In risk assessment it is highly recommended that these two characteristics are separated, although this is easier to do in quantitative risk assessment. Separating these characteristics will inform the risk managers about how much uncertainty there is associated with the final risk estimate (which could be reduced by further data collection) and also how much the risk estimate will naturally vary.

3.2.1 Qualitative risk assessment

In qualitative risk assessment the risks are predicted using descriptive terms, for example, negligible, low and high. The data requirements for a qualitative risk assessment are identical to those needed for a quantitative model. A qualitative risk assessment requires fewer mathematical resources and therefore provides a faster assessment of the risk in comparison to their quantitative counterparts. Indeed, qualitative assessments are often carried out as a pre-cursor to a quantitative assessment as the process can indicate (i) whether or not a further quantitative assessment is possible (based on data availability) and/or (ii) whether a quantitative risk assessment is even required if, for example, the risk is assessed to be negligible. The savings in time and resources gained by

developing qualitative rather than quantitative risk assessments may be especially beneficial for developing countries.

Broadly speaking, there are two methods used to combine qualitative probabilities or parameters. The first method (Non-Matrix Method) involves the risk assessor considering the probabilities/parameters to be combined, while taking into account the variability/uncertainties associated with the data, including data quality, and providing a combined assessment. Given the nature of this approach, it is often seen by some to be too subjective and lacking in transparency. Reviewers of the risk assessment should nevertheless be able to see how the risk assessor came to that particular conclusion when combining the model parameters. The Non-Matrix method allows the risk assessor to describe qualitatively the uncertainty and variability throughout the assessment. In the area of ARRA, this approach has been adopted by Wooldridge (18); Burch (19) and Snary *et al.* (20).

The second method used to combine risks within a qualitative assessment is commonly referred to as the 'matrix method'. Many risk assessors and managers prefer this method because it provides a structured approach for the combining of qualitative risks, for example see Figure 3.3, which was taken from Moutou *et al.* (21). In the area of ARRA, this approach has been used by the US Food and Drug Administration Center for Veterinary Medicine (FDA-CVM) in its guidelines for pre-approval assessment of antimicrobial resistance risks (16). Some risk assessors/managers believe that this approach provides a more transparent way of combining risks than the non-matrix method, and therefore reduces the level of subjectivity associated with the assessment. However, this approach is subject to much debate. One problem is that the bases upon which the risks (probabilities) are combined to yield the values in the matrix cells (e.g. from Figure 3.3, 'moderate' combined with 'high' yields 'high') are still arbitrary. In addition, within a risk assessment the probabilities/parameters can be additive or multiplicative and could involve combining multiple probabilities and/or probabilities and integers. A matrix as given in Figure 3.3 is not flexible enough to account for such considerations. It is also not able to distinguish between short risk pathways or long risk pathways, for example, a two-step pathway which has a 'low' probability of the event happening at each stage will have the same final risk estimate as a twenty-step pathway which has a 'low' probability at each stage.

Result of the assessment of parameter 2	Result of the assessment of parameter 1			
	Negligible	Low	Moderate	High
Negligible	Negligible	Low	Low	Moderate
Low	Low	Low	Moderate	Moderate
Moderate	Low	Moderate	Moderate	High
High	Moderate	Moderate	High	High

Negligible, when the probability of occurrence of the event is sufficiently low to be ignored, or if the event is possible only in exceptional circumstances
Low, when the occurrence of an event is a possibility in some cases
Moderate, when the occurrence of the event is a possibility
High, when the occurrence of the event is clearly a possibility

Figure 3.3 Combination of occurrence probabilities of the parameters considered in the qualitative risk assessment (21). Reproduced with permission from OIE.

However, we know that as a risk pathway increases in size, and more probabilities are combined, the magnitude of the final risk estimate should decrease. Finally, adopting the matrix approach does not allow the uncertainty and variability associated with each risk estimate to be considered when combining risks. From the perspective of best practices, it is important when using a qualitative approach (non-matrix or matrix) that there is clear definition of the terms used, and the matrix (if used) is provided, making sure that it respects rules of probability calculations.

For further information on qualitative risk assessment, including a more detailed discussion on the two qualitative risk assessment methods outlined here, see Wooldridge (22).

3.2.2 Semi-quantitative risk assessment

In semi-quantitative analysis (also known as risk ranking), a score is assigned to each of the steps in the risk pathway, for example 1–10. These are combined in a pre-determined way – for example adding or multiplying. Similarly to qualitative risk assessment, the assignment of scores to the available data can be subjective but, in the same way as the matrix method for qualitative risk assessment, the semi-quantitative method offers a formalised approach. Compared to qualitative risk assessment it has a higher degree of resolution due to a larger number of possible outcomes. An advantage of this approach is that semi-quantitative risk assessments require less time and resources compared to quantitative models, especially

since risks are being ranked so multiple models would have to be developed. However, the interpretation of the allocated scores and/or combined scores is often the subject of great debate. For example, the ranking order of the overall risks can be quite different under additive and multiplicative models. In addition, because the overall risk estimate is a number, the risk assessor/manager may wrongly interpret its meaning. For example, they may assume that a risk estimate of '8' is twice as risky as a risk estimate of '4'; which is not possible to state with confidence since the assigning of the values is subjective. Further discussion on the subjectivity and precision is available in reference (23). We are aware of no ARRA that have so far been carried out using this method.

3.2.3 Quantitative risk assessment

Using mathematical modelling techniques, quantitative risk assessments can be developed which provide a numerical estimate of risk. Two methods can be used: deterministic and stochastic, of which the latter is the more common and certainly now the more established method in the area of food safety MRA. In a deterministic model, point values are used to parameterise the risk pathway, for example, the mean or the worst-case scenario. Combining these parameters provides a point estimate for the overall risk estimate, but the uncertainty or variability associated with the estimate is not implicitly characterised within the assessment. Changes in parameter values allow 'what-if' scenarios to be investigated, and this information is extremely useful to risk managers.

An example of a deterministic ARRA is the model developed by Hurd *et al.* (24). Stochastic models allow 'chance' to be integrated into the assessment, which enables uncertainty and variability to be incorporated. The uncertainty/variability is often integrated by assigning a probability distribution to parameters within the risk pathway, which allows a range of possible values to be considered rather than, in the case of a deterministic model, a point value. Taking such an approach allows much more information to be provided to the risk manager such as, for example, confidence intervals. Also, sensitivity analyses allow the input parameters that contribute the most uncertainty to the final risk estimate to be identified; thus enabling recognition of critical data gaps/deficiencies and therefore future research needs. The handling of uncertainty and variability is extremely important as they represent two different phenomena and therefore need to be considered separately by risk managers. It is therefore recommended that the two entities be separated, and there are methods available to achieve this, including 'second order modelling' (17). Second order modelling is, however, mathematically advanced, and for practical reasons few risk assessments separate uncertainty and variability using this method.

It is important to note that quantitative risk assessment is still susceptible to subjectivity from the risk assessor. For example, similarly to the other types of ARRA there is a subjectivity associated with data quality, that is, which data sources should be included in the ARRA and which not. A degree of subjectivity unique to quantitative ARRA is the choice of a particular probability distribution in a model or modelling approach. For example, the Triangular and BetaPert distributions require the same amount of data, the minimum, mode and maximum, but even if identical parameters are used the shapes of the distributions (and hence the summary statistics) can significantly differ.

It is difficult to say whether the subjectivity associated with qualitative and quantitative ARRA are substantively different. However, it can be said that subjectivity in the assignment of qualitative probabilities to data is probably easier to detect within a qualitative ARRA. Only those knowledgeable in the methodologies used in quantitative ARRA would be able to detect subjectivity or bias relating to the choice of probability distributions or mathematical approaches.

To incorporate the probability distributions into the stochastic model, Monte Carlo simulation is often used, although other methods are gaining popularity such as Bayesian methods. Monte Carlo simulation is essentially an extension of the 'what-if' scenarios considered in deterministic modelling. Using this approach, distributions are assigned to appropriate parameters in the risk pathway, and in each run (or simulation) of the model a value from each distribution is randomly selected. Running the model for a large number of iterations will allow many scenarios to be considered and hence the final risk estimate (which is a combination of all of the distributions in the pathway) will encompass many possible scenarios, which are then summarised using a probability distribution and can be illustrated graphically. It is important to run the model for a large number of iterations as this allows the model to converge, which means reaching the point at which the summary statistics (e.g. mean) are not significantly affected by further runs of the model. There are many available software options for the development of stochastic models but the most common one is the add-in to Microsoft Excel called @Risk (Palisade). In ARRA many of the models are stochastic in nature, including those by Anderson *et al.* (14); FDA-CVM (6) and Cox and Popken (25).

3.2.4   Top–down *v* bottom–up

In the area of ARRA, the quantitative method has been much more commonly used than semi-quantitative or qualitative methods, and there are two fundamentally different approaches that have been used within it (although in theory these approaches are not limited to quantitative ARRA). These are known as the 'top–down' and the 'bottom–up' approaches.

In the bottom–up approach, the model starts from the 'source' and follows the unit of interest to the point of consumption and then the consequence of interest (e.g. infection, illness, etc.). A farm-to-consumption risk assessment is an example of the bottom–up approach (Figure 3.1), but it is not essential to start at the farm. The advantage of such an approach is that the impact of risk management interventions on the final risk estimate can be considered in the risk assessment. However, the development of such a model is extremely intensive in terms of time and data. In addition, due to the unavailability of data for many steps in the risk pathway there is often a high degree of uncertainty, which cannot always be quantified. Examples of ARRA that have used the bottom–up approach include those addressing human health impacts of fluoroquinolone use in cattle (14) and macrolide use in food animals (24).

The alternative approach is the top–down approach. This approach starts from the numbers of human cases in the population of interest, usually derived from notifiable disease reporting systems and, using epidemiological data, estimates the proportion of cases that are attributable to the source of interest. Figure 3.4 provides an example model framework for fluoroquinolone resistant *Campylobacter* from the FDA-CVM model (6). This approach is very simple and its major advantage is that it avoids the need to model areas of high uncertainty, for example, the preparation of food in the domestic kitchen, and also the amounts of data and time required are substantially reduced compared to the bottom–up approach. There are disadvantages however, including the uncertainties and

biases that may derive from epidemiological data (e.g. reporting, recall, sampling biases), and the difficulties that may arise in attribution of resistant infections (e.g. *Salmonella*) to specific food animal species. In particular, unless additional molecular epidemiological (e.g. phage typing) data are available, there may be a high degree of subjectivity in attributing exposure to a suspected source, particularly for sporadic infections.

One major disadvantage of the top–down approach is the fact that it is not amenable to investigation of risk management controls, so the choice of approach should be carried out with caution and in discussion with the risk manager. Finally, it should be noted that the top–down approach is not consistent with the risk assessment frameworks provided by Codex and OIE.

As with the choice of qualitative, semi-quantitative or quantitative type of risk assessment, there are no absolute rules for when to choose a bottom–up or top–down approach. Consequently, the merits and the drawbacks of each approach need to be considered carefully for the problem in hand and discussed with the risk manager. Again, the most important criterion is that the ARRA is deemed by the risk manager as for purpose.

3.3 Data for ARRA: requirements and sources

The availability and quality of data used in an ARRA is absolutely critical, and it is useful to bear in mind the adage 'rubbish in, rubbish out'. Unfortunately for risk managers and those who generate data, there is no standard list of data requirements for an ARRA. Such data requirements will differ between risk assessments, due to the risk question posed, scope, required resolution and whether a top–down or bottom–up approach is to be adopted.

It is important that the data requirements are identified by the risk pathway, which itself comes from the risk question. This approach allows all of the data requirements to be identified, and not just those for which data exist. Consequently, model parameters for which there are no data identified can be brought to the risk manager's attention; this can be especially important if a sensitivity analysis in a quantitative assessment identifies them as critical data gaps.

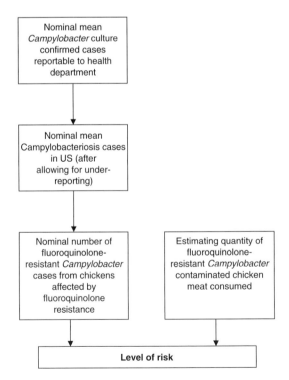

Figure 3.4 Model framework for the FDA-CVM ARRA for fluoroquinolone-resistant *Campylobacter*. Reproduced from FDA-CVM (6) with permission.

The design of the risk pathway and the data collection are independent of the type of assessment to be developed (i.e. qualitative, semi-quantitative or quantitative). However, if the data gaps are significant then it is a good idea to revisit the risk pathway, in consultation with the risk manager, and to agree on whether to continue with the agreed pathway and ARRA type.

The task of developing an ARRA is more complicated than other MRAs in the area of food safety. This is because the model needs to take into account not only whether the organism is present or not (and if present in what numbers), but also whether the organism is resistant to the antimicrobial of interest, whether the resistance is attributable to the use of the antimicrobial in the animal species of interest, and what proportion of the bacterial population are resistant. This, in turn, makes the data requirements much greater than those for a food safety risk assessment in general, especially because tra-

ditional sampling schemes for antimicrobial resistance are more focused on assessing presence/absence of the resistant organism. Other common data gaps/deficiencies encountered in ARRA relate to temporal and regional differences that exist in the microbiological methods used to identify bacteria and for susceptibility testing and interpretation, because such methodological differences make it difficult to combine data from different studies (see the review paper by Snary et al. (26) for further information). Consequently, there is a significant need for greater harmonisation of microbiological and sampling methods, including interpretation of susceptibility data, both within and between countries and between veterinary and human medicine. Thus risk assessors must exercise extreme caution when combining data from different studies. Snary et al. identified many data issues in the area of ARRA and these are given in Table 3.2.

Table 3.2 Key data limitations/issues affecting MRAs applied to the area of antimicrobial resistance. Reproduced and modified from Snary et al. (26) with permission from Oxford University Press

Data limitation/issue	Effect on MRA
Definition of resistance: • Harmonisation of minimum inhibitory concentration (MIC)/disc-diffusion breakpoints required	• Data from different sources are not comparable. May limit the amount of data available for the MRA
Microbiological methods: • Selective plating versus testing of one isolate from non-selective plate • Enrichment versus non-enrichment No. of isolates susceptibility tested, etc.	• The amount of data available for the MRA may be limited if the methods are not comparable • Cannot compare selective plating against the testing of one isolate without knowledge of the ratio of resistant to susceptible bacteria • If enriched the number of organisms is increased and therefore cannot directly be used in the MRA
Multiple levels of the sampling framework	• Large variability of sampling methods between studies. Therefore data from different sources may not be comparable; could limit the amount of data available for the MRA
Small sample sizes	• If the sample size is small at any level of the sampling framework, the uncertainty about the associated parameter will be large. This may contribute to a large uncertainty associated with the final risk estimate
Little data available on indicator organisms (resistant or susceptible) compared to pathogenic bacteria	• Surrogate organisms, and so on may be used to overcome the data gap, thus increasing the level of uncertainty in the output of the model. This uncertainty may not be quantified
Sensitivity and specificity of the tests used	• MRA may overestimate or underestimate the risk
Causality unclear	• Large assumptions made on the causality of antimicrobial resistance. This leads to a higher level of uncertainty in the model results, but which may be difficult to quantify
Lack of quantitative microbiological data	• Microbial load of resistant bacteria in/on different sources is unknown, therefore either not modelled or key assumptions made
Little information on the use of the antimicrobial agent in question for • veterinary use (at animal and farm level) • human use	• Causality difficult to consider. May lead to a large degree of uncertainty in the results of the model

They relate to many different aspects including microbiological and sampling methods and usage of antimicrobials.

There are many possible sources of data, including published literature, unpublished literature (e.g. unpublished research projects) and industry data. The best source is usually published literature as such data are subjected to a peer-review process that can increase confidence in its quality. However, ARRA often requires the raw data, rather than the summarised data usually presented in published form, and this can be difficult to obtain, particularly if the study is more than a couple of years old. Raw data is usually required for quantitative ARRA to enable proper incorporation of uncertainty and/or variability into the model. Raw data may be available from unpublished work (from industry, government or other sources), but this does have the disadvantage of not being peer reviewed and also can cause difficulties if the researchers want their data to remain confidential – therefore diminishing the transparency of the risk assessment.

Another data source is expert opinion. This is primarily used when no other data are available. Expert opinion can be one of two types (i) informal and (ii) formal. Informal expert opinion is simpler to acquire and involves contacting one or more experts and asking him/her questions. This can be used to fill data gaps or to confirm an assumption within the model. This approach has the benefit of being very quick and easy, but is highly susceptible to the biases of the experts involved, and the questioning may not be standardised. Formal solicitation of expert opinion is now quite common in risk assessment and involves the design of a standardised questionnaire and frequently the organisation of a workshop. Bywater and Casewell (13) produced a risk assessment based solely on expert opinion and Anderson *et al.* (14) used expert opinion data in their model for fluoroquinolone resistant *Campylobacter* in beef. Established methods, for example the Delphi Method (27), are sometimes used to reduce bias and to enable the existing bias to be understood. Although the use of expert opinion has been widely debated, it is important to note that such a data source does fill an otherwise unfillable data gap. In addition, further analyses (e.g. sensitivity analysis) can investigate the importance of the parameter estimated via expert elicitation on the results of the model. Other methods that can be used to overcome data gaps include the use of surrogate data, predictive mathematical modelling and limiting the model to a portion of the risk pathway (26).

3.4 Examples of ARRA

Recent reports have identified and reviewed in some detail approximately 25 published ARRAs (26, 28). Three of these are presented here as examples that illustrate a range of ARRA issues: 'bottom–up' and 'top–down' approaches; drug pre-approval and post-approval application; regulatory authority and other sponsorship; and qualitative and quantitative approaches of analysis.

3.4.1 Bottom–up qualitative ARRA: Center for Veterinary Medicine. Guidelines to evaluate the safety of new antimicrobial animal drugs with regard to their microbiological effects on bacteria of human health concern

The Center for Veterinary Medicine (CVM) produced recommended guidelines to evaluate the safety of new antimicrobial animal drugs with regard to their microbiological effects on bacteria of human health concern (16). Using these guidelines, it is intended that pharmaceutical companies perform their own qualitative risk assessment; however, the submission of quantitative risk assessments is not excluded. The 'risk' is defined as 'the probability that human food-borne illness is caused by an antimicrobial-resistant bacteria, is attributable to an animal-derived food commodity, and is treated with the human antimicrobial drug of interest'. Further discussion on the CVM guidance document and other similar qualitative systems is available in Cox *et al.* (29) and Claycamp (30).

Model framework

The guidance document uses the OIE risk analysis framework (see Table 3.1) to assess the risk described above, where the following definitions apply:

- *Release Assessment*: probability that resistant bacteria are present in target animal as a consequence of drug use.

- *Exposure Assessment:* probability for humans to ingest bacteria in question from the relevant food commodity.
- *Consequence Assessment:* probability that human exposure to resistant bacteria results in an adverse health consequence.
- *Risk Estimate:* integration of release, exposure and consequence assessments.

The scope of the release assessment is from the point of administration of the drug to the animal until the animal is slaughtered or the animal-derived food is collected (e.g. in the case of milk). This section is the most complex component, due to the many different factors that need to be considered, including information about the product and its use, the resistance mechanisms, and so on.

Data sources and availability

The pharmaceutical company develops the risk assessment and they are therefore responsible for the collection of data. Similarly, for any ARRA the amount and types of data required are significant, and the two data sources advocated in the guidance documents are primarily data from industry's internal studies and the published literature. The guidance document provides information on the types of factors that would need to be considered for the release and exposure assessments. For example, the exposure assessment includes data on contamination rates of food-borne organisms in/on food products and the amount of food products consumed per person per unit time.

Methods

The methodology described in the guidance document is a qualitative risk assessment. In the release and exposure assessments it is recommended that risks be assigned to one of the three categories: high, medium or low. The consequence assessment, which simply considers the importance of the antimicrobial or class of antimicrobials to ascertain the impact of exposure, uses the categories: critically important, highly important and important. Explanatory tables provide information on how to combine the risks using the matrix approach (see Section 3.2.1).

Impact on policy

Guidance documents such as the one described above and one in Australia (31) are extremely important in the future veterinary use of antimicrobial drugs. They enable the risks to human health to be considered prospectively (i.e. drug pre-approval), rather than retrospectively (post-approval). The CVM document also mentions risk management options or strategies (e.g. ranging from complete non-approval of the drug to approval of the drug, but with certain specified use conditions), and provides a risk-based, transparent and open approach to antimicrobial drug approvals for veterinary use in food-producing animals.

3.4.2 Bottom–up deterministic ARRA. Public health consequences of macrolide use in food animals: a deterministic risk assessment

Using the approach suggested by FDA-CVM 2003 (16), Hurd *et al.* (24) developed an ARRA for macrolide-resistant *Campylobacter* spp. and *Enterococcus faecium*. The specific risk question was: what is the risk, per year for an average individual, of an adverse therapeutic effect resulting from a prescribed macrolide treatment, due to the consumption of poultry, pork or beef that was contaminated with macrolide-resistant *Campylobacter* or *E. faecium*? The specific macrolides considered were tylosin and tilmicosin. Further information on this ARRA, the model itself and comments from other risk assessors can be obtained from Hurd *et al.* (32).

Model framework

The flow chart in Figure 3.5 describes the model structure for this risk assessment. Hurd *et al.* adopted the OIE framework and Figure 3.5 shows how the steps on the model structure conform to this. The same structure was used for all three sources (poultry, pork and non-dairy beef cattle) of macrolide-resistant *Campylobacter* and *E. faecium*. However, applying this structure to *E. faecium* is not straightforward as enterococci are considered more as a reservoir of resistance genes than a food-borne pathogen. The ARRA focused on the general population and not

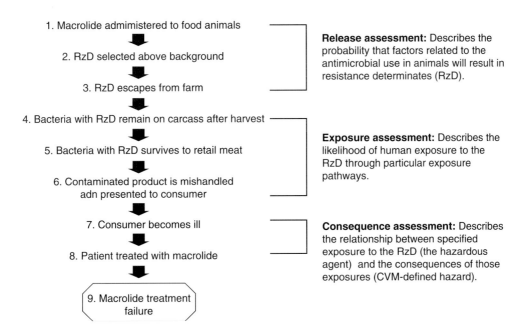

Figure 3.5 Pathway of events leading to the risk of food-borne illness with a resistant organism due to antimicrobial treatment of food animals. Reproduced from Hurd *et al*. (24). Reprinted with permission from the *Journal of Food Protection*. Copyright held by the International Association for Food Protection, Des Moines, Iowa, USA.

populations of high risk, for example the elderly and immunocompromised.

Data sources and availability

The data used in the ARRA originated from a variety of sources; these included industry drug use surveys, published scientific literature, guidelines for the medical use of antimicrobials for the treatment of food-borne infections and government documents. When data for some parameters were lacking, the authors often assigned worst-case scenario estimates.

Methods

Because data availability was limited, the authors chose to use a deterministic quantitative (binomial event) model, written in Microsoft Excel, rather than a stochastic model; the outcome was expressed as a point estimate.

For the majority of the model the approach was 'bottom–up', combining probabilities at each step of the model pathway. However, at steps 5, 6 and 7 no data

were available and therefore a 'top–down' approach was adopted to estimate the ratio between the output of steps 4 and 8 that could then be applied. This was accomplished by using two significant data sources, the contamination rates published by the US Department of Agriculture Food Safety and Inspection Service and data on numbers of human cases of *Campylobacter* infection published by the US Centers for Disease Control and Prevention (Foodnet). Combining this information with data on the number of carcasses produced, weight of dressed carcasses and serving sizes, the ratio was, essentially, the number of cases to the number of servings. This required certain implicit assumptions, for example an assumption was needed for the proportion of *Campylobacter* infections attributable to poultry, beef and pork. In addition, such an approach could not be adopted for *E. faecium*.

Results

The results suggested that the use of the macrolides tylosin and tilmicosin in poultry, pig and non-dairy beef production has a low impact on human health.

The risk, per year for an average individual, for *Campylobacter* was estimated to be approximately 1 in 10 million for all of the food types considered (Poultry: 1 in 14 million; Beef: 1 in 53 million; Pork: 1 in 236 million). Due to the uncertainty associated with two of the model parameters (probability of treatment failure if treated with macrolide; probability of significant resistance development in treated animal), the authors included a sensitivity analysis for *Campylobacter*, which showed that the model was sensitive to these parameters. The estimated combined risk for *E. faecium* was estimated to be 1 in 3 billion, which is much less than the predicted risk for *Campylobacter*. This low risk was attributable to the low values assigned to nodes 2 and 9 (Figure 3.5). However caution must be taken when considering the *E. faecium* result as the risk question, and therefore resulting ARRA, is not appropriate for this organism.

Impact on policy

This ARRA was not an official governmental risk assessment and was, in fact, funded by a pharmaceutical company. Therefore, although it was apparently not used to directly drive governmental policy, it could be used by the pharmaceutical company to support the continued use of their macrolide product in food animals. Regardless of its use to inform policy, the ARRA certainly did have merit in the identification of data gaps and in increasing the understanding of macrolide-resistant *Campylobacter* and *E. faecium* from farm-to-patient. It is also one of the first ARRA to explicitly include antimicrobial use data.

3.4.3 Top–down deterministic ARRA. Human health risks with the subtherapeutic use of penicillin and/or tetracyclines in animal feed

This quantitative risk assessment (33), published in 1989, was conducted by a committee established by the US Institute of Medicine, in response to a request by the US Food and Drug Administration (FDA) for an independent review of the human health consequences and risks associated with the use of penicillin and tetracyclines at 'subtherapeutic concentrations' (defined as administration of antibiotics in feed at 200 g/ton or less for more than 2 weeks) in animal feed. The committee was asked to address the following questions (in quotation):

- Does the subtherapeutic use of penicillin and tetracyclines in animal feed result in an increased frequency of antimicrobial resistance in pathogens, particularly food-borne pathogens? If so, can the increase in frequency be reliably estimated and compared with the increases associated with other sources of resistance?
- Does antimicrobial resistance increase (or diminish) the ability of food-borne pathogens to cause disease, change the number of food-borne pathogens (dose) needed to produce disease, or alter the severity of disease caused by food-borne pathogens?
- Does the subtherapeutic use of penicillin and tetracyclines in animal feed result in an increased prevalence of pathogens in the animals so fed and in foods derived from them?
- Does antimicrobial resistance attributable to the subtherapeutic use in feed increase the incidence of food-borne infectious disease in humans or complicate its medical management?'

The committee approached this task by developing a risk model, and limited it to *Salmonella* infections because these were the only ones among the food-borne bacterial zoonoses that were reportable in the USA for many years and for which there were disease incidence and antimicrobial susceptibility data available. This risk assessment has also been reviewed by Bailar III and Travers (28).

Model framework

The model used consisted of five quantitative estimates:

(1) the annual number of cases of salmonellosis reported annually in the USA;
(2) the fraction of human *Salmonella* infections where the isolate was resistant to penicillin/ ampicillin and/or tetracycline;
(3) the death rate associated with infection by *Salmonella* strains with different resistance patterns, including those susceptible to all antimicrobials, those resistant to any antimicrobials, and those resistant to penicillin/ampicillin and/ or tetracycline;
(4) the fraction of these deaths associated with infection of farm origin;
(5) the proportion of (4) above that arose from subtherapeutic use of antimicrobials in feed, including any antimicrobial, or penicillin and/or tetracycline.

Using data from the literature and expert opinion, low, mid-range and high numerical estimates for these elements were identified and used in the model. The five variables were multiplied together to derive low, mid-range and high numerical estimates of the number of deaths due to use of subtherapeutic antimicrobials in feed. The number of excess deaths (defined as the 'aetiologic fraction': deaths due to subtherapeutic antimicrobials that would not have occurred had the *Salmonella* strains not been resistant) was estimated by accounting for the proportion of the population taking antimicrobials at any given time and the excess risk of infection following anti-microbial administration.

Data sources and availability

Data were obtained from the published literature (reports of outbreak investigations, epidemiological and experimental studies) and national health statistics. Expert opinion was sought where data gaps or data deficiencies were identified.

Methods

The committee provided a detailed description of the scientific basis for the low, mid-range and high estimates of model variables, citing relevant literature findings and expert opinion. These variables were combined in a deterministic model. Although information on the uncertainties was not implicitly incorporated into the model, detailed description of uncertainties and limitations of the data and model were provided.

Results

Three values (high, mid-range and low) were used for each of the 5 variables in the model, therefore there were 243 different estimates of risk. The committee placed greatest reliance on estimates near the median as being 'likeliest' and were reported as point estimates. Their likeliest estimate of deaths attributed to subtherapeutic use of penicillin and/or tetracyclines in feed for both growth promotion and disease prophylaxis was 40 per year. Their likeliest estimate of deaths attributed to growth promotion use only was 15 per year. After including the aetiologic fraction, their likeliest estimates for both prophylaxis and growth promotion use, and for growth promotion use

alone, were 6 and 2 per year respectively. The committee provided a series of recommendations for strengthening databases for future risk assessments, including the implementation of antimicrobial use monitoring.

Impact on policy

In 1977, FDA proposed to withdraw the subtherapeutic use of penicillin and tetracyclines from animal feed because of their importance to human health. The US Congress held these proposals in abeyance indefinitely, and this situation was not altered by the publication of the 1989 Institute of Medicine ARRA. This assessment is important as the first example of the so-called 'top–down' approach to antimicrobial resistance risk assessment.

3.5 Future perspectives

ARRA has an important future role in support of veterinary drug regulatory decision-making and improved understanding of human health risks from antimicrobial use in animals. Its role will be enhanced by improvements in ARRA methodology that address the full range of adverse human health effects, both of a retrospective and prospective nature, the cumulative nature of antimicrobial resistance in populations, and the spread of resistance genes among populations of bacteria, including those of different genera and species. There is also a need for future risk assessments to examine non-food-borne routes of transmission, for example by direct contact with animals and by indirect contact through environmental exposure. Consideration of veterinary antimicrobial usage in such assessments should not be limited to food animals, but should also include companion animals. There is a great need for better understanding of risk assessment methodologies, strengths and limitations, and for more trained risk analysts that can undertake their own ARRA, as well as critically review those of other analysts in an open, positive and objective manner. As methods and experience improve at the national level, there is a great need for more international cooperation and standardisation of ARRA in order to protect public health and facilitate trade, better address the inherently international nature of antimicrobial resistance emergence and spread, and to increase capacity for ARRA in all countries.

3.6 Conclusions

ARRA has emerged as a promising tool for improved understanding of antimicrobial resistance risks, and for regulation of veterinary antimicrobials. It is based on Codex and OIE frameworks of risk assessment with the incorporation of several adaptations and alternative approaches in response to important data gaps and the needs of risk managers. While several ARRA have been conducted and some have contributed to regulatory policy, it cannot yet be said that ARRA is a mature, well-recognised and established part of the global effort to contain antimicrobial resistance and use antimicrobials prudently. There are, however, many reasons to be optimistic that this situation will improve in the near future. These include the ever-increasing need for evidence-based and transparent decision-making in public health, the scale of improvements in ARRA that have taken place in the past 20 years, trends at the national and international level to improve understanding of the potential role for ARRA, and the efforts by several international organisations (e.g. FAO, OIE, WHO, VICH) to improve ARRA methodologies and applications and address data and resource needs.

References

1. Advisory Committee on the Microbiological Safety of Food (ACMSF) (1999). *Advisory Committee on the Microbiological Safety of Food: microbial antibiotic resistance in relation to food safety.* HMSO, London.
2. FAO/OIE/WHO (2003). Joint FAO/OIE/WHO *Workshop on non-human antimicrobial usage and antimicrobial resistance: scientific assessment.* World Health Organization: Geneva, Switzerland, 2003; 40 pp.
3. Codex Alimentarius Commission (1999). *Principles and guidelines for the conduct of a microbiological risk assessment.* FAO, Rome. CAC/GL-30
4. Vose, D.J., Acar, J., Anthony, F. *et al.* (2001). Risk analysis methodology for the potential impact on public health of antimicrobial resistant bacteria of animal origin. *Rev. Sci. Tech. Off. Int. Epiz.* 20: 811–27.
5. World Organisation for Animal Health (2005). *OIE terrestrial animal health code.* Section 1.3 'Risk Analysis'. Available at: http://www.oie.int/eng/normes/mcode/en_titre_1.3.htm. Last accessed 8 August 2006.
6. FDA-CVM (2001). *Risk assessment on the human health impact of fluoroquinolone resistant campylobacter associated with the consumption of chicken.* Available at http://www.fda.gov/cvm/antimicrobial/Risk_asses.htm. Last accessed 8 August 2006.
7. Hopper, L.D. and Oehme, F.W. (1989). Chemical risk assessment: a review. *Vet. Hum. Toxicol.* 31: 543–54.
8. National Research Council (1994). *Science and judgement in risk assessment.* National Academy Press, Washington, DC.
9. Forsythe, S.J. (2002). *The microbiological risk assessment of food.* Blackwell Science (UK), Oxford.
10. FAO/WHO (2003). *Hazard characterization for pathogens in food and water: guidelines.* Microbiological risk assessment series; no. 3. FAO/WHO (Rome and Geneva). Available at: http://www.who.int/foodsafety/publications/micro/en/pathogen.pdf
11. WHO/FAO (2002). *Risk assessments of Salmonella in eggs and broiler chickens.* Microbiological risk assessment series 2. WHO/FAO (Rome and Geneva). Available at: http://www.who.int/foodsafety/publications/micro/en/salmonella.pdf
12. Lammerding, A. and Fazil, A. (2000). Hazard identification and exposure assessment for microbial food safety risk assessment. *Int. J. Food Microbiol.* 4: 1–11.
13. Bywater, R.J. and Casewell, M.W. (2000). An assessment of the impact of antibiotic resistance in different bacterial species and of the contribution of animal sources to resistance in human infections. *J. Antimicrob. Chemother.* 46: 639–45.
14. Anderson, S.A., Yeaton Woo, R.W. and Crawford, L.M. (2001). Risk assessment of the impact on human health of resistant *Campylobacter jejuni* from fluoroquinolone use in beef cattle. *Food Control* 12: 13–25.
15. Swann, M.M. (1969). *Report of the joint committee on the use of antibiotics in animal husbandry and veterinary medicine.* HMSO, London.
16. FDA-CVM (2003). *Evaluating the safety of antimicrobial new drugs with regard to their microbiological effects on bacteria of human health concern.* Guidance for Industry #152. Center for Veterinary Medicine. Available at: http://www.fda.gov/cvm/Guidance/fguide152.pdf. Last accessed 8 August 2006.
17. Vose, D. (2000). *Risk Analysis: A Quantitative Guide,* 2nd edn. John Wiley & Sons, UK.
18. Wooldridge, M. (1999). Qualitative risk assessment for antibiotic resistance. Case study: *Salmonella typhimurium* and the quinolone/fluoroquinolone class of antimicrobials. In *Antibiotic Resistance in the European Union Associated with the Therapeutic Use of Veterinary Medicines: Report and Qualitative Risk Assessment by the Committee for Veterinary Medicinal Products,* The European Agency for the Evaluation of Medicinal Products (EMEA) Report: Annex 1, 7 Westferry Circus, London, UK, pp. 1–41.
19. Burch, D.G.S. (2002). Risk assessment – *Campylobacter* infection transmission from pigs to man using erythromycin resistance as a marker. *Pig J.* 50: 53–8.
20. Snary, E.L., Hill, A. and Wooldridge, M. (2002). *A qualitative risk assessment for multidrug-resistant Salmonella Newport.* Report for Defra.
21. Moutou, F., Dufour, B. and Ivanov, Y. (2001). A qualitative assessment of the risk of introducing foot and mouth

disease into Russia and Europe from Georgia, Armenia and Azerbaijan. *Rev. Sci. Tech. Off. Int. Epiz.* 20: 723–30.

22. Wooldridge, M. Qualitative risk assessment. In *Microbial Risk Analysis of Foods* (ed. Schaffner, D.). American Society for Microbiology, Washington, DC, October 2007, pp. 1–29.

23. World Organisation for Animal Health (OIE) (2004). *Handbook on Import Risk Analysis for Animals and Animal Products.* Introduction and qualitative risk analysis (Volume 1). OIE, Paris, France.

24. Hurd, H.S., Doores, S., Hayes, D. *et al.* (2004a). Public health consequences of macrolide use in food animals: a deterministic risk assessment. *J. Food Prot.* 67: 980–92.

25. Cox, L.A. and Popken, D.A. (2002). A simulation model of human health risks from chicken-borne *Campylobacter jejuni. Technology* 9: 55–84.

26. Snary, E.L., Kelly, L.A., Davison, H.C., Teale, C.J. and Wooldridge, M. (2004). Antimicrobial resistance: a microbial risk assessment perspective. *J. Antimicrob. Chemother.* 53: 906–17.

27. Riggs, W.E. (1983). The Delphi Technique: an experimental evaluation. *Technol. Forecast. Soc. Change* 23: 89–94.

28. Bailar III, J.C. and Travers, K. (2002). Review of assessments of the human health risk associated with the use of antimicrobial agents in agriculture. *Clin. Infect. Dis.* 34: S135–43.

29. Cox, L.A. Jr, Babayev, D. and Huber, W. (2005). Some limitations of qualitative risk rating systems. *Risk Anal.* 25: 651–62.

30. Claycamp, H.G. (2006). Rapid benefit–risk assessments: no escape from expert judgments in risk management. *Risk Anal.* 26: 147–56.

31. National Registration Authority for Agricultural and Veterinary Chemicals (2000). *Part 10 of veterinary requirement series. Submission to working party on antibiotics.* Available at: http://www.apvma.gov.au/guidelines/vet-guideline10.pdf. Last accessed 10 July 2006.

32. Hurd, H.S., Doores, S., Hayes, D. *et al.* (2004b). *Public health consequences of macrolide use in food animals: a deterministic risk assessment.* Full technical report, model and comments. Available at: www.ifss.iastate.edu/macrolide/. Last accessed 10 July 2006.

33. Institute of Medicine (IOM) (1989). *Human Health Risks with the Subtherapeutic use of Penicillin or Tetracyclines in Animal Feed.* National Academy Press, Washington, DC.

Chapter 4

CLINICAL IMPORTANCE OF ANTIMICROBIAL DRUGS IN HUMAN HEALTH

Peter Collignon, Patrice Courvalin and Awa Aidara-Kane

4.1 Antimicrobial resistance: why is it a problem?

Antimicrobial agents are essential drugs for the health and welfare of people. Serious bacterial infections, such as bacteraemia, are associated with high mortality and morbidity rates, particularly if not treated with an effective antimicrobial. *Escherichia coli*, *Staphylococcus aureus* and *Streptococcus pneumoniae* are the most common causes of bacteraemia and other life-threatening infections in humans (1–4). The mortality rates associated with *S. aureus* and *S. pneumoniae* bacteraemia were over 80% in the pre-antimicrobial era and substantially decreased following the introduction of antimicrobial agents in human medicine (5). Life-threatening infections caused by resistant strains result in higher case-fatality rates. Multiple resistance has emerged in various bacteria causing severe infections, including *Salmonella*, *Enterococcus* (e.g. vancomycin-resistant enterococci or VRE), *Klebsiella*, *Acinetobacter baumannii* and *Pseudomonas aeruginosa* (1–4). Some of these can be resistant to all available antimicrobials. Resistance is also a problem for less serious infections such as *E. coli* urinary tract infections, where therapeutic options are limited by the high frequencies of antimicrobial resistance and the lack of readily available oral agents.

Resistance in almost all medically important bacteria and to almost all classes of antimicrobials has been

rising. The situation seems to be worse in developing countries where many people with life-threatening infections (*E. coli* bacteraemia, tuberculosis) may have no access to effective antimicrobials due to economic constraints. For many resistant bacteria, the only active antimicrobials are injectable compounds, some of which are very expensive (e.g. carbapenems for treatment of *A. baumannii* or *E. coli* infections). This means in practice that there is no available therapy for many people. In developed countries, probably because of better control on the sale, quality and use of antimicrobials, better hygiene plus good sewage and water systems, the situation is less critical in comparison to developing countries such as China (6). However, in developed countries, antimicrobial resistance is also an important public health problem as well as an economic burden to society. Wide variations in the frequency of resistance are observed between countries within the same continent. For example, Southern Europe has much higher levels of resistance compared to Scandinavian countries (7). Resistance is a particular problem in medical environments such as hospitals and tertiary care institutions, where there are large volumes of antimicrobials used and many patients are in close proximity, including immunosuppressed individuals. On some occasions, no effective antimicrobials are available for treatment of hospital-acquired infections caused by multi-resistant *A. baumannii*, *Serratia* and *Enterobacter* (8–10).

Resistant bacteria move readily from person to person and from hospital to hospital. They can also move from one ecological area to others (e.g. agriculture to people via food and water). Antimicrobials (and their classes) may often be used for different purposes in animals compared to people, so an appreciation of the 'human' perspective will be important for those who deal with animals. How and how often the spread of resistant bacteria occurs is not clear and continues to be an area of controversy, especially on the types of bacteria and the extent of any spread to people that results from antimicrobial use in agriculture. Many of the bacteria that cause infections in people are transmitted from person to person and unlikely to have an animal or food as a source. There are only a few bacterial species (e.g. *Campylobacter* and *Salmonella*) where animals are likely to be the main source for human infections, especially in developed countries with efficient water and sewage systems. However, non-pathogenic commensal such as *E. coli* and *Enterococcus*, and the resistance genes they carry, can also be transmitted to people via the food chain or by direct exposure to animals (see Chapter 2). The relative contribution by this route of transmission to antimicrobial resistance problems in humans remains controversial, but is likely to be much more substantial than currently appreciated (11–13).

The following sections outline the lack of new antimicrobial drugs (Section 4.2), the most important bacterial pathogens (Section 4.3) and clinical syndromes (Section 4.4) for which antimicrobial resistance is a problem in human medicine. Lastly, the recent classification by the World Health Organization (WHO) on the importance of the various antimicrobial classes and compounds used in human medicine is presented and discussed (Sections 4.5 and 4.6).

4.2 History of antimicrobial development: why are there so few new drugs?

One of the greatest breakthroughs in medicine in the twentieth century was the development of safe and effective antimicrobial agents that could be used for therapy of bacterial infections. The first agents that were developed were the sulfonamide-like drugs by Domagk (1935) in Germany. However, the most important discovery was that of penicillin G by Fleming in the late 1920s and then the subsequent work on benzylpenicillin by Florey and associates in 1940s, which enabled recovery of sufficient amounts of penicillin G to treat life-threatening infections caused by Gram-positive organisms, especially *S. aureus*. Penicillin G is produced by *Penicillium* (a fungus). Following the development of benzylpenicillin, major research efforts were undertaken to discover similar biological agents produced by fungi or other microorganisms that were able to kill bacteria or inhibit their growth. A large number of new and effective classes of antimicrobials became available over the following 40 years, including macrolides, tetracyclines and aminoglycosides. Research was also undertaken to develop completely synthetic antimicrobial drugs, that is drugs which were not just chemical modifications of an antimicrobial produced by microorganisms. There have been relatively few of these 'synthetic' antimicrobials however. The two more recently discovered synthetic antimicrobial classes have been the quinolones (including fluoroquinolones) and oxazolidinones (linezolid). One of the oldest classes of antimicrobials, the sulfonamides, is also synthetic.

Analogue compounds with better pharmacodynamic and pharmacokinetic properties were developed from the biologically produced antimicrobials by chemical engineering. Parent drugs were modified, often by the addition of side chains to the core structure, in order to obtain derivative drugs with a broader spectrum of activity, lower toxicity and/or able to resist inactivation by bacterial enzymes. One of the best examples of this chemical engineering resulted in the development of anti-staphylococcal penicillins. Fairly rapidly after the introduction of penicillin G, widespread penicillase production was found in *S. aureus*. The development of methicillin and other penicillinase-stable agents (e.g. dicloxacillin, oxacillin and flucloxacillin) allowed effective therapy against penicillin-resistant *S. aureus*. The discovery of new antimicrobial classes and the ability to chemically modify these agents to make them resistant to bacterial enzymes led to great optimism. Following this optimism, in the late 1960s, the Surgeon General of the USA declared that the war against infectious diseases had been won. But the war was far from being won. Unfortunately, bacteria have found many other ways of becoming resistant to antimicrobials and do not just rely on producing drug-inactivating enzymes (14, 15). Today we know that resistance can also result from modification of the drug target, synthesis of an alternative target with low affinity to the drug, or active removal of the drug from the bacterial cell by efflux pumps.

Most antimicrobial classes were discovered many decades ago. Only a few classes of antimicrobials have been developed in the last 30 years (fluoroquinolones, lipopeptides and oxazolidinones). Some antimicrobials released recently have been claimed to be new classes (e.g. the ketolides and tigecycline) but are chemically related to previously existing classes, namely macrolides and tetracyclines respectively. More precisely, they should be regarded as new generations within old classes. Discovery of new antibacterial agents is not an easy task and the situation is further complicated by variety of commercial factors. When a new antimicrobial is released on the market, its use is usually restricted to hospital life-threatening infections in order to delay development of resistance. Advertising is expensive because of a large number of 'me-too' drugs, that is compounds with very similar activity but marketed as being different to each other (e.g. fluoroquinolones). These factors have determined a poor financial return for pharmaceutical companies on developing new agents (16). Because of the relatively poor financial return, pharmaceutical companies have substantially decreased or abandoned research for development of new antimicrobial drugs. Screening for new antimicrobials has been left to small and relatively poorly resourced start-up companies. The focus of the large pharmaceutical companies has moved towards drugs against chronic diseases requiring life-long treatment (e.g. heart disease or psychiatry).

4.3 Important pathogens for which resistance is a problem

4.3.1 *Staphylococcus aureus*

S. aureus is one of the most common and virulent bacterial species that is carried by and infects people (1–5, 17–21). Indeed, one of the reasons for developing penicillin G was to combat *S. aureus* infections. In the pre-antimicrobial era, *S. aureus* bacteraemia was associated with a mortality of over 80% (5). Since antimicrobials have been developed the mortality has decreased substantially, although it still remains high with median rates of 25% and 34% for methicillin-susceptible (MSSA) and methicillin-resistant *S. aureus*

(MRSA), respectively (4). These infections are also very common. In France, it is likely that about 5000 nosocomial episodes of bacteraemia due to MRSA occurred in 2003 (18). In Australia, it is estimated that every year there are 35 cases of *S. aureus* bacteraemia per 100 000 population and 26% of cases are caused by MRSA (17). In Denmark, the annual rate of all *S. aureus* blood stream infections is approximately 28 per 100 000 inhabitants (17, 20). In the USA the rate may be as high as 50 per 100 000 inhabitants per year (17). This implies that in the USA there may be 150 000 episodes of *S. aureus* bacteraemia per year, while in Europe there are about 100 000 episodes. About two-thirds of these cases are likely to be healthcare associated, that is acquired while in hospital or as a result of a healthcare intervention (17, 20).

Antimicrobial resistance is a major problem with *S. aureus*. In some countries such as the UK and USA, close to half of *S. aureus* isolates from blood stream infections may be MRSA (2, 21). Until recently, the only effective antimicrobials available for treatment of MRSA infections were glycopeptides (mainly vancomycin, which requires i.v. administration). More recently, additional agents have become available such as linezolid, tigecycline, daptomycin and quinupristin/dalfopristin. However, resistance, associated toxicity and/or high cost have limited their use (22, 23). Various reports have documented the occurrence of *S. aureus* isolates resistant to vancomycin (24, 25). This resistance appears to have been principally through a new mechanism that makes the cell wall thicker and less penetrable by vancomycin. There has, however, also been transfer of the vanA gene cluster, encoding high-level glycopeptide resistance, from *Enterococcus* to *S. aureus* (24–26). Resistance has also emerged to more recently introduced agents such as linezolid and quinupristin/dalfopristin (22, 23), but fortunately remains uncommon.

In the past, MRSA infections were generally limited to hospitals and health care environments. However, during the last decade, MRSA have been increasingly reported to cause infections in the community (19), mainly skin and soft-tissue infections. Community-associated MRSA (CA-MRSA) are generally different from those circulating in hospitals. Because they are methicillin resistant, they are not susceptible to the most commonly used antimicrobials to treat soft-tissue infections such as β-lactams (i.e. penicillins and cephalosporins). To date, many of these infections can still be treated with agents such as tetracyclines and macrolides, as these strains, in contrast to most hospital-acquired MRSA, are usually susceptible to at least one of these drugs. However, increasing patterns of resistance have been recently observed in CA-MRSA. It can be anticipated that, with time, more and more resistance will develop. When MRSA first appeared in hospitals, strains were often susceptible to other groups of antimicrobials, but with time developed resistance to most agents, with vancomycin frequently being the only effective drug.

The recent emergence of MRSA in animals, including both food and companion animals, has also been noted (see Chapters 7, 10 and 11). Transmission of MRSA between people and animals has been reported in various countries. This gives added emphasis to the importance of limiting the use of certain drugs to human medicine, both to minimise the development and spread of these multi-resistant bacteria in animals but also to ensure, if these strains do transmit to people, that there are effective therapies still available to treat people. These considerations were important in the development of the WHO classification of critically important antimicrobial agents (Section 4.5).

4.3.2 *Streptococcus pneumoniae*

S. pneumoniae (pneumococcus) is an organism that spreads from person to person. Penicillin G used to be a reliable antibiotic to treat serious infections caused by this bacterium. However, over the last 10–20 years, increasing levels of penicillin resistance have been observed in various countries (27–30). Penicillin resistance in streptococci is mediated by modifications in the targets for penicillins – the penicillin binding proteins (PBPs). Modified PBPs have variable affinity to penicillins and for some strains treatment with penicillin is still feasible if high dosages are used. However, generally all β-lactams (including the newer penicillins and cephalosporins) are relatively ineffective as they all bind to these receptors. Serious diseases caused by pneumococci include pneumonia, bacteraemia and meningitis. It is also a frequent cause of more common but less serious infections such as otitis media. One antibiotic that can still be relied on in all circumstances to treat serious pneumococcal disease (including meningitis) is vancomycin. Other agents such as linezolid appear to be effective as resistance in pneumococcus is currently very low.

Providing resistance of pneumococcus to penicillins is only intermediate, most infections, including

episodes of bacteraemia, can still be treated effectively with penicillins if they are given intravenously. Paradoxically, most cases of intermediate penicillin-resistant pneumococci are still best treated with amoxicillin if an oral agent is used, although a higher dose is needed. This is because these organisms frequently display high-level resistance to other oral antimicrobials such as tetracyclines and macrolides. Other β-lactams such as oral cephalosporins do not achieve adequate concentrations to cure infections caused by intermediate penicillin-resistant strains.

4.3.3 *Escherichia coli*

E. coli is one of the commonest causes of bacterial infections in humans (1–3, 7, 31–33). It can cause urinary tract infections, abdominal infections (e.g. associated with appendicitis or gall bladder infections) and is also one of the most frequent causes of bloodstream infections. The rate of *E. coli* bacteraemia in developed countries is usually 35 or more per 100 000 people per year (7). Antimicrobial resistance is an increasing problem in *E. coli*. In some areas of the world, particularly developing countries (e.g. China), strains causing blood stream infections are frequently multi-resistant and in many cases there may be no effective antimicrobials to treat them with the exception of carbapenems (6, 34). Carbapenems can only be given by injection and are relatively expensive and therefore effectively unavailable to large numbers of people. Resistance mediated by enzymes able to hydrolyse all β-lactams, including carbapenems, has been increasingly reported in many areas around the world.

The main reservoir for *E. coli* is the bowel. There appears to be a large turnover of *E. coli* in the bowel each day (35). Food is an important vector for these organisms (35). Although *E. coli* is often relatively host specific, various studies have shown that resistant strains of animal origin can either colonise or cause infections in humans, for example fluoroquinolone-resistant *E. coli* of poultry origin (11, 13, 36–39). In both developed and developing countries, resistance to aminopenicillins is widespread and 50% or more of clinical isolates are usually resistant (7, 31–34). Therefore, for serious diseases, one cannot rely on these agents. In developed countries, agents such as third-generation cephalosporins, fluoroquinolones and/or aminoglycosides are usually administered for serious *E. coli* infections. Unfortunately, resistance to all these agents is widespread in developing countries. Even in developed countries resistance is increasing or high, especially in Southern Europe (7, 40). In other countries, such as Australia and Denmark, resistance to aminoglycosides, fluoroquinolones and third-generation cephalosporins remains very low in *E. coli* (32).

Community-acquired infections caused by *E. coli* strains producing extended-spectrum β-lactamases (ESBL) are being reported with increased frequency in many countries. This is despite the fact that third- and fourth-generation injectable cephalosporins are infrequently used to treat people in the community. In Spain, rising numbers of community-acquired ESBL-producing *E. coli* are being carried by the population. Carriage of ESBL-producing *E. coli* is also increasing in the USA (41). This unexpected and increasing appearance of ESBLs in community isolates of *E. coli* and other bacteria is of major concern. Food of animal origin may be an important vehicle in the spread of these bacteria, as suggested by a recent study from Spain (42) where similar bacteria were found in humans, food, animal farms and sewage. The use of third- and fouth-generation cephalosporins in food animals is likely to select for the occurrence of undesired resistance phenotypes in animal bacteria, including ESBL-producing strains (43). A worldwide epidemic of these resistant bacteria and their genes, for example those encoding for CTX-M and CMY β-lactamases, has been hypothesised (44, 45).

4.3.4　Other Gram-negative bacteria

There are various Gram-negative bacteria that cause serious diseases and where antimicrobial resistance is a major problem. These include *Enterobacter, P. aeruginosa, Serratia, Klebsiella* and *Acinetobacter* (8–10). Many of these organisms are multiresistant by nature. In patients with cystic fibrosis, it is common to find strains of *P. aeruginosa* and *Burkholderia cepacia* for which there are no effective antimicrobials (46). These isolates are 'intrinsically resistant' to most antimicrobials and rapidly acquire resistance to the remaining antimicrobials that may still be active. In some cases, therapy with alternative agents such as the polymixins is tried, but with variable and often poor clinical outcomes and with significant associated toxicity. In some genera belonging to the family Enterobacteriaceae, particularly *Klebsiella* and *Enterobacter*, resistance to β-lactams, including third-generation cephalosporins, is mediated by

ESBLs encoded by transmissible plasmids (47). As a consequence, this unwanted resistance mechanism may diffuse not only by clonal spread but also by horizontal transfer. One of the major reasons for concern is the recent emergence of metallo β-lactamases, which confer resistance to carbapenems. Such resistance can be difficult to detect in clinical laboratories. The responsible genes have been found in various Gram-negative species (48).

4.3.5　*Enterococcus*

Enterococcus species, in particular *Enterococcus faecium*, are intrinsically resistant to a large number of antimicrobials. Most enterococcal infections in people are associated with *E. faecalis* (about 90%) (49). In medical practice, the main agents that are used to treat enterococcal infections are ampicillin (and derivatives) or vancomycin. Aminoglycosides are often used in combination with ampicillin in serious infections such as endocarditis and bacteraemia for their synergistic activity, as otherwise enterococci cannot be killed if ampicillin or vancomycin are used alone. Other agents such as macrolides and tetracyclines appear to have relatively poor activity against enterococci. Quinupristin/dalfopristin is a recently developed combination of two streptogramins that is active against most strains of *E. faecium*. However, most strains of *E. faecalis* are resistant to quinupristin/dalfopristin, probably due to an efflux mechanism. Linezolid, another recently released agent, is active against most enterococci, including *E. faecium* (49, 50).

The importance of *Enterococcus* as a hospital pathogen is increasing, particularly in the USA, where vancomycin-resistant strains (VRE) are common (49). The increasing spread of resistant enterococci is very problematic as there are very limited options for treating serious infections caused by these bacteria. If a patient has endocarditis caused by enterococci, antimicrobial options are very limited. This condition is associated with a high case fatality rate. Usually, penicillins such as ampicillin need to be combined with an aminoglycoside, and 4–6 weeks of intravenous antimicrobials are needed. Unfortunately, prolonged aminoglycoside therapy often leads to renal and eighth nerve damage. If ampicillin resistance is present, most often in *E. faecium*, then vancomycin with an aminoglycoside needs to be used. If the strain displays high-level aminoglycoside resistance, it can be almost impossible to cure infection and the mortality rate is high. Quinupristin/dalfopristin remains one of few available therapics for the treatment of infections due to multi-drug resistant *E. faecium*, particularly following the emergence of linezolid-resistant strains.

4.3.6 Food-borne pathogens

Antimicrobial resistance is also increasing in food-borne pathogens such as *Salmonella* and *Campylobacter* (51–53). *Salmonella typhi* is a human-adapted *Salmonella* that spreads from person to person, usually via contaminated food and water (54). Most of the non-typhoid *Salmonella*, particularly in developed countries, are typically spread via food and water with the source often being food animals. Outbreaks of multi-resistant non-typhoid *Salmonella* have occurred in both Europe and the USA. In some cases there has been no effective antimicrobial therapy available. Most cases of *Salmonella* diarrhoea do not require antimicrobial therapy (54). Indeed, antimicrobial therapy may prolong excretion of the organism. However, there are also episodes where invasive disease occurs with *Salmonella*, like bloodstream infections and/or signs of systemic infection. In these cases, antimicrobial therapy is needed, and currently the most effective antimicrobials are fluoroquinolones and third-generation cephalosporins (54). Resistance is a particular problem for children, as fluoroquinolones are contra-indicated because of potential joint damage, and third-generation cephalosporins are often the only effective therapy available (54).

Campylobacter is one of the commonest causes of bacterial diarrhoea (53). On most occasions, *Campylobacter* infections do not need antimicrobial therapy and resolve spontaneously. However, antimicrobial therapy is needed when there is evidence of invasive disease or prolonged symptomatic disease with some systemic reaction. In these cases, either macrolides (erythromycin) or fluoroquinolones are the drugs of choice. Increasing resistance is seen to these latter agents, particularly to the fluoroquinolone ciprofloxacin (51,55,56). Available evidence suggests that much of this resistance is related to the use of fluoroquinolones in food animals. Countries where fluoroquinolones are either banned in food animals or else used fairly sparingly (e.g. Sweden, Norway and Australia) have a very low prevalence of fluoroquinolone resistance in *Campylobacter* (52). In countries where fluoroquinolones are frequently used in food animals (e.g. Spain, China, USA), resistance is commonly observed in both animal and human isolates (53). Macrolides are widely used in food animal production and are known to select for macrolide-resistant *Campylobacter* in animals. These antibiotics are the drugs of choice for treating serious *Campylobacter* infections in humans, especially children, where the use of fluoroquinolones is not recommended. Given the high incidence of human disease due to *Campylobacter*, the absolute number of serious cases is substantial (53, 57). Most disease in people is caused by *C. jejuni*, which is the most common species occurring in poultry. However, the species frequently isolated from pigs, *C. coli*, also causes infections in people.

4.4 Common clinical syndromes for which resistance is a problem

When a patient presents with a clinical infectious syndrome, for example pneumonia, meningitis, abdominal sepsis, or urinary tract infection, it is often not clear which bacterial species is involved. The physician needs to diagnose what organ system is involved but also to predict the most likely bacterium causing the infection. Once the diagnosis has been made, the most appropriate antimicrobial can be administered on the basis of the likely resistance profile of the causative organism. This is particularly important for life-threatening infections such as *S. aureus* bacteraemia or pneumococcal meningitis.

Usually, empiric antimicrobial therapy is given for the first 24–48 h until culture and antibiogram results are available. Empiric therapy for conditions such as bacteraemia usually consists of an anti-staphylococcal agent along with an aminoglycoside. This combination covers most of the likely causative bacteria, unless resistant strains are involved. For a hospital-acquired infection, the anti-staphylococcal agent would usually be vancomycin, as the prevalence of MRSA can be high in some hospitals/countries. Until recently, for a community-acquired infection, an agent such as flucloxacillin with an aminoglycoside would have sufficed. However, as a consequence of the increasing frequency of CA-MRSA infections, vancomycin with an aminoglycoside may be used. In most developed countries either the use of an aminoglycoside or a third-generation cephalosporin could be assumed to be effective against most Gram-negative pathogens.

The problem with just using a third-generation cephalosporin by itself is that its anti-staphylococcal activity is relatively poor compared to other agents, and if the organism is a MRSA it will be ineffective. If agents such as carbapenems (e.g. meropenem) are used empirically, this will also be problematic, as this class of antimicrobials does not cover MRSA. In addition, if these agents are used for all infections empirically, then resistance will inevitably arise as a consequence. The likely problem of widespread resistance to vancomycin as a consequence of frequent usage, is that vancomycin is not as effective as β-lactams against β-lactam susceptible *S. aureus*. With MSSA, if vancomycin is used for blood stream infections instead of flucloxacillin, there is a much higher case fatality rate (58). Thus, if vancomycin is used as empiric therapy for all suspected *S. aureus* infections and the majority of infections are caused by MSSA, this would result in a poorer outcome.

For meningitis, many now recommend using vancomycin, often in combination with a third-generation cephalosporin because of increasing resistance to glycopeptides. For abdominal infections the recommended drugs are still usually ampicillin, gentamicin and metronidazole. However, there are variations on these recommendations in various antimicrobial guidelines (54). Problems with aminoglycosides include renal and eighth nerve toxicity and this means that other agents, like cephalosporins, are frequently used in their place.

4.5 The WHO classification on the critical importance of antimicrobials used in human medicine

4.5.1 The Canberra meeting 2005

There is growing concern about the use of large volumes of antimicrobials in agriculture and in veterinary medicine, some of which may be of 'critical' importance to human medicine (59–63). Generally, there is a lack of information on the importance of different classes of antimicrobial agents used in human medicine. WHO organised a working group consultation in Canberra in 2005 with the scope to develop a list of critically important antimicrobial agents in human medicine (59). In developing the list, no antimicrobial or class of antimicrobials used in human medicine were considered unimportant and three categories were defined: *critically important, highly important* and *important* agents. The tables drafted in this meeting were raised in the following. WHO Consultation in Copenhagen (Section 4.5.2) (Tables 4.1 to 4.3). Comments were included in the tables where it was recognised that regional factors might affect the ranking, but these comments were not meant to be exhaustive, and other regional factors may be relevant. Each antimicrobial agent (or class) was assigned to one of the three categories on the basis of two criteria: (1) sole therapy, or one of few alternatives to treat serious human disease; and (2) antimicrobial used to treat diseases caused by organisms that may be transmitted via non-human sources, or diseases causes by organisms that may acquire resistance genes from non-human sources. *Critically important* antimicrobials are those that meet both criteria 1 and 2. *Highly important* antimicrobials are those that meet criteria 1 or 2. *Important* antimicrobials are those that meet neither criteria 1 nor 2.

In relation to criterion 1, it is self-evident that antimicrobials that are the sole or one of few alternatives for treatment of serious infections in humans have an important place in human medicine. It is of prime importance that the utility of such antimicrobial agents should be preserved, as loss of efficacy in these drugs due to emergence of resistance would have an important impact on human health. In the Comments section of the table, the WHO panels included examples of the diseases for which the given antimicrobial (or class of selected agents within a class) was considered one of the sole or limited therapies for specific infection(s). This criterion does not consider the likelihood that such pathogens may, or have been proven to, transmit from non-human source to humans.

According to criterion 2, antimicrobial agents used to treat diseases caused by bacteria that may be transmitted to man from non-human sources are considered of higher importance. In addition, commensal organisms from non-human sources may transmit resistance determinants to human pathogens and the commensals may themselves be pathogenic in the immunosuppressed. The link between non-human sources and the potential to cause human disease appears greatest for the above bacteria. The WHO panels included, in the Comments section of the table (where appropriate), examples of the bacterial genera or species of concern. The panel did not consider that transmission of such organisms or their genes must be proven, but only the potential for such transmission to occur.

Table 4.1 'Critically important' antimicrobials for human health (64)

Drug name	Criterion 1	Criterion 2	Comments
Aminoglycosides Amikacin Arbekacin Gentamicin Netilmicin Tobramycin Streptomycin	Yes (Y)	Yes (Y)	Limited therapy as part of treatment of enterococcal endocarditis and multidrug-resistant (MDR) tuberculosis Potential transmission of *Enterococcus*, *Enterobacteriaceae* (including *Escherichia coli*), and *Mycobacterium* from non-human sources
Ansamycins Rifabutin Rifampin Rifaximin	Y	Y	Limited therapy as part of therapy of mycobacterial diseases including tuberculosis and single drug therapy may select for resistance Potential transmission of *Mycobacterium* from non-human sources
Carbapenems and other penems Ertapenem Faropenem Imipenem Meropenem	Y	Y	Limited therapy as part of treatment of disease due to MDR Gram-negative bacteria Potential transmission of *Enterobacteriaceae* including *E. coli* and *Salmonella* from non-human sources
Cephalosporins (third and fourth generation) Cefixime Cefoperazone Cefoperazone/sulbactam Cefotaxime Cefpodoxime Ceftazidime Ceftizoxime Ceftriaxone Cefepime Cefoselis Cefpirome	Y	Y	Limited therapy for acute bacterial meningitis and disease due to *Salmonella* in children Additionally, fourth generation cephalosporins provide limited theraphy for empirical treatment of neutropenic patients with persistent fever Potential transmission of *Enterobacteriaceae* including *E. coli* and *Salmonella* from non-human sources
Glycopeptides Teicoplanin Vancomycin	Y	Y	Limited therapy for infections due to MDR *Staphylococcus aureus* and *Enterococcus* Potential transmission of *Enterococcus* spp. and MDR *S. aureus* from non-human sources
Lipopeptides Daptomycin	Y	Y	Limited therapy for infections due to MDR *S. aureus* Potential transmission of *Enterococcus* and MDR *S. aureus* from non-human sources
Macrolides including 14-,15-,16-membered compounds, ketolides Azithromycin Clarithromycin Erythromycin Midecamycin Roxithromycin Spiramycin Telithromycin		Y	Limited therapy for *Legionella*, *Campylobacter,* and MDR *Salmonella* infections Potential transmission of *Campylobacter* from non-human sources (see text section immediately following this table for further explanation)

Continued

Table 4.1 (Continued)

Drug name	Criterion 1	Criterion 2	Comments
Oxazolidinones Linezolid	Y	Y	Limited therapy for infections due to MDR *S. aureus* and *Enterococcus*
			Potential transmission of *Enterococcus* spp. and MDR *S. aureus* from non-human sources
Penicillins, natural aminopenicillins and antipseudomonal Ampicillin Ampicillin/sulbactam Amoxicillin Amoxicillin/clavulanate Azlocillin Carbenicillin Mezlocillin Penicillin G Penicillin V Piperacillin Piperacillin/tazobactam Ticarcillin Ticarcillin/clavulanate	Y	Y	Limited therapy for syphilis (natural penicillins) *Listeria*, *Enterococcus* (*aminopenicillins*) and MDR *Pseudomonas* (*antipseudomonal*)
			Potential transmission of *Enterococcus*, *Enterobacteriaceae* including *E. coli* as well as *Pseudomonas aeruginosa* from non-human sources
			(see text section immediately following this table for further explanation)
Quinolones Cinoxacin Nalidixic acid Pipemidic acid Ciprofloxacin Enoxacin Gatifloxacin Gemifloxacin Levofloxacin Lomefloxacin Moxifloxacin Norfloxacin Ofloxacin Sparfloxacin	Y	Y	Limited therapy for *Campylobacter*, invasive disease due to *Salmonella*, and MDR *Shigella* infections
			Potential transmission of *Campylobacter* and *Enterobacteriaceae* including *E. coli* and *Salmonella* from non-human sources
Streptogramins Quinupristin/dalfopristin, pristinamycin	Y	Y	Limited therapy for MDR *Enterococcus faecium* and *S. aureus* infections
			Potential transmission of *Enterococcus* and MDR *S. aureus* from non-human sources
			(see text section immediately following this table for further explanation)
Tetracyclines (glycylcyclines) Tigecycline	Y	Y	Limited therapy for infections due to MDR *S. aureus*
Drugs used solely to treat tuberculosis or other mycobacterial diseases Cycloserine Ethambutol Ethionamide Isoniazid *Para*-aminosalicylic acid Pyrazinamide	Y	Y	Limited therapy for tuberculosis and other *Mycobacterium* spp. disease and for many of these drugs, single drug therapy may select for resistance
			Potential transmission of *Mycobacterium* from non-human sources

Table 4.2 'Highly important' antimicrobials for human health (64)

Drug name	Criterion 1	Criterion 2	Comments
Amidinopenicillins Mecillinam	No (N)[a]	Yes (Y)	Potential transmission of *Enterobacteriaceae* including *E. coli* from non-human sources [a]MDR *Shigella* spp. infections may be a regional problem
Aminoglycosides (other) Kanamycin Neomycin Spectinomycin	N	Y	Potential transmission of Gram-negative bacteria that are cross resistant to streptomycin from non-human sources
Amphenicols Chloramphenicol Thiamphenicol	N[b]	Y	[b]May be one of limited therapies for acute bacterial meningitis, typhoid fever and respiratory infections in certain geographic areas
Cephalosporins, first and second generation Cefaclor Cefamandole Cefuroxime Cefazolin Cefalexin Cefalothin Cephradine Loracarbef	N	Y	Potential transmission of *Enterobacteriaceae* including *E. coli* from non-human sources
Cephamycins Cefotetan Cefoxitin	N	Y	Potential transmission of *Enterobacteriaceae* including *E. coli* from non-human sources
Clofazimine	Y	N	Limited therapy for leprosy
Monobactams Aztreonam	N	Y	Potential transmission of *Enterobacteriaceae* including *E. coli* from non-human sources
Penicillins (antistaphylococcal) Cloxacillin Dicloxacillin Flucloxacillin Oxacillin Nafcillin	N	Y	*S. aureus* including MRSA can be transferred to people from animals
Polymixins Colistin	Y	N	Polymixins may be the only available therapy for therapy of some MDR Gram-negative infections e.g. *Pseudomonas*
Polymixin B	Y	N	Limited therapy for MDR Gram-negative bacterial infections, e.g. those caused by *Acinetobacter* and *Pseudomonas aeruginosa*
Sulfonamides, DHFR inhibitors and combinations[c] *Para*-aminobenzoic acid Pyrimethamine Sulfadiazine Sulfamethoxazole Sulfapyridine Sulfisoxazole Trimethoprim	N[c]	Y	[c]May be one of limited therapies for acute bacterial meningitis and other infections in certain geographic areas Potential transmission of *Enterobacteriaceae* including *E. coli* from non-human sources

Continued

Table 4.2 (Continued)

Drug name	Criterion 1	Criterion 2	Comments
Sulfones Dapsone	Y	N	Limited therapy for leprosy
Tetracyclines Chlortetracycline Doxycycline Minocycline Oxytetracycline Tetracycline	Y	N	Limited therapy for infections due to *Chlamydia* and *Rickettsia*

Table 4.3 'Important' antimicrobials for human health (64)

Antimicrobial class/drug	Criterion 1	Criterion 2	Comments
Cyclic polypeptides Bacitracin	No (N)	No (N)	
Fosfomycin	N[a]	N	[a]May be one of limited therapies for Shiga-toxin producing *E. coli* O157 in certain geographic areas
Fusidic acid	N[b]	N	[b]May be one of limited therapies to treat MDR *S. aureus* infections in certain geographic areas
Lincosamides Clindamycin Lincomycin	N	N	
Mupirocin	N	N	
Nitrofurantoins Furazolidone Nitrofurantoin	N	N	
Nitroimidazoles Metronidazole Tinidazole	N[c]	N[d]	[c]Evaluation based on antimicrobial properties only [d]May be one of limited therapies for some anaerobic infections including *C. difficile* in certain geographic areas

Tables 4.1–4.3 outline how antimicrobials were grouped. The tables list only the generic drug names of antimicrobials and only those used in people. They show examples of members of each drug class, and it is not meant to be inclusive of all drugs. In most groups, similar drugs are used in animals, for example enrofloxacin as a fluoroquinolone and tylosin as a macrolide. It is important to appreciate that if resistance develops to one chemical group of antimicrobial, then generally all the other antimicrobials in that group are also affected due to cross-resistance. The WHO classification should be considered a core list of the most 'critical' antimicrobials agents globally (59). However, considerations such as cost and availability of antimicrobials in various geographic areas, as well as local resistance rates, could cause the list of *critically important* agents to be altered for regional use (e.g. an antimicrobial agent ranked *highly important* may become *critically important* in a particular region). It is of prime importance that the utility of such antimicrobial agents should be preserved, as loss of efficacy in these drugs due to emergence of resistance would have an important impact on human health.

The WHO classification was mainly conceived to guide decisions in risk management strategies of antimicrobial use. Cost was not a primary consideration in developing the list of *critically important* antimicrobial agents as there is little choice regarding cost when an antimicrobial is the sole or one of few available alternatives to treat a disease. The list should be updated regularly as new information becomes available, including data on resistance patterns, new and emerging diseases and the development of new drugs. The history of the development of antimicrobial resistance shows that resistance may appear after a long period of usage. As an example, vancomycin resistance in *Enterococcus* was first detected after the drug had been in use for over 40 years. Conversely, however, it can also develop and disseminate rapidly, like penicillinase production in *S. aureus*. Even if resistance has not developed to date in particular groups of bacteria, it does not mean that it will not develop in the near future.

The WHO criteria were developed solely with regard to the importance of these antimicrobials in human medicine. Drug classes that are not used in humans, and are currently only used in animal medicine, include arsenicals, bambermycins, ionophores, orthosomycins, quinoxalines and others. The OIE (Office International des épizooties which is French for 'International Epizootic Office' but now known as the World Organisation for Animal Health) has taken a similar initiative to define critically relevant antimicrobial agents in veterinary medicine. There will be further meetings between the WHO, FAO and OIE to allow appropriate discussion on how best to use drugs considered '*critically important*' in both human and veterinary medicine, especially macrolides and penicillins.

4.5.2 The Copenhagen meeting 2007

A second meeting to evaluate the classification of antimicrobials was held in Copenhagen in 2007 (64). Relatively few changes were needed to update the classification tables resulting from the Canberra meeting (Tables 4.1 to 4.3). Such changes are listed below:

- Tigecycline (a new tetracycline derivative with activity against multi-resistant *S. aureus* and Gram-negative bacteria) was released in 2005, and it was categorised as *critically important*.
- All penicillins (other than anti-staphylococcal penicillins) were grouped together and remain as *critically important*.
- The anti-staphylococcal penicillins were moved from *important* to *highly important*, as there is now more evidence of the potential transfer of *S. aureus*, including MRSA, from animals to humans.
- Because of the evidence of transfer of *flo* genes and chloramphenicol-resistant *Salmonella* from

animals to humans, the amphenicols were moved from *important* to *highly important*.
- Because of different resistance mechanisms, the aminoglycosides were divided into two groups. As a result, two aminoglycosides (kanamycin, neomycin) were moved from *critically important* to *highly important*.
- The classification of third- and fourth-generation cephalosporins was not changed, but they were combined in the tables as their mechanisms for antimicrobial resistance are similar and the criteria for their classifications were the same. The first- and second-generation cephalosporins were also combined in the tables for similar reasons. This is consistent with the grouping of other classes like quinolones.

4.6 Comments on the WHO classification of antimicrobial agents

The WHO classification in 2005 was the first important attempt to classify antimicrobial agents based on their importance in human medicine. The conclusions of the WHO panel were unanimous on all the drug classifications with one exception (59). There was significant discussion regarding the classification of natural penicillins and aminopenicillins. After thorough discussion, the consensus was that these drugs are used as therapy with few other options for serious human disease such as invasive enterococcal infections. This view was reinforced at the 2nd 2007 WHO meeting in Copenhagen (64).

It may be unclear why streptomycin was classified as 'critical important' since its use has become very rare in human medicine and, to the best of our knowledge, this compound does not cross-select for resistance to important aminoglycosides in human medicine, such as gentamicin. Similarly, within β-lactams, it can be argued as to whether penicillin G and ampicillin should be considered as important as third- or fourth-generation cephalosporins. The main reason that streptomycin is on the 'critical' list is for the therapy of rare types of enterococcal infections caused by strains with high-level resistance to gentamicin that have retained susceptibility towards streptomycin. In the same way, the reason that penicillins and aminopenicillins are on the 'critical' list is for the therapy of enterococcal infections. These agents are among the few available for therapy for invasive enterococcal and *Listeria* infections. Both enterococci and *Listeria* can be transmitted from animals to humans. This is why, according to the criteria used, natural penicillins and aminopenicillins were classified as being *critically important* for human health (59).

Macrolides are widely used in food animal production and are known to select for macrolide-resistant *Campylobacter* in animals. Macrolides are one of few available therapies for treatment of serious *Campylobacter* infections, particularly in children in whom quinolones are not recommended for treatment. Given the high incidence of human disease due to *Campylobacter*, the absolute number of serious cases is substantial. In the case of quinupristin/dalfopristin, this streptogramin combination remains one of few available therapies for treatment of infections due to multidrug-resistant *E. faecium*, particularly given the emergence of linezolid-resistant strains. A related streptogramin, virginiamycin, is known to select for quinupristin/dalfopristin resistance in *E. faecium* in food animals.

There is still need for discussion to further improve the current classification of critically important antimicrobials in human medicine. While some drug groups listed as *critically important* should not be controversial (e.g. fluoroquinolones), for others it may be less clear why they were placed in this category (e.g. aminopenicillins). Some groups may also need to be subdivided and/or separated (e.g. streptomycin from aminoglycosides and older quinolones from fluoroquinolones). Furthermore, the likely contribution to resistance problems in human medicine consequent to usage of a certain antimicrobial drug in any particular animal sector (aquaculture, food animal production, companion animal medicine, etc.) needs to be taken into account. As an example, macrolides were classified as *critically important* because they are used in the therapy of campylobacteriosis and thus macrolide resistance in this pathogen is of concern. However, if the target pathogen is not present in certain animals or types of production (e.g. aquaculture), it should be considered that macrolide usage is less likely to select for resistant bacteria that can be transmitted to humans. In some situations, such as aquaculture, transmission of enterococci via the food chain may not occur with any frequency.

4.7　Concluding remarks

Humans can be infected with various microorganisms that include viruses, bacteria, protozoa, fungi and worms. The focus in this chapter has been on the clinical importance of antibacterial drugs in human medicine and on the main bacterial pathogens for which resistance is a problem. However, it is important to note that the same principles apply for other agents including antifungals. We also need to acknowledge that most of our research and studies have been on organisms that cause disease directly, neglecting important contributions by commensal bacteria, which carry antimicrobial resistance genes. These cause disease relatively infrequently, but can transfer antimicrobial resistance to pathogenic bacteria. This phenomenon may have occurred with various pathogenic bacteria including *S. aureus*, where the gene encoding methicillin resistance (*mecA*) is likely to originate from low-virulent coagulase-negative staphylococci. Horizontal transfer may occur relatively infrequently, but once the gene is established in a successful virulent clone, then the clone and the carried gene are able to spread in individual countries and worldwide, as in the case of multi-resistant *S. aureus* and pneumococci.

References

1. Decousser, J.W., Pina, P., Picot, F. *et al.* (2003). Frequency of isolation and antimicrobial susceptibility of bacterial pathogens isolated from patients with bloodstream infections: a French prospective national survey. *J. Antimicrob. Chemother.* 51(5): 1213–1222.

2. Diekema, D.J., Pfaller, M.A., Jones, R.N. *et al.* (2000).Trends in antimicrobial susceptibility of bacterial pathogens isolated from patients with bloodstream infections in the USA, Canada and Latin America. SENTRY Participants Group. *Int. J. Antimicrob. Agents* 13(4): 257–271.

3. McGregor, A.R. and Collignon, P.J. (1993). Bacteraemia and fungaemia in an Australian general hospital–associations and outcomes. *Med. J. Aust.* 158(10): 671–674.

4. Cosgrove, S.E., Sakoulas, G., Perencevich, E.N. *et al.* (2003). Comparison of mortality associated with methicillin-resistant and methicillin-susceptible *Staphylococcus aureus* bacteremia: a meta-analysis. *Clin. Infect. Dis.* 36: 53–59.

5. Finland, M., Jones, W.F. Jr. and Barnes, M.W. (1959). Occurrence of serious bacterial infections since introduction of antibacterial agents. *J. Am. Med. Assoc.* 170: 2188–2197.

6. Wang, H. and Chen, M. (2005). China Nosocomial Pathogens Resistance Surveillance Study Group. Surveillance for antimicrobial resistance among clinical isolates of gram-negative bacteria from intensive care unit patients in China, 1996 to 2002. *Diagn. Microbiol. Infect. Dis.* 51: 201–208.

7. European Antimicrobial Resistance Surveillance System Annual Report. Available at: http://www.rivm.nl/earss/results/monitoring-reports, Accessed November 13th 2007.

8. Coelho, J.M., Turton, J.F., Kaufmann, M.E. *et al.* (2006). Occurrence of carbapenem-resistant *Acinetobacter baumannii* clones at multiple hospitals in London and Southeast England. *J. Clin. Microbiol.* 44(10): 3623–3627.

9. Hujer, K.M., Hujer, A.M., Hulten, E.A. *et al.* (2006). Multi-drug resistant *Acinetobacter* spp. isolates from military and civilian patients treated at the Walter Reed Army Medical Center: analysis of antibiotic resistance genes. *Antimicrob. Agents Chemother.* 50(12): 4114–4123.

10. Li, J., Nation, R.L., Turnidge, J.D. *et al.* (2006). Colistin: the re-emerging antibiotic for multidrug-resistant gram-negative bacterial infections. *Lancet Infect. Dis.* 6(9): 589–601.

11. Collignon, P. and Angulo, F.J. (2006). Fluoroquinolone-resistant *Escherichia coli*: food for thought. *J. Infect. Dis.* 194(1): 8–10.

12. Heuer, O.E., Hammerum, A.M., Collignon, P. and Wegener, H.C. (2006). Human health hazard from antimicrobial-resistant enterococci in animals and food. *Clin. Infect. Dis.* 43(7): 911–916.

13. Johnson, J.R., Kuskowski, M.A., Menard, M. *et al.* (2006). Similarity of human and chicken *Escherichia coli* isolates with relation to ciprofloxacin resistance status, Accessed November 13th 2007. *J. Infect. Dis.* 194: 71–78.

14. Opal, S. and Medeiros, A. (2005). Molecular mechanisms of antibiotic resistance in bacteria. In: *Principles and practice of infectious diseases* (eds. Mandell, G.L., Bennett, J.E. and Dolin, R.), 6th edn. Elsevier Churchill Livingstone, Philadelphia, pp. 252–270.

15. Jacoby, G.A. and Munoz-Price, L.S. (2005). The new beta-lactamases. *N. Engl. J. Med.* 352: 380–391.

16. Power, E. (2006). Impact of antibiotic restrictions: the pharmaceutical perspective. *Clin. Microbiol. Infect.* 12 (Suppl 5): 25–34.

17. Collignon, P., Nimmo, G.R., Gottlieb, T. and Gosbell, I.B. (2005). Australian Group on Antimicrobial Resistance. *Staphylococcus aureus* bacteremia, Australia. *Emerg. Infect. Dis.* 11(4): 554–561.

18. van der Mee-Marquet, N., Domelier, A.S., Girard, N., Quentin, R. (2004). Bloodstream Infection Study Group of the Relais d'Hygiene du Centre. Epidemiology and typing of *Staphylococcus aureus* strains isolated from bloodstream infections. *J. Clin. Microbiol.* 42(12): 5650–5657.

19. Collignon, P., Gosbell, I., Vickery, A. *et al.* (1998). Community-acquired meticillin-resistant *Staphylococcus aureus* in Australia. *The Lancet* 352: 146–147.

20. Danish *Staphylococcus aureus* bacteremia group. (2002). Annual report on *Staphylococcus aureus* bacteremia in Denmark. Statens Serum Institut. Copenhagen. Available at: http://www.ssi.dk/graphics/dk/overvagning/Annual02.pdf. Accessed November 13th 2007.

21. Anonymou (2002). *Staphylococcus aureus* bacteraemia: England, Wales and Northern Ireland, January to December. Available at: http://www.hpa.org.uk/cdr/PDFfiles/2004/staph_ann_1604.pdf. Accessed November 13th 2007.

22. Roberts, S.M., Freeman, A.F., Harrington, S.M. *et al.* (2006). Linezolid-resistant *Staphylococcus aureus* in two pediatric patients receiving low-dose linezolid therapy. *Pediatr. Infect. Dis. J.* 25(6): 562–564.

23. Livermore, D.M. (2000). Quinupristin/dalfopristin and linezolid: where, when, which and whether to use? *J. Antimicrob. Chemother.* 46(3): 347–350.

24. Courvalin, P. (2006). Vancomycin resistance in gram-positive cocci. *Clin. Infect. Dis.* 42 (Suppl 1): S25–S34.

25. Tenover, F.C. and McDonald, L.C. (2005). Vancomycin-resistant staphylococci and enterococci: epidemiology and control. *Curr. Opin. Infect. Dis.* 18(4): 300–305.

26. Whitener, C.J., Park, S.Y., Browne, F.A. *et al.* (2004). Vancomycin-resistant *Staphylococcus aureus* in the absence of vancomycin exposure. *Clin. Infect. Dis.* 38(8): 1049–1055.

27. Collignon, P.J. and Turnidge, J.D. (2000). Antibiotic resistance in *Streptococcus pneumoniae*. *Med. J. Aust.* 173 (Suppl): S58–S64.

28. Turnidge, J.D., Bell, J.M. and Collignon, P.J. (1999). Rapidly emerging antimicrobial resistances in *Streptococcus pneumoniae* in Australia. *Med. J. Aust.* 15: 152–155.

29. Pallares, R., Liñares, J., Vadillo, M. *et al.* (1995). Resistance to penicillin and cephalosporin and mortality from severe pneumococcal pneumonia in Barcelona, Spain. *N. Engl. J. Med.* 333: 474–480.

30. Hsueh, P.-R., Teng, L.-J., Lee, L.-N. *et al.* (1999). Dissemination of high-level penicillin-, extended-spectrum cephalosporin-, and erythromycin-resistant *Streptococcus pneumoniae* clones in Taiwan. *J. Clin. Microbiol.* 37: 221–224.

31. Waisbren, B.A. (1951). Bacteremia due to gram-negative bacilli other than the *Salmonella*; a clinical and therapeutic study. *Am. Med. Assoc.'Arch. Int. Med.* 88(4): 467–488.

32. Turnidge, J., Bell, J., Pearson, J. and Franklin, C. (2004). *Gram-negative survey 2004 Antimicrobial susceptibility report.* The Australian Group on Antimicrobial Resistance. Available at: http://antimicrobial-resistance.com. Accessed 14 October 2006.

33. Beidenbach, D.J., Moet, G.J. and Jones, R.N. (2004). Occurrence and antimicrobial resistance patterns comparisons among bloodstream infection isolates from the SENTRY antimicrobial surveillance programme (19972002–). *Diagn. Microbiol. Infect. Dis.* 50: 59–69.

34. Kumar, S., Rizvi, M., Vidhani, S. and Sharma, V.K. (2004). Changing face of septicaemia and increasing drug resistance in blood isolates. *Indian J. Pathol. Microbiol.* 47: 441–446.

35. Corpet, D.E. (1988). Antibiotic resistance from food. *N. Engl. J. Med.* 318: 1206–1207.

36. Garau. J., Xercavins, M., Rodriguez-Carballeira, M. *et al.* (1999). Emergence and dissemination of quinolone-resistant *Escherichia coli* in the community. *Antimicrob. Agents Chemother.* 43(11): 2736–2741.

37. Zhao, S., White, D.G., McDermott, P.F. *et al.* (2001). Identification and expression of cephamycinase *bla*(CMY) genes in *Escherichia coli* and *Salmonella* isolates from food animals and ground meat. *Antimicrob. Agents Chemother.* 45: 3647–3650.

38. Brinas, L., Moreno, M.A., Zarazaga, M. *et al.* (2003). Detection of CMY-2, CTX-M-14, and SHV-12 betalactamases in *Escherichia coli* fecal-sample isolatesfrom healthy chickens. *Antimicrob. Agents Chemother.* 47: 2056–2058.

39. Shiraki, Y., Shibata, N., Doi, Y. and Arakawa, Y. (2004). *Escherichia coli* producing CTX-M-2 beta-lactamase in cattle, Japan. *Emerg. Infect. Dis.* 10: 69–75.

40. Oteo, J., Lazaro, E., Abajo, F.J. *et al.* (2005). Antimicrobial-resistant invasive *Escherichia coli*, Spain. *Emerg. Infect. Dis.* 11: 546–553.

41. Lautenbach, E., Fishman, N.O., Metlay, J.P. *et al.* (2006). Phenotypic and genotypic characterization of fecal *Escherichia coli* isolates with decreased susceptibility to fluoroquinolones: results from a large hospital-based surveillance initiative. *J. Infect. Dis.* 194(1): 79–85.

42. Mesa, R.J., Blanc, V., Blanch, A.R. *et al.* (2006). Extended-spectrum beta-lactamase-producing Enterobacteriaceae in different environments (humans, food, animal farms and sewage). *J. Antimicrob. Chemother.* 58(1): 211–215.

43. Tragesser, L.A., Wittum, T.E., Funk, J.A. *et al.* (2006). Association between ceftiofur use and isolation of *Escherichia coli* with reduced susceptibility to ceftriaxone from fecal samples of dairy cows. *Am. J. Vet. Res.* 67(10): 1696–1700.

44. Shiraki, Y., Shibata, N., Doi, Y. and Arakawa. Y. (2004). *Escherichia coli* producing CTX-M-2 beta-lactamase in cattle, Japan. *Emerg. Infect. Dis.* 10: 69–75.

45. Brinas, L., Moreno, M.A., Zarazaga, M. *et al.* (2003). Detection of CMY-2, CTX-M-14, and SHV-12 beta-lactamases in *Escherichia coli* fecal-sample isolates from healthy chickens. *Antimicrob. Agents Chemother.* 47: 2056–2058.

46. Dobbin, C., Maley. M, Harkness, J. *et al.* (2004). The impact of pan-resistant bacterial pathogens on survival after lung transplantation in cystic fibrosis: results from a single large referral centre. *J. Hosp. Infect.* 56(4): 277–282.

47. Piddock, L.J., Walters, R.N., Jin, Y.F. *et al.* (1997). Prevalence and mechanism of resistance to '3rd-generation' cephalosporins in clinically relevant isolates of Enterobacteriaceae from 43 hospitals in the UK, 1990–1991. *J. Antimicrob. Chemother.* 39(2): 177–187.

48. Walsh, T.R., Toleman, M.A., Poirel, L. and Nordmann, P. (2005). Metallo-beta-lactamases: the quiet before the storm? *Clin. Microbiol. Rev.* 18(2): 306–325.

49. Moellering, R. (2005). *Enterococcus* species, *Streptococcus bovis* and *Leuconostoc* species. In *Principles and practice of infectious diseases* (eds. Mandell, G.L., Bennett, J.E. and Dolin, R.), 6th edn, Elsevier Churchill Livingstone, Philadelphia, pp. 2411–2422.

50. Eliopoulos, G.M. (2003). Quinupristin-dalfopristin and linezolid: evidence and opinion. *Clin. Infect. Dis.* 36(4): 473–481.

51. Gupta, A., Nelson, J.M., Barrett, T.J. *et al.* (2004). Antimicrobial resistance among *Campylobacter* strains, United States, 1997–2001. *Emerg. Infect. Dis.* 10(6): 1102–1109.

52. Unicomb, L., Ferguson, J., Riley, T.V. and Collignon, P. (2003). Fluoroquinolone resistance in *Campylobacter* absent from isolates, Australia. *Emerg. Infect. Dis.* 9(11): 1482–1483.

53. Centers for Disease Control and Prevention (CDC) (2004). Preliminary FoodNet data on the incidence of infection with pathogens transmitted commonly through food – selected sites, United States, 2003. *MMWR* 53(16): 338–343.

54. Pegues, D., Ohl, M. and Miller, S. (2005). *Salmonella* species including *Salmonella typhi*. In *Principles and practice of infectious diseases* (eds. Mandell, G.L., Bennett, J.E. and Dolin, R.), 6th edn, Elsevier Churchill Livingstone, Philadelphia, pp. 2636–2654.

55. Mead, P.S., Slutsker, L., Dietz, V. *et al.* (1999). Food-related illness and death in the United States. *Emerg. Infect. Dis.* 5: 607–625.

56. Iovine, N.M. and Blaser, M.J. (2004). Antibiotics in animal feed and spread of resistant *Campylobacter* from poultry to humans. *Emerg. Infect. Dis.* 10(6): 1158 1159.

57. Anonymous (2006). *DANMAP 2005 – Use of antimicrobial agents and occurrence of antimicrobial resistance in bacteria from food animals, foods and humans in Denmark.* Statens Serum Institut, Danish Veterinary and Food Administration, Danish Medicines Agency and Danish Institute for Food and Veterinary Research; Copenhagen. http://www.danmap.org/pdfFiles/Danmap_2005.pdf Accessed 14 October 2005.

58. Gonzalez, C., Rubio, M., Romero-Vivas, J. *et al.* (1999). Bacteremic pneumonia due to *Staphylococcus aureus*: A comparison of disease caused by methicillin-resistant and methicillin-susceptible organisms. *Clin. Infect. Dis.* 29(5): 1171–1177.

59. WHO (2005). *Critically important antibacterial agents for human medicine for risk management strategies of non-human use: report of a WHO working group consultation*, 15–18 February 2005, Canberra, Australia. World Health Organization, Geneva 2005. Available at: http://www.who.int/foodborne_disease/resistance/amr_feb2005.pdf. Accessed November 13th 2007.

60. Anonymous (2003). *Joint FAO/OIE/WHO expert workshop on non-human antimicrobial usage and antimicrobial resistance: scientific assessment.* Geneva, 1–5 December. WHO, Geneva. Available at: http://www.who.int/foodsafety/publications/micro/nov2003/en/. Accessed November 13th 2007.

61. JETACAR (1999). *Report on antibiotic use in Australia in animals and people.* Canberra. Available at: http://www.health.gov.au/internet/wcms/Publishing.nsf/Content/health-pubs-jetacar.htm. Accessed November 13th 2007.

62. Mellon, M. and Fondriest S. (2001). *Hogging it. Estimates of antimicrobial abuse in livestock.* Union of Concerned Scientists 23(1). Cambridge, MA. Available at: http://www.ucsusa.org/food_and_environment/antibiotics_and_food/hogging-it-estimates-of-antimicrobial-abuse-in-livestock.html. Accessed November 13th 2007.

63. WHO (1998). *Use of quinolones in food animals and potential impact on human health.* Report of a WHO Meeting Geneva, Switzerland 2–5 June 1998. Available at: http://whqlibdoc.who.int/hq/1998/WHO_EMC_ZDI_98.10.pdf. Accessed 16 March 2006.

64. WHO (2007). Critically important antibacterial agents for human medicine: catergorization for the development of risk management strategies to contain antimicrobial resistance due to non-human use. Report of the second WHO Expert Meeting, Copenhagen, 29–31 May 2007. World Health Organization, Geneva 2007. Available at: http://www.who.int/foodborne_disease/resistance/en/index.html. Accessed 27 September 2007.

Chapter 5

GEOGRAPHICAL DIFFERENCES IN MARKET AVAILABILITY, REGULATION AND USE OF VETERINARY ANTIMICROBIAL PRODUCTS

Angelo A. Valois, Yuuko S. Endoh, Kornelia Grein
and Linda Tollefson

Antimicrobial products intended for use in animals undergo extensive testing prior to marketing. The testing determines if the products are efficacious for their intended use and confirms that they are safe when used according to the labelled directions. The safety evaluation encompasses safety to the animal, the human user of the product and the environment. Products for use in food-producing animals undergo additional safety testing to ensure safety to humans consuming food products from the treated animals.

Veterinary antimicrobial products must be produced with reliable quality in order to ensure the safety and efficacy of the product. Product consistency is required, and also that the product fulfils the established specifications to the end of the authorized shelf life. Therefore, all veterinary medicinal products (VMPs) are required to be manufactured to the appropriate quality and purity and are produced in compliance with the provisions of Good Manufacturing Practices.

The registration requirements for VMPs, including antimicrobials, have been largely harmonized at the international level under the International Cooperation on Harmonization of Technical Requirements for Registration of Veterinary Medicinal Products (VICH), which was established in 1996 under the auspices of the World Organisation for Animal Health/Organization International Epizooties (OIE)

with representation of government and industry of the participating countries. VICH has developed harmonized guidelines on data requirements, criteria and standards for the registration of new pharmaceutical and immunological veterinary products in respect of their quality, safety and efficacy, which have been implemented in the participating countries (Table 5.1). The original VICH members, the EU, Japan and the USA, have been joined by observers from Australia, Canada and New Zealand.

This chapter describes the regulatory authorities and registration procedures relevant to the approval and regulation of veterinary antimicrobial agents in Australia, the EU, Japan and the USA, the general data requirements for establishing safety and efficacy and additional requirements for addressing the issue of antimicrobial resistance. Where possible, the reasons underlying differences are explained.

5.1 Regulatory authorities and registration principles

Veterinary medicinal products (VMPs) (in some countries called 'veterinary chemical products' or 'veterinary drugs') have to be registered (also called 'authorized') before they are allowed to be marketed or used. In some

Table 5.1   VICH harmonized guidelines for registration of veterinary medicinal products most relevant for safety of antimicrobials[a]

Guideline number and date	Guideline name and topic
GL6 – 2001	Environmental Impact Assessment for Veterinary Medicinal Products – Phase I
GL22 – 2001	Studies to Evaluate the Safety of Residues of Veterinary Drugs in Human Food: Reproduction Toxicity Testing
GL23 – 2001	Studies to Evaluate the Safety of Residues of Veterinary Drugs in Human Food: Genotoxicity Testing
GL27 – 2003	Pre-Approval Information for Registration of New Veterinary Medicinal Products for Food Producing Animals with Respect to Antimicrobial Resistance
GL28 – 2002	Studies to Evaluate the Safety of Residues of Veterinary Drugs in Human Food: Carcinogenicity Testing
GL31 – 2002	Studies to Evaluate the Safety of Residues of Veterinary Drugs in Human Food: Repeat-Dose (90 Day) Toxicity Testing
GL32 – 2002	Studies to Evaluate the Safety of Residues of Veterinary Drugs in Human Food: Developmental Toxicity Testing
GL33 – 2004	Studies to Evaluate the Safety of Residues of Veterinary Drugs in Human Food: General Approach to Testing
GL36 – 2004	Studies to Evaluate the Safety of Residues of Veterinary Drugs in Human Food: General Approach to Establish a Microbiological ADI
GL37 – 2003	Studies to Evaluate the Safety of Residues of Veterinary Drugs in Human Food: Repeat-Dose (Chronic) Toxicity Testing
GL38 – 2003	Environmental Impact Assessment for Veterinary Medicinal Products – Phase II

[a] All can be accessed at http://www.vichsec.org/en/guidelines.htm

countries, legislation and registration procedures for veterinary medicines for therapeutic use and disease prevention are separate from registration of feed additives (FA) (EU and Japan), while in others they follow the same legislation (Australia and the USA).

Following scientific assessment of the data provided with an application, and providing adequate quality, safety and efficacy of the product has been proven, the registration or marketing authorization issued allows the use of the product according to the approved conditions. In particular the indication(s), target species, dosage regime including frequency and duration of treatment, administration route(s), indicated withdrawal period (for products for food-producing animals), specific advice, warnings or restrictions for handling, storage and waste disposal or any other conditions are specified in the product specification and labelling. Changes to the registration or marketing authorization, such as extension to additional species, changes or adding of indications, dosage, administration form or conditions of use require a similar approval process and registration before the product is allowed to be sold and used.

5.1.1   Australia

Under the *Agricultural and Veterinary Chemicals Code Act 1994* (Agvet Code), the Australian Pesticides and

Veterinary Medicines Authority (APVMA) is responsible for the evaluation, registration and review of agricultural and veterinary chemicals, and their control up to the point of retail sale. Registered products can only be used for those approved purposes that are specified on the label. A product is only registered if the APVMA is satisfied that it does not pose an undue risk to human health and safety, is safe for the environment, will not affect international trade through residue problems and is effective for its intended use. The APVMA may only grant an application for the registration of a product, once it approves each active constituent for the product. The registration of new or significant variations (e.g. new dosage forms, extensions to use that are likely to result in a significant increase in the volume of usage or may pose an increased risk to public health) to currently registered antimicrobial active constituents and veterinary antimicrobial products require applicants to submit additional information.

Submissions for veterinary antimicrobial agents are required to be in the form of a qualitative risk assessment and supported by scientific evidence. The ranking of the antimicrobials with respect to their importance to the human public (see Section 5.3.1 for further information), and proposed use in food-producing versus non-food-producing animals, may be used as a guide to the need to supply data and/or scientific argument.

The APVMA's Manual of Requirements and Guidelines (MORAG) is a web-based interactive form providing information on data requirements and guidelines for applications to register chemical products, labels, active constituents and permits (1). Special data requirements and guidelines for veterinary antimicrobial products are contained in Volume 3 of the Manual (2).

5.1.2 European Union

In the EU any VMP, that is a product for treating or preventing disease in animals, must be authorized in accordance with the EU legislation, Directive 2001/82/EC (3) and Regulation (EC) No 726/2004 (4), before it is allowed to be sold or used. The legal basis of the authorization requirements is laid down in Directive 2001/82/EC. Annex I to this Directive provides detailed descriptions of the data that need to be provided with an application for a marketing authorization in relation to quality, safety and efficacy of the product.

The body that is responsible for the authorization procedure can be either the European Medicines Agency (EMEA) and the European Commission, or national competent authorities in EU Member States, depending on the procedure chosen for the marketing authorization application. In the centralized procedure, which is optional for new chemical entities and innovative products and mandatory for products derived by biotechnological processes, the application for a marketing authorization is submitted to the EMEA, and the EMEA's Committee for Medicinal Products for Veterinary Use (CVMP) carries out the scientific evaluation. Following the evaluation, on the basis of a positive opinion reached by the CVMP, the European Commission issues a marketing authorization. Such a centralized marketing authorization is binding on all EU Member States. The other procedures are the mutual recognition procedure and the decentralized procedure, where the scientific evaluation is carried out by the Member States in which the product is intended to be marketed, with one country, the reference Member State, taking the lead. The aim is to agree on a joint assessment and identical conditions for the marketing authorization in all countries involved. If no agreement can be reached or a serious risk is identified by one or more Member States, the matter of concern is referred to the CVMP for arbitration. The marketing authorizations resulting from these procedures are issued by the Member States concerned. National

marketing authorizations, that is, individual marketing authorizations issued by Member States, exist for VMPs that were on the market in the EU before the system described above was introduced into the legislation in 1995, and can be issued today if a product is intended for one single EU Member State only.

FAs are regulated by separate legislation to that applying to VMPs (5). The scientific assessment of applications for FA authorizations is carried out by the European Food Safety Authority (EFSA). With the ban of avoparcin (January 1997), ardacin (January 1998), and bacitracin zinc, virginiamycin, tylosin phosphate and spiramycin (December 1998), only four antibiotic FA (flavophospholipol, salinomycin sodium, avilamycin, monensin sodium, all which are not used in medicines for humans) were remaining. These four remaining antimicrobial FA were phased out from 1 January 2006. The use of coccidiostats, even if of antibiotic origin, as FA is at present still allowed. However, stricter rules for the authorization and use of coccidiostats apply and the phasing out of coccidiostats as FA has been planned by the current regulation (5).

5.1.3 Japan

Veterinary medicinal products, which include antimicrobial products used for prophylaxis and therapy, are regulated by the Pharmaceutical Affairs Law (6). The purpose is to regulate matters pertaining to drugs, quasi-drugs and medical devices so as to ensure their quality, efficacy and safety at each stage of development, manufacturing (importing), marketing, retailing and usage. The Ministry of Agriculture, Forestry and Fisheries (MAFF) regulates VMPs and special regulations are set for antimicrobial agents (see Section 5.3.3).

FAs are regulated by the Law Concerning Safety Assurance and Quality Improvement of Feed (7). Antimicrobial agents used for growth promotion are designated under this law and are controlled by MAFF. At the present time, 26 antimicrobial agents including anticoccidials are designated as FA. Antimicrobial growth promoters cannot be used for milking-cows, laying-hens, pigs and chickens during the seven days preceding slaughter for human consumption. A list of Japan's designated FAs is available online (8).

5.1.4 United States

In the USA, the regulatory authority for approval of VMPs is the Food and Drug Administration (FDA)

(9). The legal basis is set in the *Federal Food, Drug and Cosmetic Act of 1906* and associated regulations. In order for a veterinary drug to be legally marketed in the USA, it must have an approved new animal drug application. Veterinary drugs include all VMPs regardless of the intended use of the product, that is, growth promotion, prevention or therapy.

New veterinary antimicrobial products and significant variations to an existing approval, such as new dosage forms or for use in new species, must be shown to be efficacious and safe by adequate tests under the conditions prescribed, recommended or suggested in the proposed labelling.

5.2 Data requirements to establish safety and efficacy and assessment principles

Veterinary medicinal products undergo comprehensive testing for efficacy and for safety to the target animals, the users of the product, the consumers and to the environment prior to receiving marketing approval. Detailed requirements for the review and approval of veterinary drugs are available (10–12). A package of pharmacological and toxicological data, based on studies in laboratory animals, is required for all pharmacologically active substances in veterinary products. The requirements are more extensive if the substance is intended for use in food-producing animals and include setting maximum residue limits (MRLs) (Table 5.1) as well as assessing the potential to contribute to resistant pathogens that may infect humans.

The standard battery of safety studies to be provided includes studies that examine the effect of the product on systemic toxicity, reproductive toxicity, genotoxicity, developmental toxicity, carcinogenicity and, specifically for antimicrobials, effects on the human intestinal flora (Table 5.1). The toxicology studies are designed to show a dose that causes a toxic effect and a dose that causes no observed effect. Once the no-observed-effect level is established for all the toxicity endpoints, the most sensitive effect in the species most predictive of humans is identified. This no-observed-effect level is divided by an uncertainty factor to account for uncertainty in extrapolating from animals to humans and for variability, that is, the difference among individuals, to calculate an acceptable daily intake (ADI) for drug residues. Additionally, for antimicrobials, a microbiological ADI in accordance with the VICH GL 36, which assesses the effect of

the antimicrobial substance on the human gut flora, including its capacity to increase resistant bacterial populations, is also required.

In some countries (EU) data on the impact of the antimicrobial agent on food processing, that is, on yoghurt starter cultures, is also required. A pharmacological ADI can also be required for certain substances. In any case, the relevant ADI is the lowest one established. The ADI represents the amount of drug residue that can be safely consumed daily for a lifetime. Based on the ADI and metabolism and residue depletion studies, taking into account an estimate of dietary exposure, and analytical methods for measuring the residue, MRLs or tolerances (the latter term is used in the US) are established in the different target tissues. The MRL is the highest concentration of a residue for a particular chemical that is legally permitted in a food. An appropriate withdrawal period is then established to ensure that the residues are depleted below the MRL (Australia, EU, Japan) or ADI (US).

An exposure threshold approach is generally used to determine when environmental fate and effect studies are needed according to the VICH guidelines 6 and 38 on environmental impact assessment (Table 5.1). Environmental studies are not necessary for compounds that have limited environmental introductions, for example, antimicrobial products that are only used for individual dogs. When an environmental exposure of the VMP is not limited and further environmental impact assessment is required, the drug sponsor conducts physical-chemical properties studies, environmental fate studies and effect (toxicity) studies with algae, invertebrates, plants, fish and soil microorganisms representative of the environmental compartment of concern. The toxicity endpoints of these studies are no-observed-effect concentration, EC_{50} (median effective concentration) or LC_{50} (median lethal concentration), and the difference in rates of nitrate formation in the case of soil microorganisms. No-observed-effect concentration, EC_{50} or LC_{50} are divided by an assessment factor to arrive at a Predicted Environmental No Effect Concentration (PNEC). When the Predicted Environmental Concentration (PEC)/PNEC ratio is less than one, significant environmental effects are not predicted to occur due to the use of the animal drug product.

Specific data are requested to demonstrate the therapeutic efficacy of an antimicrobial substance for a given indication using a therapeutic regimen that aims to minimize the risk of selecting antimicrobial resistant bacteria. These are specific pharmacodynamic and pharmacokinetic data and address the detection of any developing antimicrobial resistance. Guidance is available, which includes the description of the pharmacokinetic–pharmacodynamic (PK–PD) analysis aimed at finding the best correlation between clinical cure and bacterial killing and how to conduct the clinical efficacy trials (13, 14).

5.2.1 Australia

Following an application to register an antimicrobial product, the APVMA undertakes a detailed, independent assessment of all data to ensure that high standards of quality, safety and efficacy are met, and that the product will have no unacceptable adverse impact on public health, occupational health and safety, trade or the environment. In undertaking its assessment, the APVMA receives specialist advice from various government agencies, including the Department of Health and Ageing (assessment of toxicology and public health data), the Department of Environment and Water Resources (assessment of environmental implications), the State/Territory Agriculture Departments (assessment of efficacy data for food-producing animals), and the National Health and Medical Research Council's Expert Advisory Group on Antimicrobial Resistance (assessment of human public risk from the development of antimicrobial resistance).

A summary of APVMA's data requirements for submissions relating to antimicrobial products is provided in Table 5.2.

5.2.2 European Union

Antimicrobial VMPs can be authorized in the EU only for the treatment and prevention of infectious animal diseases. To determine the food safety for an antimicrobial substance the applicant is required to submit the safety data as outlined in the introduction to this section, including the establishment of a microbiological ADI according to VICH GL 36 (Table 5.1) and addressing the impact of food processing (11).

In the EU the evaluation of the safety of residues and establishment of MRLs is a procedure separate from the marketing authorization, with the scientific assessment always undertaken by the CVMP. Before a marketing authorization for a VMP intended for a food-producing animal can be granted, the pharmacological active substances contained in the product have to be included in Annex I, II or III of Regulation (EEC) 2377/90, laying down a Community procedure

for the establishment of MRLs for VMPs in foodstuffs of animal origin (15). Annex I lists all substances for which final MRLs have been established including these MRLs, Annex II lists all substances for which it has not been considered necessary to establish MRLs in order to protect consumer health, and Annex III contains all substances with provisional MRLs.

The food safety data submitted with an application for a marketing authorization are largely the same, and have already been assessed in the preceding MRL application.

The specific data requested in the EU to demonstrate the therapeutic efficacy of an antimicrobial substance are summarized in the introduction to this section.

5.2.3 Japan

The characteristics of an antimicrobial substance in a VMP must be clearly described in the dossier. The period of administration is generally restricted to not more than one week. The data are evaluated by the expert meeting of the Pharmaceutical Affairs and Food Sanitation Council (PAFSC), which is an advisory organization to the Ministry of Health, Labour and Welfare (MHLW) and MAFF. The data on VMPs used in food-producing animals are also evaluated by the Food Safety Commission (FSC). PAFSC evaluates the quality, efficacy, safety and residue levels in food-producing animals of the VMP. If the VMP satisfies all requirements, the Minister of MAFF approves the VMP.

5.2.4 United States

To determine the food safety of residues of an antimicrobial agent, the drug sponsor submits general information similar to that required by Australia (see Table 5.2) and conducts a standard battery of toxicology tests.

Usually, the FDA establishes a withdrawal time to allow the drug residues to deplete below the calculated ADI (16).

A microbiological ADI in accordance with the VICH GL 36 (Table 5.1) is also required in the USA. Perturbation of the barrier effect and changes in enzymatic activity are potential impacts of antimicrobial agent residues on the human intestinal microflora that are of public health concern. A perturbation in the barrier effect is of concern because the gut microflora provide protection against the overgrowth and invasion of pathogenic bacteria.

Table 5.2 Data requirements for APVMA antimicrobial risk assessment

Item	Elements
Description of the antibiotic constituent/s of the product	• Name and identification of antimicrobial class. • Mechanism and type of antimicrobial action. • Antimicrobial activity of the antibiotic (antimicrobial spectrum, post-antibiotic and other anti microbial effects, minimum inhibitory concentrations (MICs) of target pathogens and organisms). • Antimicrobial resistance mechanisms and genetics. • Occurrence and rate of transfer of antimicrobial resistance genes. • Occurrence of cross-resistance. • Occurrence of co-resistance/co-selection. • *In vitro* mutation frequency studies. • Other animal studies.
Description of the product(s)	• Attributes (distinguishing name(s), formulation type(s)/pharmaceutical dosage form(s), pack sizes, claims, poisons scheduling, draft product label). • Pharmacokinetic/pharmacodynamic profile of the active constituent after administration of the product(s). • Antimicrobial agent activity in the intestinal tract. • Registration status in Australia and overseas.
Proposed maximum residue limits (MRLs) for food-producing species	• Proposed MRLs and microbiological acceptable daily intake (ADI). • Include CVMP technical reports, other regulatory agency reports or Joint FAO/WHO Expert Committee on Food Additives (JECFA) technical reports, if available and where applicable. • Refer to VICH guideline number 36: Studies to Evaluate the Safety of Residues of Veterinary Drugs in Human Food: General Approach to Establish a Microbiological ADI. • Address the risk of susceptible humans developing antimicrobial resistant infections as a result of exposure to antimicrobial residues in food commodities (as distinct from transferred microorganisms or genetic material).

When an antimicrobial agent destroys this barrier, overgrowth of pathogenic bacteria may occur.

5.3 Assessment of the public health risk associated with antimicrobial resistance

In order to assess the risk of transfer of resistant bacteria or resistance determinants from foodstuff of animal origin to humans, a harmonized VICH guideline, GL 27, on data requirements to study this risk for all antimicrobial VMPs that are intended for use in food-producing animals was developed (Table 5.1). The data that need to be provided include information on target animal pathogens, food-borne pathogens and commensal organisms. These data are assessed in terms of the exposure of food-borne pathogens and commensal organisms of the intestinal microflora of the target animal species to the product itself, under the proposed conditions of use. Guidelines for analysing the risks to animal and

public health from antimicrobial resistant microorganisms of animal origin have also been developed by the OIE in their Terrestrial Animal Health Code (17).

Some countries have approached the assessment of risk to public health from use of antimicrobial agents in animals by attempting to stratify regulatory requirements based on how important the drug is to public health. This results in stricter use of conditions on those products of relatively more importance to human medicine. National rankings of the importance of antimicrobial agents to public health will naturally reflect the needs and practices of that geographical area. Acknowledging the need for a universal ranking, the WHO held a consultation in February 2005 in Canberra, Australia to develop the criteria for ranking critical antimicrobials for human medical therapy (see Chapter 4). Similarly, the OIE, through its *ad hoc* Group on antimicrobial resistance, organized a worldwide consultation and issued a list of antimicrobials of veterinary importance based on this consultation. Furthermore, the WHO/FAO/OIE held a similar consultation meeting to find an appropriate balance between animal health needs and public health considerations, taking into account the overlap of the two lists of critically important antimicrobials (CIAs) developed by WHO and OIE, in November 2007 in Rome, Italy.

Work at the international level is also going on within the Codex Alimentarius. The Codex Alimentarius Committee on Residues of Veterinary Drugs in Food developed a Code of Practice to Minimize and Contain Antimicrobial Resistance. The Codex Alimentarius Commission adopted the Code in July 2005 (18). In addition, in 2006, the Codex Alimentarius Commission agreed to set up an Ad Hoc Intergovernmental Task Force on antimicrobial resistance to consider risk assessment and risk management options. The first meeting of this Codex Task Force was convened in October 2007 in Seoul, Korea.

The outcome of these activities, with respect to the risk assessment and risk management approach for antimicrobials used in veterinary medicines, is reported by the different organizations concerned.

5.3.1 Australia

In 1999, the Joint Expert Technical Advisory Committee on Antibiotic Resistance (JETACAR) recommended 'that all antibiotics for use in humans and animals (including fish) be classified as S4 (prescription only)' (19). The Australian Government accepted this recommendation with the proviso that exemptions from S4 scheduling could be considered on a case-by-case basis (20). Such exemptions could be considered in cases where the risk of promoting antimicrobial resistance was considered minimal, and where third party audited industry codes of practice are established.

For an assessment of the public health risk from the development of antimicrobial resistance in human pathogens associated with the use of antimicrobials in animals, the APVMA seeks advice from the Expert Advisory Group on Antimicrobial Resistance (EAGAR), including advice on risk management options. EAGAR is a committee under the Australian Government's National Health and Medical Research Council (NHMRC). A key output for EAGAR is the importance rating and summary of antibiotic uses in humans in Australia. EAGAR uses this information as a guide for providing advice to regulatory agencies and government committees. The information also serves as a guide to clinicians and the pharmaceutical industry, both human and animal, about the importance

of various antimicrobial agents available for human use in Australia. EAGAR ratings can change over time as antimicrobial resistance levels change, new antimicrobial agents are introduced and optimum drug choices alter because of new medical evidence. It is not an exhaustive list, but aims to include all agents of significant antimicrobial activity (21).

5.3.2 European Union

In the EU, it is a requirement to assess the risk of all antimicrobial VMPs that are intended for use in food-producing animals in accordance with VICH GL 27 (Table 5.1) and described in the introduction to Section 5.3. The Summary of Product Characteristics (SPC) of antimicrobial products should contain the necessary information making it possible to use the product effectively and safely while at the same time minimizing the risk of development of antimicrobial resistance. The efficacy data provided are summarized in the SPC, which includes the pharmacodynamic properties such as resistance information, pharmacokinetic properties, indications of the use of the product and contraindications, the target animal species, special warnings for use and appropriate recommendations to decrease the risk of development of antimicrobial resistance, and instructions on the posology and method of administration. Specific guidance has been developed in the EU for this purpose, which includes examples of standard phrases for such warnings and instructions (22).

The CVMP Scientific Advisory Group on Antimicrobials (SAGAM) was established in 2004, implementing new legal provisions under Regulation (EC) 726/2004 requiring that the EMEA (CVMP) provide scientific advice on the use of antimicrobial agents in food-producing animals in order to minimize the occurrence of bacterial resistance (4). The SAGAM is composed of acknowledged experts selected by the CVMP with expertise in antimicrobial resistance, efficacy of antimicrobials and use of antimicrobial agents in different target animal species (especially poultry, pigs, cattle) and molecular biology. The tasks of the SAGAM are to provide advice to the CVMP to specific questions raised by the Committee on all matters regarding authorization and use of veterinary medicines containing antimicrobial substances. The SAGAM is routinely involved with the evaluation of centralized marketing authorization applications of antimicrobial products for food-producing animals and specific cases for non-food-producing animals.

The SAGAM's mandate includes advising on the need to exercise certain controls on those classes of compounds of greater importance to human medicine, for example, third- and fouth-generation cephalosporins and fluoroquinolones. A position statement regarding the use of fluoroquinolones was published in 2007 (23). It included a series of actions proposed by the CVMP aimed at maintaining the efficacy of fluoroquinolones containing VMPs and, *inter alia*, promoting prudent use of antimicrobials, and especially fluoroquinolones, by requiring appropriate conditions of use in the marketing authorizations to be reflected in the SPC. These are planned to be implemented by the EU Member States authorities and animal health industry.

The CVMP's strategy and its accomplished work on antimicrobials is summarized in the *CVMP Strategy on Antimicrobials for 2006–2010* (24). The strategy focuses in particular on prudent use, ensuring appropriate conditions for marketing authorizations of antimicrobial VMPs in respect to the dossier assessment and conditions of use of the products as well as contributions to international activities in the field of antimicrobial resistance.

5.3.3 Japan

There are specific requirements for approval of antimicrobial VMPs related to important human medical products in Japan, for example, fluoroquinolones and third- and later generation cephalosporins. Data concerning the antimicrobial spectrum; the antimicrobial susceptibility tests of recent field isolates of targeted bacteria, indicator bacteria and food-borne bacteria; and the resistance acquisition test, are attached to the application for consideration of public and animal health issues. The application for approval of agents that are considered particularly important for public health is not accepted until the end of the re-examination period of the corresponding agent for use in humans. Furthermore, the drug may not be considered as the first-choice drug. For the approval of VMPs for food-producing animals, data concerning the stability of the antimicrobial substances under natural circumstances are also attached. After marketing, monitoring data on the sales amount and the appearance of antimicrobial resistance in target pathogens and food-borne pathogens must be submitted to MAFF.

The Food Safety Basic Law (25) was established to comprehensively promote policies to ensure food safety by establishing basic principles, by clarifying the responsibilities of the State, local governments and food-related business operators, as well as the roles of consumers, and by establishing a basic direction for policy formulation. The risk assessment for antimicrobial resistance in bacteria arising from the use of antimicrobials, especially those that are common to human medicine, is performed by the FSC, at the request of MAFF. The FSC undertake risk assessments independent from MAFF and MHLW, which undertake risk management. The risk assessment for antimicrobial resistance arising in bacteria from the use of antimicrobial agents in animals is undertaken on the basis of new guidelines based on the OIE guidelines of antimicrobial resistance. The risk assessments of antimicrobial resistance, with the exception of an assessment for one FA in food-producing animals, have not yet been completed by the FSC. To perform appropriate risk-management on antimicrobial resistance, the benefits/risks of antimicrobial VMPs should be scientifically evaluated. This should take into consideration the existence and emergence of resistance to CIAs.

In 2006, the FSC established a list of CIAs in human medicine: 14–15 member-ring macrolides (except erythromycin), ketolides, oxazolidinones, arbekacin, carbapenems, glycopeptides, anti-tuberculosis, streptogramins, the third- and fourth-generation cephalosporins, fluoroquinolones and mupirocin and new antimicrobials active against bacteria causing severe diseases, were ranked as the first class of CIAs. Of these antimicrobials, only third-generation cephalosporins and fluoroquinolones have been approved as VMPs.

5.3.4 United States

In order to better manage and mitigate the risk to humans from development of resistant organisms due to use of antimicrobials in animals, the FDA published guidance in 2003 that outlines an evidence-based approach (26). The guidance provides a scientific process for assessing the likelihood that an antimicrobial drug used to treat a food-producing animal may cause an antimicrobial resistance problem in humans consuming milk, eggs, honey, meat or other edible tissue from that animal. The essential components include a release assessment, which determines the probability that resistant bacteria will be present in animals as a result of the use of the antimicrobial new agent; an exposure assessment, which gauges the likelihood that humans would ingest the antimicrobial resistant bacteria; and the consequence assessment, which assesses the chances that human exposure to the resistant bacteria would result in adverse public health consequences (Chapter 3).

Items to be considered for the release assessment are essentially identical to those required in Australia (Table 5.2). For assessment of exposure, the evaluation considers both the frequency of bacterial contamination (e.g. *Salmonella*) of food products and *per capita* consumption of animal-derived food categories from treated animals. Thus, the exposure assessment is independent of the use of the antimicrobial agent under review. These two factors are integrated to estimate the probability in terms of high, medium or low likelihood of human exposure to the hazardous agent.

The consequence assessment involves placing the drug into 'critically important', 'highly important' and 'important' categories based on the usefulness of the drug in food-borne infections, availability of alternative therapies, the ease with which such resistance develops and other factors. This process is essentially identical to that used in Australia (EAGAR ratings). However, the criteria used in the USA to categorize the drugs based on importance to human medical therapy is somewhat different than that used in Australia, and therefore the rankings also differ, as both also differ from the WHO rankings (see Chapter 4).

Antimicrobials agents are ranked as *critically important* if they meet both criteria 1 and 2; *highly important* if they meet either criterion 1 or 2; and *important* if they meet either criterion 3 and/or 4 and/or 5 (Table 5.3).

Finally, the risk estimation step of the qualitative risk assessment process integrates the results from the release, exposure and consequence assessments into an overall risk estimation associated with the proposed conditions of use of the drug. This process classifies the drug as high, medium or low risk. These risk rankings represent the potential for public health to be adversely impacted by the selection or emergence of antimicrobial resistant food-borne bacteria associated with the use of the drug in food-producing animals.

If the qualitative risk assessment shows that the risks are significant, the FDA can deny the application for marketing authorization, thus preventing the use of the drug in food animals, or the FDA can approve the drug but place conditions on its use designed to ensure it would not pose a public health risk. Table 5.4 illustrates the risk management options available, stratified by the level of risk. These include prescription or non-prescription status of the antimicrobial, approval in only certain species of animals or only certain routes of administration (e.g. via feed or water versus injectable-only products), and the need for external consulting groups to provide advice.

5.4 Post-marketing monitoring of antimicrobial resistance and drug usage

5.4.1 Australia

Recommendations 3 and 11 of JETACAR called for a comprehensive monitoring and audit system for

---

Table 5.3 Criteria considered in the US ranking of antimicrobial drugs according to their importance in human medicine

Critically Important: Antimicrobial drugs which meet BOTH criteria 1 and 2
Highly Important: Antimicrobial drugs which meet EITHER criteria 1 or 2
Important: Antimicrobial drugs which meet EITHER criterion 3 and/or 4 and/or 5.

1. *Antimicrobial drugs used to treat enteric pathogens that cause food-borne disease*

2. *Sole therapy or one of few alternatives to treat serious human disease or drug is essential component among many antimicrobials in treatment of human disease.*

    Serious diseases are defined as those with high morbidity or mortality without proper treatment regardless of the relationship of animal transmission to humans.

3. *Antimicrobials used to treat enteric pathogens in non-food-borne disease*

4. *No cross-resistance within drug class and absence of linked resistance with other drug classes*

    Absence of resistance linked to other antimicrobials makes antimicrobials more valuable.

5. *Difficulty in transmitting resistance elements within or across genera and species of organisms*
    Antimicrobials to which organisms have chromosomal resistance would be more valuable compared to those antimicrobials whose resistance mechanisms are present on plasmids and transposons.

Table 5.4 Examples of risk management options in the USA based on the level of risk identified (High, Medium or Low)

Approval conditions	Category 1 (High Risk)	Category 2 (Medium Risk)	Category 3 (Low Risk)
Marketing status[a]	Rx	Rx/VFD	Rx/VFD/OTC
Extra-label use (ELU)	ELU Restrictions	Restricted in some cases	ELU permitted
Extent of use[b]	Low	Low, medium	Low, medium, high
Post-approval monitoring (e.g. NARMS[c])	Yes	Yes	In certain cases
Advisory committee review considered	Yes	In certain cases	No

[a]Prescription (Rx), Veterinary Feed Directive (VFD), Over-the-counter (OTC).
[b]Number of animals to be treated and duration of use.
[c]National Antimicrobial Resistance Monitoring System.

antimicrobial agents from the importer to the end-user, and that aggregated information on import quantities be made publicly available (19). As no anti-microbial agents are manufactured in Australia, all antimicrobials used must be imported. The Office of Chemical Safety within the Australian Government Department of Health and Ageing issues permits and collects end-use data to monitor the antimicrobials imported into Australia.

In March 2005, the APVMA released a report on antimicrobials sold for veterinary use in Australia from 1999 to 2002 (27). The report covers therapeutic/ prophylactic, growth promotants and anticoc-cidial products. According to the report, 552 407 and 540 tonnes of antimicrobial active ingredients were imported for veterinary use in 1999/2000, 2000/2001 and 2001/2002 respectively. Of these amounts, 161, 175.5 and 199 tonnes respectively, were sold for therapeutic/prophylactic purposes. The APVMA is continuing to collect sales volume data and is expected to issue reports for later years on a regular basis.

Australia has recently finalized a *Pilot Surveillance Program for Antimicrobial Resistance in Bacteria of Animal Origin* and plan to release in 2008. The pilot program was based on the analysis of bacterial isolates recovered from caecal specimens collected from healthy livestock (cattle, pigs, chickens) follow-ing their slaughter in commercial establishments.

5.4.2 European Union

Data on the use of antimicrobials in the late 1990s are compiled in the EMEA report on *Antibiotic Resistance in the European Union Associated with Therapeutic use of Veterinary Medicines* (28). Specific national

surveillance programmes to monitor consumption of antimicrobials and antimicrobial resistance develop-ment have been set up by many European countries, for instance Denmark (DANMAP), Finland (FINRES-Vet), France (FARM), The Netherlands (MARAN), Norway (NORM/NORM-Vet) and Sweden (SVARM/ SWEDRES). Other countries with surveillance schemes are Germany, Spain and the UK. The Community system for monitoring and collecting information on zoonoses was established in 1992. Directive 2003/99/EC obliges Member States, since 2005, to monitor antimicrobial resistance at least in *Salmonella* and *Campylobacter* (29). The European Food Safety Authority (EFSA) has been assigned the tasks of examining the data collected and preparing the Community Summary Report. The EFSA's first and second *Community Summary Report on Trends and Sources of Zoonoses, Zoonotic Agents and Antimicrobial Resistance* in the European Union in 2004 and 2005 are available online (30).

In order to standardize the susceptibility testing performed in the different European countries, an EU funded concerted action with the participation of 19 Member States (Antibiotic resistance in bacteria of animal origin – II (ARBAO-II)) was created. The objectives are to create a network of national veteri-nary reference laboratories in the EU Member States, to harmonize the susceptibility testing of bacteria from food animals in European veterinary reference laboratories, to collect and evaluate the susceptibility data from these laboratories and to make comparable results available for the public and decision-makers. The project focuses on monitoring of the zoonotic agents and commensal bacteria *Salmonella* spp., *Campylobacter jejuni, Campylobacter coli, Enterococcus* spp. and *Escherichia coli* in cattle, pigs, poultry and food of animal origin.

5.4.3 Japan

The Japanese Veterinary Antimicrobial Resistance Monitoring System (JVARM) (31) started in 1999 and conforms to the OIE standards on antimicrobial resistance. In the JVARM program, the 47 prefectures are divided into four groups selected evenly on the basis of geographical difference from northern to southern areas (11 or 12 prefectures per group). Sampling and bacterial isolation were carried out at livestock hygiene service centres. Bacteria for resistance testing are collected continuously and include zoonotic bacteria (*Salmonella* and *Campylobacter*) and indicator bacteria (*E. coli* and *Enterococcus* spp.) isolated from the excrement of healthy animals. Animal pathogens are selected annually to balance the consideration of public and animal health. Antimicrobial susceptibility of the *Salmonella* species, *Staphylococcus aureus, Actinobacillus pleuropne-umoniae*, the *Streptococcus* species and *Mannheimia haemolytica,* has been examined as these are significant animal pathogens.

Furthermore, therapeutic use of antimicrobial agents for animals on farms where faecal samples are collected are recorded at the time of sampling. JVARM subsequently analyses and evaluates the association between antimicrobial usage and the antimicrobial resistant population. As for monitoring of antimicrobial agent consumption, pharmaceutical companies that produce and import antimicrobial agents for animals are required to submit data to the NVAL annually in accordance with Pharmaceutical Affairs Law. MAFF publishes these data in a yearly report entitled the 'Amount of medicines and quasi-drugs for animal use'. After 2001, sales amounts of antimicrobial agents by animal species have been estimated using the annual reports from pharmaceutical companies. MAFF analyses sales amounts for each class of antimicrobial agents and the appearance of antimicrobial resistance to these antimicrobial agents, using JVARM data.

For example, in 2001, the total sales of antimicrobial VMPs used for animal health purposes was 1059 tonnes, including: tetracyclines (456 tonnes, 43%), sulfonamides group (175 tonnes, 17%), macrolides (142 tonnes, 13%) and penicillins (103 tonnes, 10%). The sales of fluoroquinolones and cephalosporins accounted for 0.6% (approximately 6.3 tonnes) and 0.2% (approximately 1.7 tonnes) respectively, of the total sales of antimicrobial agents for animal health purposes. These antimicrobial VMPs were mainly used for pigs (54%), fish (20%), broiler chickens (11%), cattle (8%) and laying chickens (4%). Of the total sales amount of antimicrobial VMPs for pigs, tetracyclines accounted for 51.1% (292 tonnes). The total sales amount of FAs was 260 tonnes in 2001.

5.4.4 United States

Currently, in the USA, there is no national system for monitoring antimicrobial use in either animals or humans. However, published information states that almost 90% of the antimicrobial agents used in livestock and poultry in the USA are admini-stered at subtherapeutic levels, at concentrations usually less than 200 g/tonne of feed, for disease prevention or growth promotion (32). The subtherapeutic use of penicillin, tetracycline and other feed-additive antimicrobials provides considerable pressure for selection of antimicrobial resistant microorganisms.

Antimicrobial resistance among enteric zoonotic pathogens is monitored in isolates from humans, at federally inspected slaughter plants for food-producing animals and for retail meat in the National Antimicrobial Resistance Monitoring System (33).

5.5 Availability of veterinary antimicrobial products

The APVMA PUBCRIS database (34) contains details of agricultural and veterinary chemical products that are registered for use in Australia. The database is updated continuously and, at the time of writing, there were 395 registered veterinary antimicrobial (and related) products, 83% (328) of which are classified as S4 (prescription only). Similarly, the FDA maintains a database of veterinary drugs that are approved for use in the USA. Due to the structure of the EU and an authorization scheme with marketing authorizations at both national and community wide level, there is currently no one spot database on the authorized veterinary antimicrobial agents in the EU. Depending on the authorization scheme, lists of authorized VMPs in the EU could be found at the EMEA website (11) for centralized marketing authorizations, the Member States' Heads of Agencies website (35) or the websites of the national agencies, which can be accessed through the EMEA or Heads of Agencies website.

Table 5.5 summarizes the approved uses of the antimicrobial classes that are used in the main food-producing species in Australia, the EU, Japan and the USA. Table 5.6 summarizes the approved uses

Table 5.5 Antimicrobials used for therapeutic, prophylactic or growth promotion purposes in food-producing animals

Antimicrobial class	Animal species	Approved use		
		Therapy[a]	Prophylaxis[b]	Growth promotion[c]
Tetracyclines	Cattle	AU, EU, J, US	AU, US	J, US
	Pigs	AU, EU, J, US	AU, US	J, US
	Sheep	AU, EU, US	US	US
	Chickens	AU, EU, J, US	AU, US	J, US
	Fish	EU, J, US		
Polypeptides	Cattle	AU, EU, J	US	J
	Pigs	EU, J	US	J
	Sheep	AU, EU		
	Chickens	AU, EU, US	AU, US	AU, J, US
β-Lactams	Cattle	AU, EU, J, US	J, US	US
	Pigs	AU, EU, J, US	US	US
	Sheep	AU, EU, US	US	US
	Chickens	AU, EU, J, US	US	US
	Fish	EU, J, US		
Macrolides	Cattle	AU, EU, J, US	AU, US	US
	Pigs	AU, EU, J, US	AU, US	AU, J, US
	Sheep	AU, EU, US		US
	Chickens	AU, EU, J, US	AU, US	US
	Fish	J, US		
Streptogramins	Cattle		AU, US	US
	Pigs		US	J, US
	Sheep		AU, US	US
	Chickens		AU, US	J, US
Trimethoprim/sulfonamides	Cattle	AU, EU, J		
	Pigs	AU, EU, J		
	Sheep	AU, EU		
	Chickens	AU, EU, J	J	
	Fish	EU, J		
Aminiglycosides	Cattle	AU, EU, J, US	AU, J, US	
	Pigs	AU, EU, J, US	US	AU, J, US
	Sheep	AU, EU, US	US	US
	Chickens	AU, EU, J, US	AU, US	
Lincosamides	Cattle	EU, US		
	Pigs	AU, EU, J, US	US	AU, US
	Sheep	EU		
	Chickens	AU, EU, J	US	US
	Fish	J		
Pyridone carboxylic acids[d]	Cattle	EU, J, US		
	Pigs	EU, J	J	
	Chickens	EU, J		
	Fish	EU, J		

AU, Australia; EU, European Union (veterinary medicinal product authorized in at least one EU Member State); J, Japan; US, United States.

[a] For treatment and control of disease.

[b] For prevention of disease; no information provided for EU.

[c] For growth promotion and improving feed efficiency; no use of antimicrobials for growth promotion in the EU.

[d] Quinolones or fluoroquinolones.

Table 5.6 Antimicrobials used for therapeutic or prophylactic purposes in companion animals

Antimicrobial class	Animal species	Approved use	
		Therapy[a]	Prophylaxis[b]
Tetracyclines	Dogs	AU, EU, J, US	J, US
	Cats	AU, EU, US	J, US
	Horses	EU, US	
Polypeptides	Dogs	AU, EU, US	
	Cats	AU, EU, US	
	Horses		
β-Lactams	Dogs	AU, EU, J, US	J, US
	Cats	AU, EU, J, US	J, US
	Horses	EU, J, US	US
Macrolides	Dogs	AU, EU, J, US	J
	Cats	AU, EU, J, US	J
	Horses	EU, J	
Streptogramins	Dogs		
	Cats		
	Horses		AU
Trimethoprim/sulfonamides	Dogs	AU, EU, J, US	J, US
	Cats	AU, EU, J, US	J, US
	Horses	EU, J, US	
Aminiglycosides	Dogs	AU, EU, J, US	J
	Cats	AU, EU, J, US	AU
	Horses	AU, EU, J, US	
Lincosamides	Dogs	AU, EU, J, US	J
	Cats	AU, EU, J, US	J
	Horses		
Pyridone carboxylic acids[c]	Dogs	EU, J, US	
	Cats	EU, J, US	

AU, Australia; EU, European Union (veterinary medicinal product authorized in at least one EU Member State);
J, Japan; US, United States.
[a] For treatment and control of disease.
[b] For prevention of disease; no information provided for the EU.
[c] Quinolones or fluoroquinolones.

and routes of administration of the antimicrobial classes that are used in the main companion animals in Australia, the EU, Japan and the USA. Although horses are listed in this table, they are treated as food animals in the EU and Japan.

5.6 Control of use and off-label use

The control of use of VMPs, including antimicrobials, is normally governed by the directions for use provided in the product label instructions. Off-label or extra-label use of antimicrobial agents are defined as use of the product in any manner not specified on the label. This includes use in a different species, use for a different indication, or use at a dosage different to that on the label.

5.6.1 Australia

Responsibility for the control of use, including off-label use of agricultural and veterinary chemical products, lies with the State and Territory Governments. This is underpinned by legislation enacted by each of the States and Territories (except the Australian Capital Territory). A summary of the control of use principles for veterinary medicines is provided below. However, this information should not be relied upon

---

Box 5.1   Summary of control of use of veterinary medicines in Australia.

- Veterinarians cannot use unregistered products except with an APVMA permit.
- The use of registered products must comply with the directions for use provided in the container/product label instructions.
- Persons other than veterinarians must adhere to written use instructions from a veterinarian. In addition, the animal(s) must be under the care of that veterinarian.
- Veterinarians are permitted to give directions for off-label use under certain conditions:
  ○ Products registered for use in one major food-producing species can be used in another food-producing species.
  ○ Off-label use is permitted in minor-food-producing species. Note: no restrictions in New South Wales and Victoria but some restrictions apply in other jurisdictions.
- For major food-producing species, the use of a veterinary medicine contrary to label instructions or the use of an unregistered product requires a written advice note from a veterinarian. Veterinarian supply and treatment records must be kept. Treated animals must be identified up to the point of slaughter and withholding periods must be adhered to. Liabilities apply to veterinarians and farmers that breach any of these requirements.
- Label restraints (DO NOT statements) must be adhered to. In some cases, the treatment of a single animal contrary to restraints is permitted for example if the animal is not slaughtered.
- In the case of companion animals (non-food-producing species), off-label use is generally permitted. However, provisions do apply. The exception is New South Wales, which requires registered products to be used according to label directions.
- The use of unregistered products in companion animals is permitted, provided that use is not in breach of any other legislation, for example, for cruelty.
- Jurisdictions, to the extent possible, have nationally agreed restrictions for the use of veterinary medicines. Each jurisdiction also has powers to further restrict use for example 'Restricted Chemical Products'.
- Pharmacy medicines may be used as long as their use does not contravene any restraints.

---

to explain every situation that may be encountered in dealing with use controls (Box 5.1).

The legislation for each State or Territory differs to a varying degree and should therefore be consulted for specific details.

In practice, situations often arise where chemicals are needed for a use not specified on the label. The AVPMA has a Permit Scheme in place that allows for the legal use of chemicals in ways different to the uses set out on the product label. These are called 'off-label' permits (OLPs). Generally, permits to allow off-label uses can be viewed as additional, or an addendum, to the use pattern or instructions on an approved label. The APVMA will only consider granting OLPs for a use that contradicts a label instruction if a 'strong' case can be presented. Permits can only be issued in response to an application for a minor use, an emergency use or research purposes.

5.6.2   European Union

The control of the appropriate use of veterinary medicines in accordance with the conditions of marketing authorizations lies with the Member States' competent authorities. In the EU any VMP is only allowed to be used in accordance with the marketing authorization conditions specified in the SPC and labelling. A veterinary prescription is required for VMPs for food-producing animals containing antimicrobials. The exceptional off-label use of authorized medicines is allowed under specified conditions described in Directive 2001/82/EC as amended, which are often referred to as the 'cascade'. EU Member States are obliged to take measures that, if there is no authorized VMP in a Member State for a specific condition, the responsible veterinarian may, under his/her direct personal responsibility and in particular to avoid causing unacceptable suffering, treat the animal concerned with a VMP authorized in the Member State concerned for another animal species or for another condition in the same species. If there is no such product authorized, a medicinal product authorized for human use in the Member State concerned, or a VMP authorized in another Member State for use in the same species, or in another species for the condition in question or for another condition may be used. If, however, there is no such product a VMP prepared extemporaneously by a person legally authorized to do so following a veterinary prescription may be used.

For food-producing animals, these provisions apply to animals on a particular holding only, the pharmacologically active substances in the medicinal product used must be listed in Annex I, II or III to Regulation 2377/90, and the veterinarian must specify an appropriate withdrawal period, which shall be at least 7 days for eggs, 7 days for milk, 28 days for meat from poultry and mammals, including fat and offal, and 500 degree-days for fish meat.

5.6.3 Japan

In Japan, no person shall provide unapproved anti-microbial agents to livestock animals (cattle, pigs or other animals specified by the MAFF Ministerial Ordinance, which are provided as food). This provision does not apply when antimicrobial agents are intended for use in research and development, or in a case where it is specified by the MAFF Ministerial Ordinance. One of these cases is 'off-label' use of antimicrobial VMPs when occurring under the direction of a veterinarian. The veterinarian should be responsible for setting an appropriate prohibition period to prevent antimicrobial residue beyond MRLs in livestock products provided under the Food Sanitation Law by MHLW (36).

Since most of the antimicrobial VMPs (except those for external use and those used for aquaculture) have been approved as drugs requiring directions or prescriptions by a veterinarian, these VMPs cannot be used without diagnosis and instruction by a veterinarian. VMPs for aquaculture are used under the technical guidance of Prefectural Fisheries Experimental Stations etc. The distribution and use of VMPs, including veterinary antimicrobial agents, is routinely inspected by the regulatory authority (MAFF and prefectural governments) to promote proper use of VMPs.

The amount of antimicrobial VMPs sales for dogs and cats was 3.3 tonnes (0.3%) in 2001. However, little is known about 'off-label' use of antimicrobial agents (mainly for human use) for companion animals, including dogs and cats. Horses are not regarded as companion animals in Japan. As few VMPs are approved for companion animals other than dogs and cats, antimicrobial VMPs are used 'off-label' to treat bacterial disease in other companion animals.

5.6.4 United States

The choice of an alternative product or therapeutic regimen should be based, whenever possible, on the results of valid scientific information demonstrating efficacy for the condition and safety for the

---

Box 5.2 Off-label drug use has several constraints or conditions in the USA, including.

- For food animals, such use is not permitted if a drug exists that is labelled for the food animal species and contains the needed ingredient, is in the proper dosage form, is labelled for the indication and is clinically effective.
- Off-label drug use is permitted for therapeutic purposes only when an animal's health is suffering or threatened. Extra-label drug use is not permitted for food production drugs (e.g. growth promotion).
- Off-label drug use is not permitted if it results in a violative food residue, or any residue that may present a risk to public health.
- Off-label drug use requires scientifically based drug-withdrawal times to ensure food safety.

Box 5.3 A VCPR exists when *all* of the following conditions have been met.

- The veterinarian has assumed the responsibility for making clinical judgments regarding the health of the animal(s) and the need for medical treatment, and the client has agreed to follow the veterinarian's instructions.
- The veterinarian has sufficient knowledge of the animal(s) to initiate at least a general or preliminary diagnosis of the medical condition of the animal(s). This means that the veterinarian has recently seen and is personally acquainted with the keeping and care of the animal(s) by virtue of an examination of the animal(s) or by medically appropriate and timely visits to the premises where the animal(s) are kept.
- The veterinarian is readily available for follow-up evaluation, or has arranged for emergency coverage, in the event of adverse reactions or failure of the treatment regimen.

---

species concerned. In the USA, veterinary oversight is required for the use of approved antimicrobials in an off-label manner (Box 5.2). This direction may only take place within the context of a veterinarian–client–patient relationship (VCPR, Box 5.3).

5.7 Pharmacovigilance, prudent use guidelines and codes of practice

The VICH is developing guidelines for the pharmacovigilance of VMPs (10). The Codex Alimentarius Committee on Residues of Veterinary Drugs in Food developed a Code of Practice to Minimize and Contain Antimicrobial Resistance. The Code was adopted by the Codex Alimentarius Commission in July 2005 (18). Guidelines for the responsible and prudent use of antimicrobial agents in veterinary medicine have been developed by the OIE (17). National guidelines are described in the following sections.

5.7.1   Australia

The APVMA seeks to identify and act promptly on adverse experiences through the Adverse Experience Reporting Program for veterinary medicines (AERP Vet). This is a quality assurance initiative established to facilitate responsible management of veterinary chemical products throughout their lifecycle. Reports received by the APVMA are assessed to determine whether the adverse experience is related to the product formulation, manufacturing processes, use practices or product labelling. The APVMA publishes an annual report summarising all adverse experiences, including outcomes of investigations and the course of action taken. The reports are available on the APVMA website (37). The importance of prudent use guidelines and codes of practice were identified in Recommendations 15–17 of JETACAR (19). The responsibility for developing and supporting these is shared between veterinary peak bodies, learned societies, professional organizations, producer organizations, pharmaceutical companies, veterinary registration boards and the federal and State and Territory governments.

The Australian Veterinary Poultry Association released a code of practice for the use of antimicrobial agents in the poultry industry in 2001. The code of practice is endorsed by the Australian Chicken Meat Federation and the Australian Egg Industry Association (37). The Australian Veterinary Association (AVA) has developed and published Policies on the Use of Veterinary Medicines, which includes Guidelines for Prescribing and Dispensing in Veterinary Medicine and a Code of Practice for the Use of Antimicrobial Drugs in Veterinary Practice. The policy covers professional intervention, veterinary care and Prescription Animal Remedy (PAR) medications. The AVA has published other relevant codes and guidelines in Section 2 of their Policy Compendium (38). In 2003, Australian Pork Limited released a series of six Technical Notes for Australian pork producers to provide guidance on practices and management regimes that can be used

to reduce the risk of increasing antimicrobial resistant bacteria in pigs (39).

5.7.2   European Union

The surveillance of VMPs under the EU pharmacovigilance system collects suspected adverse reactions in animals and in human beings relating to the use of VMPs under normal conditions, but also takes into account other available relevant information arising from the use of the product, which may have an impact on the risk–benefit balance of the product, for instance information related to the lack of expected efficacy. This is particularly important in relation to the detection of potential antimicrobial resistance development, off-label use, investigations of the validity of the withdrawal period and the potential environmental problems arising from the use of the product, which may have an impact on the risk–benefit balance of the product.

The marketing authorization holders are obliged to collect and assess all suspected adverse reactions reported for their VMPs and submit to the competent authority for the product concerned, that is, either a Member State authority or the EMEA, dependent on the marketing authorization procedure.

All pharmacovigilance data are to be reported electronically, and a database has been established by the EMEA in cooperation with Member States that ensures that comprehensive safety information is available to the EMEA and all Member States in order to allow appropriate and harmonized regulatory decisions for all products authorized in the EU. Based on the assessment of pharmacovigilance data and considering the risk–benefit balance of a product, the marketing authorization conditions may be amended or the authorization may be suspended or withdrawn.

The CVMP's strategy on antimicrobial agents for 2006–2010 (24) focuses on prudent use instructions, which are considered an efficient way for controlling resistance development through the authorization of veterinary medicines. The Federation of Veterinarians in Europe (FVE), together with its 38 national federations of veterinary surgeons in Europe and four specialized European associations, issued a leaflet on antimicrobial resistance including guidance on prudent use of antibiotics (40).

Initiatives exist also at a national level aimed to maximize communication on the prudent use guidance. As an example, the Responsible Use of Medicines in Agriculture Alliance (RUMA), which is dedicated to promote the standards of food safety, animal health and animal welfare in British livestock farming, has published guidelines for the 'Responsible Use of Antimicrobials' in the main farm animal species including: dairy and beef cattle, sheep, pigs and poultry (41).

5.7.3   Japan

Although there have not been guidelines for prudent use in Japan, MAFF accepts the guidelines for the responsible and prudent use of antimicrobial agents in veterinary medicine developed by the OIE (17) and a Code of Practice to Minimize and Contain Antimicrobial Resistance developed by the Codex Alimentarious Commission (18).

MAFF introduced the translated Japanese version of the OIE guidelines (42). The risk management policy of MAFF is almost in line with these guidelines.

5.7.4   United States

The USA requires pharmacovigilance reports of all marketed VMPs. The American Veterinary Medical Association (AVMA) has led the effort to develop guidelines for judicious therapeutic use of antimicrobials for several animal species, including aquatic species, cats, dogs, horses, beef cattle, dairy cattle, poultry and swine (43).

Acknowledgements

Japan – The author gratefully acknowledges Dr Tetsuo Asai for his considerable support and valuable advice. Australia – The author gratefully acknowledges Ms Robyn Leader for her support, advice and revision of the Australian text.

References

1. Australian Pesticides and Veterinary Medicines Authority (APVMA). *Manual of Requirements and Guidelines (MORAG).* Available at: http://www.apvma.gov.au/MORAG_vet/MORAG_vet_home.shtml

2. Australian Pesticides and Veterinary Medicines Authority (APVMA). Part 10, Special Data: Antibiotic Resistance. Available at: http://www.apvma.gov.au/MORAG_vet/vol_3/part_10_antibiotic_resistance.pdf

3. European Parliament and Council (2001). Directive 2001/82/EC of the European Parliament and the Council of 6 November 2001. *Off. J. Eur. Comm.* L311: 28.11.2004, pp. 01–66, as amended by Directive 2004/28/EC of the European Parliament and the Council of the 31 March 2004 amending Directive 2001/82/EC on the Community code relating to veterinary medical products. *Off. J. Eur. Comm.* L136: 30.04.2004, 58–84. Available at: http://ec.europa.eu/enterprise/pharmaceuticals/eudralex/homev5.htm

4. European Parliament and Council (2004). Regulation (EC) No 726/2004 of the European Parliament and of the Council of 31 March 2004 laying down Community procedures for the authorisation and supervision of medicinal products for human and veterinary use and establishing a European Medicines Agency. *Off. J. Eur. Comm.* L136: 30.4.2004, 1–33. Available at: http://ec.europa.eu/enterprise/pharmaceuticals/eudralex/homev5.htm

5. European Parliament and Council (2003). Regulation (EC) No 1831/2003 of the European Parliament and of the Council of 22 September 2003 on additives for use in animal nutrition. *Off. J. Eur. Comm.* L268: 18.10.2003, 29–43. Available at: http://eur-lex.europa.eu/LexUriServ.do?uri=CELEX: 32003R1831:EN:NOT

6. The Government of Japan. The Pharmaceutical Law. (Law No.145 of 1960).

7. The Government of Japan. The Law Concerning Safety Assurance and Quality Improvement of Feed. (Law No.35 of 1953). Available at: http://www.famic.go.jp/ffis/feed/obj/sianhou_eng.pdf

8. Food and Agricultural Materials Inspection Center (FAMIC). List of Feed Additives. Available at: http://www.famic.go.jp/ffis/feed/sub3_feedadditives_en.html

9. U.S. Food and Drug Administration. Available at: www.fda.gov/cvm. Last accessed: November 23, 2007.

10. VICH. VICH Guidelines. Cooperation on Harmonisation of Technical Requirements for Registration of Veterinary Medicinal Products. Available at: http://www.vichsec.org/index.htm. Last accessed November 23, 2007.

11. EMEA. Veterinary Medicinal Products. European Medicines Agency, London. Available at: http://www.emea.europa.eu/index/indexv1.htm; http://www.emea.europa.eu/htms/vet/vetguidelines/background.htm

12. U.S. Food and Drug Administration, Center for Veterinary Medicine. Information and requirements for review and approval. Available at: www.fda.gov/cvm/nadaappr.htm. Last accessed: November 23, 2007.

13. EMEA (2002). *Guideline for the demonstration of efficacy for veterinary medicinal use containing antimicrobials.* EMEA/CVMP/627/01. European Medicines Agency, London. Available at: http://www.emea.europa.eu/pdfs/vet/ewp/062701en.pdf

14. EMEA (1999). *Guidelines for the conduct of efficacy studies for intramammary products for use in cattle.* EMEA/CVMP/344/99. European Medicines Agency, London. Available at: http://www.emea.europa.eu/pdfs/vet/ewp/034499en.pdf

15. European Council (1990). Council Regulation (EEC) No 2377/90 of 26 June 1990 laying down a Community procedure for the establishment of maximum residue limits for veterinary medicinal products in foodstuffs of animal origin. *Off. J. Eur. Comm.* L224: 18.8.90, 1–8. Available at: http://ec.europa.eu/enterprise/pharmaceuticals/mrl/conspdf/01990r237720050711--en.pdf

16. Friedlander, L.G., Brynes, S.D. and Fernandez, A.H. (1999). In chemical food borne hazards and their control. *Vet. Clin. North. Am. Food. Anim. Pract.* 15: 1–11.

17. OIE (2006). *Terrestrial animal health code*. World Organisation for Animal Health, Paris. Available at: http://www.oie.int/eng/normes/mcode/en_chapitre_3.9.3.htm

18. Codex Alimentarius Commission (2006). ALINORM 05/28/31, Appendix VIII. Available at: http://www.codexalimentarius.net/web/index_en.jsp. Last accessed: November 23, 2007.

19. Joint Expert Technical Advisory Committee on Antibiotic Resistance (JETACAR) (1999). *The use of antibiotics in food-producing animals: antibiotic-resistant bacteria in animals and humans.* Commonwealth Departments of Health and Aged Care, and Agriculture, Fisheries and Forestry, Canberra Australia. Available at: http://www.health.gov.au/internet/wcms/publishing.nsf/content/health-pubs-jetacar-cnt.htm/$FILE/jetacar.pdf

20. The Commonwealth Government Response to the Report of the Joint Expert Technical Advisory Committee on Antibiotic Resistance (JETACAR) (2000). Commonwealth Departments of Health and Aged Care, and Agriculture, Fisheries and Forestry, Canberra Australia. Available at: http://www.health.gov.au/internet/wcms/publishing.nsf/content/health-pubhlth-publicat-document-jetacar-cnt.htm/$FILE/jetacar.pdf

21. Australian Government National Health and Medical Research Council. Available at: http://www.nhmrc.gov.au/about/committees/expert/eagar/_files/antirate.pdf

22. EMEA (2007). *Revised guideline on the SPC for antimicrobial products.* EMEA/CVMP/SAGAM/38344/2005. European Medicines Agency, London. Available at: http://www.emea.europa.eu/pdfs/vet/sagam/3834410.enfin.pdf

23. EMEA (2007). *Public statement on the use of (Fluoro) quinolones in food-producing animals in the European Union: development of resistance and impact on the human and animal health.* EMEA/CVMP/SAGAM/184651/2005. European Medicines Agency, London. Available at: http://www.emea.europa.eu/pdfs/vet/srwp/18465106en.pdf

24. EMEA (2006). *CVMP strategy on antimicrobials for 2006–2010 and status report on activities on antimicrobials.* EMEA/CVMP/353297/2005. European Medicines Agency, London. Available at: http://www.emea.europa.eu/pdfs/vet/swp/35329705.pdf

25. The Government of Japan. The Food Safety Basic Law. (Law No. 48 of 2003). Available at: http://www.fsc.go.jp/sonota/fsb_law1807.pdf

26. U.S. Food and Drug Administration, Center for Veterinary Medicine. (2003). Guidance for Industry #152: Evaluating the safety of antimicrobial new animal drugs with regard to their microbiological effects on bacteria of human health concern. Available at: www.fda.gov/cvm/Guidance/fguide152.DOC.

27. Australian Pesticides and Veterinary Medicines Authority (APVMA). Available at: http://www.apvma.gov.au/registration/downloads/antibiotics_1999_2002.pdf

28. EMEA (1999). *Antibiotic resistance in the European Union associated with therapeutic use of veterinary medicines: report and qualitative risk assessment by the Committee for Veterinary Medicinal Products.* EMEA/CVMP/342/99. European Medicines Agency, London. Available at: http://www.emea.europa.eu/pdfs/vet/regaffair/034299en.pdf

29. European Parliament and Council (2003). Directive 2003/99/EC of the European Parliament and of the Council, of 17 November 2003 on the monitoring of oonoses and zoonotic agents, amending Council Decision 90/424/EEC and repealing Council Directive 92/117/EEC. *Off. J. Eur. Comm.* L325: 12.12.2003, 31–40. Available at: http://eur_lex.europa.eu/LexWriServ.do?uri=CELEX:32003L0099:EN:NOT

30. EFSA (2006). *The community summary reports on trends and sources of zoonoses, zoonotic agents and antimicrobial resistance in the European Union in 2004 and 2005.* European Food Safety Authority, Parma. Available at: http://www.efsa.europa.eu/en/science/monitoring_zoonoses/reports.html

31. The National Veterinary Assay Laboratory, MAFF (NVAL). Available at: http://www.nval.go.jp/taisei/etaisei/JVARM (text%20and%20Fig)%Final.htm

32. Institute of Medicine, Committee on Human Health Risk Assessment of Using Subtherapeutic Antibiotics in Animal Feeds (1989). *Human health risks with the subtherapeutic use of penicillin or tetracyclines in animal feed.* National Academy Press, Washington, DC.

33. National Antimicrobial Resistance Monitoring System. Available at: http://fda.gov/cvm/narms_pg.html

34. Australian Pesticides and Veterinary Medicines Authority (APVMA). Available at: http://services.apvma.gov.au/PubcrisWebClient/welcome.do

35. The Heads of Medicines Agencies website. Available at: http://www.hma.eu/

36. The Government of Japan. The Food Sanitation Law. (Law No.233 of 1947). Available at: http://www.jetro.go.jp/en/market/regulations/pdf/food-e.pdf

37. Australian Chicken Meat Federation and the Australian Egg Industry Association. Available at: http://www.jcu.edu.au/school/bms/avpa/code_of_prac_jul_2001.pdf

38. Australian Veterinary Association (AVA). Use of antimicrobial drugs in veterinary practice, 1999; Safe use of veterinary medicines on farms, 1997; Code of practice for the use of prescription animal remedies (schedule 4 substances) in the pig industry, 1997; and Code of practice for the use of prescription animal remedies (schedule 4 substances) in the poultry industry, 2001. Available at: http://www.ava.com.au

39. Australian Pork Limited Technical Notes. Available at: http://www.australianpork.com.au/index.cfm?menuid=D912DD189027–E5331–F749DF794A6BC9E

40. FVE Antibiotic Resistance and Prudent Use of Antibiotics in Veterinary Medicine. Federation of Veterinarians in Europe, Brussels. Available at: http://fve.org/papers/pdf/vetmed/position_papers/antibioen.pdf

41. RUMA (2004). *Guidelines for the 'Responsible Use of Antimicrobials' in poultry, pigs, cattle, sheep and fish.* Responsible Use of Medicines in Agriculture Alliance, Welwyn, UK. Available at: http://www.ruma.org.uk/

42. NVAL. Available at: http://www.nval.go.jp/taisei/oie/OIEguide2.htm

43. The American Veterinary Medical Association (AVMA) guidelines. Available at: www.avma.org/reference/defalut.asp

Chapter 6

STRATEGIES TO MINIMISE THE IMPACT OF ANTIMICROBIAL TREATMENT ON THE SELECTION OF RESISTANT BACTERIA

Peter Lees, Ove Svendsen and Camilla Wiuff

The success (or failure) of antimicrobial prophylaxis, metaphylaxis or therapy depends on the assessment criteria used and end-points adopted. Total success or absolute failure, with a spectrum of possibilities between these extremes, may be gauged using one or more of three criteria: *clinical signs, bacteriological outcome* and *emergence of resistance*. In many cases, clinical cure does not guarantee bacteriological cure. For example, in a 'heavy' infection the number of colony forming units (CFU) at the infection site may be as high as 10^9 CFU/ml. If the combined effect of an antimicrobial drug and immune defences reduces this to 10^2 CFU/ml, the decrease is massive in absolute and percentage terms. The clinical response is likely to be excellent, but not all organisms have been eradicated. Thus, a small number of organisms may remain, insufficient in number to provide any persisting clinical signs, but nevertheless creating the possibilities of resurgence of infection at a later stage and/or transfer of microorganisms to humans and other animals. In case of clinical cure without microorganism eradication, the animal patient obviously feels better (cured in fact) *but* the outcome is clearly less than optimal. Therefore, from the standpoint of assessing efficacy, the gold standard must be bacteriological cure at the infection site.

When there is a *true* bacteriological cure, all organisms are killed and therefore resistance does not emerge (at least not in the now eradicated population of pathogens) and cannot therefore spread. However,

two caveats must be made here. First, *apparent* bacteriological cure, whilst reducing the number of organisms to below detectable levels, may involve persistence of a small population and these organisms may have reduced susceptibility to antimicrobial drugs. Some recent studies indicate that avoidance of resistance may sometimes require administration of such high doses of an antimicrobial drug as to create problems of host toxicity or to render therapy with that drug impractical from an economic perspective (Figure 6.1). Second, even assuming successful therapy (with both clinical and bacteriological cures), resistance may have arisen in commensal organisms and the genetic elements responsible may then spread by horizontal transfer to pathogenic bacteria.

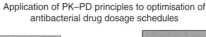

Application of PK–PD principles to optimisation of antibacterial drug dosage schedules

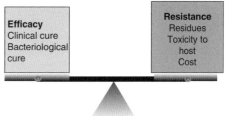

Figure 6.1 Balance of factors in selecting antimicrobial dosage.

Pharmacokinetics and pharmacodynamics in antimicrobial chemotherapy

Setting dosage schedules:

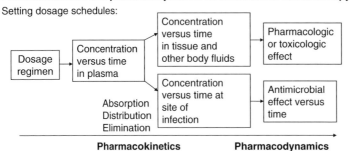

Pharmacokinetics   Pharmacodynamics

Figure 6.2 Pharmacokinetic and pharmacodynamic considerations in relation to dosing regimens.

It is widely accepted that antimicrobial resistance emerges according to the classic Darwinian principle of selective pressure, in which antimicrobial agents inhibit the most susceptible organisms, with regrowth of the remaining less susceptible organisms initially occurring in very small numbers. Antimicrobial drugs do not create but select for resistant mutants and/or strains that have acquired resistance genes prior to or during treatment. It is also widely acknowledged that the most important single factor leading to antimicrobial resistance selection is exposure to insufficient drug concentrations at the infection site. In broad terms, the success or failure of antimicrobial therapy depends on two factors: (a) achieving penetration of the drug to the infection site in a sufficient concentration (pharmacokinetics) and (b) the potency and efficacy of the drug against infecting microorganisms at the infection site (pharmacodynamics) (Figure 6.2). A third factor, often ignored but of considerable potential importance in regard to the emergence of resistance, is compliance with administration of the prescribed drug according to the recommended dosage schedule. The balance of the many factors (often conflicting) determining dosage is summarised in Figure 6.3.

The aims of this chapter are to review: (a) the mechanisms by which resistance arises in both pathogenic and commensal microorganisms; (b) how resistance may spread; (c) the pharmacological (pharmacokinetic and pharmacodynamic) factors which determine the outcome of therapy; and (d) the ways in which pharmacokinetic and pharmacodynamic principles and data can be used to optimise dosing schedules, with particular reference to the goal of minimising the emergence of resistance.

Rational dosing of antimicrobial drugs

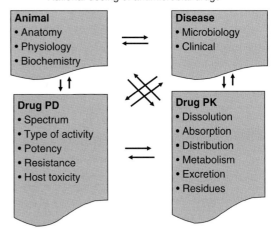

Figure 6.3 Rational design of dosing schedules depends on factors relating to the animal, the disease, drug pharmacokinetics, drug pharmacodynamics and complex potential interactions between these factors.

6.1 Mechanisms of selection for resistance

Mutations and other genetic changes in the bacterial genome generate the basis of antimicrobial resistance by decreasing the susceptibility of the affected bacteria. Genetic changes in the bacterial genome can be generated in a number of ways, including spontaneous mutation and acquisition of genetic mobile elements such as plasmids and integrons. Chromosomal mutations typically lead to modification of the antimicrobial drug target molecules involved in vital processes of the bacterial cell (Table 6.1). Though chromosomal in origin, many of these resistance genes can be integrated into mobile genetic elements such as

Table 6.1 Classification of antimicrobial drugs according to mechanism of action and as bacteriostatic or bactericidal agents

Mechanism of action

Either inhibit cell wall synthesis or activate enzymes which disrupt the cell wall.	Act on cell (plasma) membrane to modify permeability causing loss of intracellular molecules to the external environment.	Inhibit synthesis of nucleic acids.	Inhibit enzymes involved in DNA metabolism, including DNA gyrase and DNA-dependent RNA polymerase or cause disruption of the DNA template.	Bind to 50S subunit of ribosomes causing inhibition of bacterial protein synthesis.	Bind to 30S ribosomal subunit of ribosomes leading either to misreading of mRNA code or to inhibition of the first step of protein synthesis.
Drug classes					
Penicillins Cephalosporins Bacitracin Glycopeptides	Polymixins	Diaminopyrimidines Sulfonamides	Fluoroquinolones Nitrofurans Nitroimidazoles Rifamycins	Macrolides[a] Triamilides[a] Lincosamides Phenicols[a] Fusidic acid	Tetracyclines Aminocyclitols Aminoglycosides
Bacteriostatic or bactericidal action					
Bactericidal	Bactericidal	Bacteriostatic but bactericidal when one drug from each group is combined.	Bactericidal	Bacteriostatic	Bacteriostatic (tetracyclines[a]) or bactericidal (aminoglycosides and aminocyclitols).

[a]Some drugs in these classes are bactericidal against some species.

integrons and transposons and be readily transferred to new hosts and combined with other resistance genes. Other genetic changes lead to enzymatic degradation (1) and reduced uptake or increased efflux of antimicrobials (2, 3).

In growing populations of most bacterial species, resistant mutants emerge spontaneously at rates of 10^6 to 10^{10} per gene per generation. However, often more than one molecular mechanism contributes to lowering the susceptibility of bacteria. In that case, the resulting frequency of resistant mutants will be a function of the multiple of the mutation rates in all the different genes that affect the susceptibility to a given drug (4). The immune system of the host plays a very important role in minimising the emergence of resistance by reducing the bacterial population size, which in turn decreases the likelihood of mutation to resistance and inhibits the growth of the resistant mutants themselves (5, 6).

Selective pressure refers to the environmental conditions that allow organisms with novel mutations or newly acquired characteristics to survive and proliferate (7). In nature, the environment within a host is very heterogeneous and contains many sub-environments (compartments) in which particular selective forces are exerted. When treating animals or humans with antimicrobial drugs, concentration gradients are created within the body. Along such gradients the numerous sub-environments create selective compartments in which bacteria encounter particular selective forces (8). The selection of a resistant bacterial population within a particular compartment is dependent on various factors: (i) the type and concentration of drug; (ii) the time period for which the organism is exposed to the drug selective forces; (iii) the species and population sizes of the microorganisms present at the infection site; and (iv) the general composition of the environment (9). During antimicrobial therapy, new drug gradients are continuously created within the body of the treated host due to the distribution, elimination, metabolism and inactivation of the drug, and this is followed by creation of new selective compartments.

The normal flora, in particular those organisms which possess antimicrobial inactivating enzymes, also contribute to the gradient formation (5).

The selection for resistance is most intense in narrow concentration ranges, referred to as *selective windows*, in which the antimicrobial inhibits the growth of one (or more) subpopulations while it has no antimicrobial effect on other subpopulations (Figure 6.4).

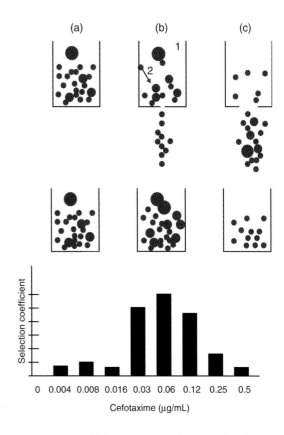

Figure 6.4 Principle of concentration-specific selection in selective windows. Small balls represent susceptible sub-populations and larger balls represent intermediate and resistant sub-populations. The size of the hole at the bottom represents the concentration of the inhibitor (the antimicrobial agent). The first row shows the effect of piercing holes of different sizes in three compartments (treating with various concentrations); (a) if the hole is very small (low antimicrobial concentration) no balls are dropped (no bacteria are killed), (b) if the hole is of intermediate size (intermediate concentration) only the small balls are dropped (only the susceptible sub-populations are killed and the resistant sub-populations survive), (c) and if the hole exceeds a critical diameter (high concentrations), all types of balls are dropped (both susceptible and resistant sub-populations are killed). The second row shows what happens when the holes are closed (i.e. the antimicrobial agent is eliminated) and all surviving balls (bacteria) multiply at the same rate; in this scenario the highest frequency of resistant bacteria will be found in (b), which corresponds to the compartment of the body that is exposed to selecting concentrations of the antimicrobial agent, the selective window. In the diagram at the bottom the mutant selection coefficient *in vitro* was highest at intermediate cefotaxime concentrations of 0.03–0.12μg/ml. From Baquero, *Drug Resistance Updates*, 4, 93–105, 2001.

This typically happens at concentrations above the minimum inhibitory concentration (MIC) of the more susceptible strains (subpopulations) and below the MIC of the more resistant variants. Selective pressure favours the growth of one population over another on the basis of very small, nearly undetectable, differences in MIC between those populations (10). Repeated exposure to selective drug concentrations can broaden the selective window by gradually enriching the less susceptible sub-population (10, 11) so that increasingly higher drug concentrations are needed for bacteriological cure. The stepwise evolution towards higher resistance levels can occur in a single host or in distinct hosts and environments. It is exposure, and especially repeated exposure, to sub-optimal drug concentrations that is the most important single factor in resistance emergence and its subsequent spread (12). As exposure is dose related, there is a direct link between administered dose and resistance development. These fundamental principles apply to commensal as well as pathogenic organisms, so that even with adequate exposure of pathogens, commensals may be underexposed. This situation may lead to development of resistance in the commensal flora and transfer of resistance genes to pathogenic organisms at a later stage (13).

Newly mutated resistant bacteria tend to grow more slowly than their ancestors, because the resistance conferring mutations may disrupt some normal physiological processes, which in turn can impose a fitness cost on the bacteria (14). However, the fitness cost imposed by resistance mutations can be overcome by compensatory mutations occurring either in the affected gene (intragenic), or in other genes (extragenic) elsewhere in the genome (15–22) or by gene amplification (copying of genes) (23). Several experimental and theoretical studies have shown that the cost of resistance and degree of compensation are the main determinants of the rate and extent of resistance development both whilst under selective pressure and whenever the antimicrobial agent use is reduced or terminated (24). In addition, recent studies have identified resistant mutants with no (or very little) fitness cost, enabling them to persist when the antimicrobial agent is no longer present (25–29). It is not only the fitness of a pathogen that will determine its fate; its virulence and transmissibility are also essential to the survival and proliferation of resistant clones (17, 30).

It is important to emphasise that for some antimicrobial agents (e.g. quinolones), the evolution of resistance is a progressive process in which small changes in susceptibility can lead through stepwise changes to high-level drug resistance. It has been observed *in vitro* that exposure to low antimicrobial concentrations selects for strains with a much broader variety of genetic changes and biochemical mechanisms of resistance than exposure to higher concentrations (5), although this phenomenon does not apply to all drugs. Changes in expression levels and mutations in housekeeping genes, outer membrane proteins, lipopolysaccharide, efflux pumps, enzymes and other physiological changes can result in low-level resistance, which might be the first step towards high-level resistance. A range of such changes, leading to multiresistant phenotypes, has been shown to precede and accelerate the evolution of high-level fluoroquinolone resistance in *Escherichia coli* and *Salmonella* mediated by specific target mutations (31–34). Recently, new modes of plasmid-mediated fluoroquinolone resistance have been described in multi-drug resistant clinical isolates of *Klebsiella pneumoniae* and *Enterobacteriaceae* conferred by *qnr* genes, which encode gyrase-protecting proteins and antimicrobial agent-degrading enzymes (35–38). Gene products of the *qnr* genes reduce the susceptibility to quinolones but do not confer clinical resistance.

The stepwise evolution of TEM β-lactamases is another example of how small stepwise changes in susceptibility can progressively lead to high levels of resistance to a broad spectrum of agents (39). ESBL-producing *Salmonella* and *E. coli* (of the related enzyme types CTX-M and SHV) have recently been observed in foods and food-producing animals (40–43) as well as in companion animals (44–46). Thus, there is a real risk that these resistance mechanisms are selected by antimicrobial use in animals and subsequently transferred to humans by food consumption or direct exposure to animals.

In conclusion, the drug concentration achieved and resultant antimicrobial activity at the site of infection are of major importance, both in determining the efficacy of treatment regimens and the risk of selecting resistant pathogens. The recurring theme of this chapter is that achieving and maintaining adequate drug concentrations at the site of infection is essential both to eradicating the infecting bacterial population and to preventing the emergence of resistant strains.

6.2 Pharmacodynamics of antimicrobial drugs

At the molecular level, antimicrobial agents produce inhibition of growth or kill microorganisms by several mechanisms. A classification of the major antimicrobial groups based on chemical structure is presented in Table 6.1. As well as the mechanism of action as a basis for classification, antimicrobial drugs may be categorised as bactericidal (kill bacteria) or bacteriostatic (inhibit cell division at concentrations achievable with therapeutic doses). Bacteriostatic drugs have greater dependence on the animal's innate immune mechanisms of defence for cure of infections. In fact, at low concentrations, all antimicrobial agents are bacteriostatic and bacteriostatic drugs may have bactericidal effects at high concentrations. The distinction

is therefore artificial, but is retained because bacteriostatic agents may not achieve a significant reduction in cell numbers at concentrations achieved *in vivo* at sites of infection. A third approach is to classify drugs according to the type of killing action as time-dependent, concentration-dependent or co-dependent (Table 6.2). This nevertheless useful system also oversimplifies antimicrobial drug actions because, for individual drugs, the killing action may be time, concentration or co-dependent, depending on species and even strain for a given species.

Selecting antimicrobial drugs for clinical use and determining dosage thus requires knowledge of how drugs act, of whether they are -static or -cidal and of the type of killing action. In addition, drug selection, dosage determination and the outcome of therapy also depend on: (1) the spectrum of activity,

Table 6.2 Classification of antimicrobial drugs according to type of killing action[a]

Action types	Chemical groups	Drug examples	Integrated PK–PD variables correlating with bacteriological effect
Concentration-dependent killing, usually exerting significant post-antibiotic effect.	Fluoroquinolones	Enrofloxacin, Danofloxacin, Marbofloxacin, Difloxacin, Ibafloxacin	AUC/MIC; C_{max}/MIC
	Aminoglycosides	Streptomycin, Neomycin, Gentamicin, Amikacin, Tobramycin	C_{max}/MIC
	Nitroimidazoles	Metronidazole	AUC/MIC; C_{max}/MIC
	Polymixins	Colistin	AUC/MIC
Time-dependent killing with either no or limited post-antibiotic effect.	Penicillins	Benzylpenicillin, Cloxacillin, Ampicillin, Amoxicillin, Carbenicillin	$T>MIC$
	Cephalosporins	Ceftiofur, Cefalexin, Cefapirin	$T>MIC$
	Macrolides and triamilides	Aivlosin, Tylosin, Erythromycin, Tilmicosin, Tulathromycin	$T>MIC$[b]
	Lincosamides	Clindamycin	$T>MIC$
	Phenicols	Chloramphenicol, Florphenicol	$T>MIC$
	Sulfonamides	Sulfadoxine, Sulfadiazine	$T>MIC$
	Diaminopyrimidines	Trimethoprim	$T>MIC$
Co-dependent killing that is killing action dependent on both duration of exposure and maintained drug concentration.	Tetracyclines	Oxytetracycline, Chlortetracycline, Doxycycline	AUC/MIC
	Ketolides	Azithromycin, Clarithromycin	AUC/MIC
	Glycopeptides	Vancomycin	AUC/MIC

[a]This general classification holds true for most drugs cited and most organisms BUT type of action can be both 'drug and bug specific'. Moreover, for many drugs data available are limited or absent.
[b]For some macrolide and triamilide drugs AUC/MIC best correlates with efficacy; for others no correlations have been established.

which defines the range of susceptible organisms; (2) the levels of resistance that may either be innate or may have emerged during prior use of the drug; and (3) the immune status of the host. If infections are both life threatening and at infection sites where immune defences are minimal, for example in cerebrospinal fluid, the use of a bactericidal drug is preferred. Once the drug is selected, it is necessary to choose a suitably formulated product and route of administration and then administer a dosage schedule which, with the aid of natural body defences, provides a bacteriological (and not only a clinical) cure.

The universally recognised variable, which provides a quantitative index of drug efficacy and potency, is the *minimum inhibitory concentration* (MIC). MIC is determined *in vitro* and is defined as the lowest concentration, measured in liquid broth or on agar plates, which under defined conditions completely inhibits bacterial growth. When many strains of a single bacterial species are examined, MIC values differ and the distribution may be normal, lognormal or even polymodal. It is therefore common to express activity as MIC_{50} or MIC_{90}, corresponding to the percentage of strains affected. EMEA/CVMP Guidelines on data required to support dosage claims for Marketing Authorisation applications, indicate that the reported MIC_{50} should be based on all organisms evaluated, whilst MIC_{90} should relate solely to susceptible strains. Minimum bactericidal concentration (MBC) is an alternative, but less frequently used, measure of potency. It is the drug concentration that produces a 99.9% reduction in bacterial count.

Another pharmacodynamic variable, used specifically in relation to antimicrobial resistance acquired by mutation (e.g. quinolone resistance), is *mutant prevention concentration* (MPC), which is defined as the concentration that does not allow any mutant to be recovered from a population of more than 10^{10} microorganisms (47). During or following administration of an antimicrobial drug, concentrations may decrease to sub-inhibitory levels, that is, no sub-population is inhibited. The concentration range between the MPC and the concentration inhibiting no organisms is generally regarded as the *mutant selection window* (MSW) (47, 48). Ideally, antimicrobial therapy should eradicate bacteria before concentrations decrease below the MPC and reach the MSW. However, as this can never be guaranteed in all circumstances, the MSW should be kept as short as possible, by appropriate selection of drug dosage and product formulation.

Fluoroquinolone resistance in Gram negatives develops by two successive mutations, the first on gyrase and the second on topoisomerase IV. The concentration window between the MIC of wild-type bacteria and the MPC prevents the growth of first step mutants. When concentrations are greater than the MPC, it is highly improbable that a wild-type sub-population will undergo the two mutations (11). However, poor correlations between MPCs and MICs have been observed in a variety of clinical isolates including *E. coli*, *Salmonella enterica* and *Staphylococcus aureus* (49). Clinical isolates can potentially contain many mutant subpopulations that vary considerably in relative number and susceptibility, which will contribute to a wide variation in MIC and MPC. In addition, some mutations have a much larger effect on MPC than on MIC. Consequently, therapeutic strategies aimed at the prevention of resistant mutants require measurement of the MPC for the specific strains causing infection in individual patients and are difficult to determine under clinical conditions.

There are several limitations in using MIC values measured *in vitro* together with pharmacokinetic data to determine dosing schedules for clinical use. First, as indicated above, use of the doubling dilution technique involves overestimation of the true MICs for individual strains. Second, the conditions for bacterial growth in artificial media, in respect of pH and nutrient, electrolyte and protein concentrations, differ from those in biological fluids, so that MICs determined in artificial media and natural body fluids may differ from *in vivo* MICs. This is particularly likely if binding of drug to plasma proteins is high, as only the non-protein bound fraction is microbiologically active. Third, MIC determination involves exposing organisms to a fixed drug concentration for a fixed period (18–24 h), while during antimicrobial therapy plasma concentrations either fall, for example after IV bolus dosing, or first increase to a peak and then fall, when administration is by a non-vascular route. In addition, under clinical circumstances, microorganisms are exposed for much longer periods than 24 h with most dosing strategies. Thus, MIC is a static endpoint rather than a dynamic measure of concentration as a function of time. Finally, immune defence mechanisms are normally absent *in vitro*, whereas they normally play a significant role in curtailing infections *in vivo*.

For antimicrobial agents with a concentration-dependent killing action, MIC determined *in vitro* may underestimate *in vivo* efficacy because of the potential contributions to bacterial growth inhibition or eradication by *post-antimicrobial effect* (PAE), *post-antimicrobial sub-MIC effect* (PASME) and *post-antimicrobial leucocyte enhancement* (PALE) mechanisms. PAE is defined as the period of inhibition of bacterial growth occurring after exposure to concentrations greater than MICs, when the drug is removed or neutralised. PASME similarly defines the persistent period of growth inhibition when organisms have been previously exposed to drug concentrations lower than MIC. PALE describes the enhancement of the killing action of leucocytes following bacterial exposure to the drug. However, it is not clear that these several *in vitro* indices of drug activity operate *in vivo* in the same manner. For example, PAE is generally short, and its significance for drugs administered in a long-acting formulation or with a repeat dose administration is questionable when treating disease.

Non-inherited resistance, also known as *phenotypic tolerance or persistence*, is another phenomenon that complicates the prediction of antimicrobial treatment outcome (50–52). During exposure to an antimicrobial agent the killing rate of bacteria gradually decreases with time and a fraction of the bacteria may survive, even in the presence of antimicrobial agent. These surviving cells, present in all bacterial populations, are phenotypic variants of the wild type, supposedly without any genetic changes. *In vitro* studies and mathematical modelling suggest that the presence of such tolerant populations may lead to clinical treatment failure (53).

Attempts to resolve some of these concerns regarding the use of MIC in dosage selection have involved measurement of MIC in body fluids such as serum, and accuracy can be improved by use of several overlapping sets of doubling dilutions (54–58). Other approaches have involved the use of more sophisticated *in vitro* models, in which drug concentrations are not fixed but simulate those obtained *in vivo* by continuous infusion of a drug, followed by infusion of a drug-free growth medium (59). Quantitative efficacy assessment *in vitro* may also be based on time–kill curves, which by definition not only describe the final outcome quantitatively (indicated by change in bacterial count from the initial inoculum count), but also the time course of change in inoculum count. Other studies have involved determination of time–kill curves *ex vivo*, and these may be regarded as more clinically relevant than most *in vitro* approaches.

For example, time–kill curves for fluoroquinolones have been reported in which antimicrobial action has been established in natural body fluids such as serum, exudate and transudate (in a tissue cage model) after administration of drugs to target species at recommended dose rates (54–56). In addition, there have been many *in vivo* approaches to studies of efficacy, based either on disease models or evaluation in clinical trials. In these studies the end points all too often are, unfortunately but sometimes necessarily, based solely on clinical outcome.

In some instances, optimisation of antimicrobial therapy may be further complicated by *the Polyanna phenomenon*: a drug providing a complete bacteriological cure may not fully resolve clinical signs, whereas another drug achieving incomplete bacteriological cure rate may result in a good clinical response. This was shown for ceftiofur in the treatment of colibacillosis in neonatal pigs (60); there was little difference in reduction in mortality between dosage groups, but a positive correlation between dose and bacterial shedding was established. More recently, the same phenomenon has been described for the fluoroquinolone, pradofloxacin, in canine urinary tract infections (Fraatz and Griefe, per. commun.). Hence, total bacteriological cure is the gold standard for optimising efficacy and minimising resistance emergence. The Polyanna phenomenon also accounts for the commonly encountered difficulty of pharmaceutical companies in demonstrating the improved efficacy of new agents in comparison with established drugs. For example, this problem may arise when spontaneous resolution from infection is high, as well as for drugs which possess non-antimicrobial actions contributing to the clinical outcome, as in the case of some quinolones, macrolides and tetracyclines possessing anti-inflammatory and/or immunomodulatory properties (61–63) (see Section 6.6).

In clinical practice, veterinarians sometimes prescribe combinations of antimicrobial drugs or combinations of drugs with chemical (non-drug) synergy. The objective of this therapeutic approach is to enhance antimicrobial pharmacodynamics, and various commercially available products based on this principle are available. The best examples are: (1) sulfonamides combined with tetrahydrofolate inhibitors such as trimethoprim (the combinations achieve synergism reflected in bactericidal effect, extended antimicrobial spectrum and much reduced dosage required of each constituent); and (2) the use of potassium clavulanate as an inhibitor of β-lactamase enzymes (to extend the spectrum of activity to organisms with either innate or acquired production of β-lactamase). These types of antimicrobial combinations may be regarded as both rational and advantageous in terms of reducing the likelihood of resistance emergence.

Combination of antimicrobial agents with non-antimicrobial drugs is also common in veterinary practice and includes: (1) the administration of antimicrobial drugs to animals receiving therapy for non-infectious conditions (e.g. heart failure); and (2) the selected use of non-antimicrobial drugs to modulate the actions of an antimicrobial agent (e.g. concomitant use of non-steroidal anti-inflammatory drugs in the therapy of calf and piglet pneumonia). In both circumstances, interactions may be beneficial or deleterious and involve either pharmacodynamics or pharmacokinetics of the two drugs. However, not all combinations, either in single products or as two products co-prescribed, have a sound scientific basis and their practice should never be undertaken in the absence of a sound rationale. Because of a general lack of published data to justify either use or non-use of particular combinations of drugs, it is difficult to offer firm guidance. Nevertheless, it seems prudent to avoid combining two drugs with similar toxicity profiles (e.g. renotoxicity of aminoglycosides, polymixins and some loop diuretics at high dose rates) or to use drugs in combination that might interact pharmacokinetically. Thus, drugs that either induce (phenobarbitone) or inhibit (chloramphenicol) drug metabolising hepatic microsomal enzymes, may decrease or increase respectively the body clearance of drugs of other classes which are metabolised by these enzymes.

6.3 Pharmacokinetics of antimicrobial drugs

Pharmacokinetics is the science of drug absorption into, fate within and elimination from, the body: dissolution, absorption, distribution, metabolism and excretion. Together, metabolism and excretion comprise elimination of the parent drug, although it should be noted that, in a few instances, metabolites retain antimicrobial activity. An example is the *in vivo* conversion of enrofloxacin into ciprofloxacin. Antimicrobial pharmacokinetics is partly dependent on intrinsic properties of the drug such as clearance

and volume of distribution, and other properties depending on extrinsic factors such as route of administration and/or product formulation. For example, both rate and extent of absorption derived from both oral dosing and non-vascular injection may be significantly modified by formulation changes. The intrinsic pharmacokinetic properties of drugs are generally not determined by their detailed chemical structure but by simple physico–chemical properties, including water and lipid solubility and molecular size. The latter is generally of little significance, as all drug molecules are sufficiently small to traverse capillary endothelial cells to enter interstitial fluid, but sufficiently large to fail to penetrate most cells through the small pores in their membranes by filtration. Therefore, passage of all membranes, when it occurs, is usually by passive diffusion (*vide infra*). Based on relative solubility, antimicrobial drugs may be broadly categorised into (1) water-soluble (polar) and usually lipid-insoluble compounds and (2) non-polar and usually lipid-soluble drugs (Table 6.3). The differences are not absolute since many antimicrobial drugs have intermediate properties.

Water solubility is important because water is the universal biological solvent. Therefore, drugs must be in aqueous solution in order to (1) be absorbed from the gastrointestinal tract or from non-vascular injection sites; (2) distribute from plasma into the bacterial biophase; and (3) penetrate into bacterial cells. However, because most drugs are potent, being effective in μg or ng/ml concentrations, water solubility does not have to be high in order to ensure antibacterial activity. *Lipid solubility* is a key determinant of antimicrobial pharmacokinetics because high solubility enables drugs to cross cell membranes by passive diffusion – literally by dissolving in the lipid component of the membrane and thereby traversing it down the concentration gradient. The many pharmacokinetic implications associated with the degree of lipid solubility of antimicrobial drugs are summarised in Table 6.3.

After absorption, drug distribution to the infection site is a key factor in determining the level and duration of antimicrobial exposure of microorganisms. As many bacterial infections are confined to extracellular fluids (plasma and interstitial fluid), the limited ability of poorly lipid-soluble molecules to cross cell membranes does *not* impair their penetration to sites of infection. This is because penetration from plasma to interstitial fluid is rapidly achieved irrespective of lipid solubility through the large channels in

Table 6.3 Relationship of lipid solubility of antimicrobial drugs to pharmacokinetic properties (ADME)[a]

Drugs with high lipophilicity	Drugs with moderate to high lipophilicity			Drugs with low lipophilicity	
	Weak acids	Weak bases	Amphoteric	Strong acids	Strong bases or polar bases[b]
Lipophilic tetracyclines • Minocycline • Doxycycline Fluoroquinolones Phenicols Nitroimidazoles Rifamycins	Sulfonamides	Diaminopyrimidines Macrolides Lincosamides Ketolides Triamilides	Most Tetracyclines • Oxytetracycline • Chlortetracycline	Penicillins Cephalosporins	Aminoglycosides Aminocyclitols Polymixins
Cross cell membranes very readily and therefore penetrate into intracellular and transcellular fluids, for example, synovial and prostatic fluids and bronchial secretions. Also penetrate well into CSF, except tetracyclines and rifampin. Generally well absorbed from g.i.t. in monogastric species. Termination of activity dependent on a high proportion of the administered dose being metabolised, for example, in the liver but also at other sites, for example, kidney, enterocytes. Some drugs actively secreted into bile.	Readily cross cell membranes. Therefore, effective concentrations achieved in intra- and trans-cellular as well as extracellular fluids. Ability to penetrate into CSF and ocular fluids depends on plasma protein binding, for example, most sulfonamides and diaminopyrimidines penetrate well but penetration of macrolides, lincosamides and tetracyclines is more variable. Weak acids are ion trapped in fluids alkaline relative to plasma, such as herbivore urine. Weak bases are ion trapped in fluids acidic relative to plasma, for example, prostatic fluid, milk, intracellular fluid, carnivore urine. Moderate to good absorption from g.i.t. but species dependent. Commonly dependent on biotransformation for termination of activity but may also be excreted unchanged in urine and/or bile. Some drugs actively secreted into bile.			Unable to readily penetrate cell membranes. Distribution therefore limited mainly to extracellular fluids. Concentrations in intracellular fluid, CSF, milk, and ocular fluids are usually very low, but effective concentrations may be reached in synovial, peritoneal and pleural fluids. Some penicillins are actively transported out of CSF into plasma. Limited or no significant absorption from g.i.t., except the acid stable aminopenicillins, which have moderate but species variable absorption. Generally excreted, usually in urine, in high concentrations as the parent molecule. Some drugs actively secreted into bile. Biotransformation (e.g. in the liver) usually slight or absent.	

[a] Absorption, distribution, metabolism and excretion.
[b] Polymixins are strong bases, whereas aminoglycosides and aminocyclitols are weak bases, but nevertheless they are polar and poorly lipid soluble because of the presence of sugar residues in the molecules.

capillary membranes, which permit transfer of the free concentration of virtually all antimicrobial drugs. In other words, penetration across the endothelial cell membrane occurs rapidly and readily in most vascular beds by a simple process of ultrafiltration. For most extracellular fluid infections, it is the non-protein bound (i.e. free) plasma drug concentration that determines concentration in the biophase. However, when infections are present in transcellular (e.g. synovial, intraocular, etc.), cerebrospinal and prostatic fluids or in the epithelial lining fluid in the lungs, highly or moderately lipid soluble drugs are most likely to achieve therapeutic concentrations (Table 6.3). Similarly, intracellular (e.g. *Mycoplasma*, *Salmonella*, *Rhodococcus equi*, *Actinobacillus pleuropneumoniae*, *Anaplasma phagocytophilum*, etc.) infections cannot be treated effectively by lipid insoluble drugs due to failure to penetrate the host cell membrane, even if the pathogens involved are fully susceptible. An extension of this phenomenon can arise for drugs that do enter intracellular fluid but then fail to enter that intracellular compartment (e.g. the phagolysosome) in which some microorganisms may reside.

In diseased animals, blood flow, epithelial permeability and volumes of extracellular fluid may be altered, possibly causing reduced drug concentration at the infection site. In pigs infected with *Salmonella* Typhimurium the antimicrobial concentrations of danofloxacin in plasma were higher in infected animals than in controls even though the actual tissue concentrations were lower, presumably due to reduced intestinal blood flow and inability of the intestinal mucosa to secrete the drug (64). In contrast, in some infections the inflammatory process might increase drug concentrations at an infection site by increasing blood flow to the affected area.

Some antimicrobial agents are either weak bases or weak acids and at the pH of physiological fluids (e.g. 7.4 for plasma) they exist in equilibrium between ionised and un-ionised forms, the relative proportions of which are determined by both pH and acidic or basic strength. Generally, antimicrobials are lipid soluble only in their un-ionised forms. Therefore, when pH on opposite sides of a cell membrane differs, only the un-ionised moiety traverses the membrane down its concentration gradient, giving rise to the phenomenon of *ion trapping*. Weak acids are trapped in media alkaline to plasma (e.g. the urine of herbivores), whereas weak bases are trapped in acid environments (e.g. milk, prostatic fluid and urine of carnivores). Ion trapping explains the accumulation of macrolides (weak bases) in milk and the ready excretion of sulfonamides (weak acids) in the alkaline urine of herbivores. On the other hand, strong acids and bases, being wholly ionised at physiological pH, are polar lipid insoluble molecules that do not cross cell membranes readily and result in excretion at high concentrations in urine, as most or all of the drug filtered at the glomerulus, being poorly lipid soluble, is excreted in urine. Examples include aminoglycosides and penicillins (Table 6.4).

Table 6.4 Clearance, elimination half-life and volume of distribution of antimicrobial agents in the dog

Drug	Clearance Cl_B (ml/min kg)	Elimination half-life $T\frac{1}{2}\beta$ (h)	Volume of distribution Vd area (ml/kg)
Ticarcillin[a]	4.30	0.95	340
Benzylpenicillin[a]	3.60	0.50	156
Gentamicin[a]	3.10	1.25	335
Amikacin[a]	2.61	1.10	245
Sulfadiazine[b]	0.92	5.63	422
Erythromycin[b]	18.20	1.72	2700
Enrofloxacin[b]	8.56	3.35	2454
Norfloxacin[b]	5.53	3.56	1770
Trimethoprim[b]	4.77	4.63	1849
Metronidazole[b]	2.50	4.50	948
Marbofloxacin[b]	1.66	12.40	1900

[a]Poorly lipid soluble molecules with high urine concentrations, short elimination half-life and low volume of distribution.
[b]Molecules with medium to high lipid solubility with generally longer half-life, higher volume of distribution.
Clearance values vary widely, ranging from low (marbofloxacin) to relatively high (erythromycin).

For most antimicrobial drugs, biotransformation is of importance primarily because it normally reduces or abolishes activity. Biotransformation, together with renal excretion, is the mechanism whereby antimicrobial activity is terminated. Examples of the pharmacokinetic consequences of varying degrees of drug lipid solubility on biotransformation are given in Table 6.4. The liver is the main organ responsible for drug biotransformation, although it is now recognised that many other organs, tissues and cells, for example kidney and enterocytes, can metabolise some drugs. It should be noted that species variation in the rate of metabolism is the rule rather than the exception, so that there are profound inter-species differences in clearance and terminal half-life for individual drugs (Table 6.5). This phenomenon determines major species differences in both dose requirements and half-life, determining dose intervals. Moreover, mechanisms and pathways of hepatic metabolism and renal excretion are not fully developed in neonates, leading to slower clearance and a longer elimination half-life. Reduced hepatic and renal functions may also occur in aged animals. Finally, in fish, clearance and elimination rates vary markedly with body temperature, and drugs such as sulfadimidine, trimethoprim and oxytetracycline have up to three-fold longer half-life values at low (10–12°C) compared to high (20–25°C) environmental (and body) temperatures.

A further consideration in relation to antimicrobial pharmacokinetics is the existence of active transport mechanisms for some antimicrobial drugs. These can either enhance or retard absorption from the gastrointestinal tract (and hence affect bioavailability), depending on whether the drug is actively taken up by enterocytes or extruded from enterocytes back into the gastrointestinal liquor. Drug transporters also exist in other tissues and are responsible, for example, for active secretion of penicillins and cephalosporins by renal proximal tubular cells into tubular fluid and thence into urine, and active extrusion of penicillins from CSF into plasma. There is increasing recognition that for some antimicrobial drugs, transporters can influence both intestinal absorption and penetration to sites of action.

As some antimicrobial drugs (e.g. most aminoglycosides, penicillins and cephalosporins) are rapidly cleared and have short elimination half-lives (Tables 6.4 and 6.5), therapeutic concentrations are maintained for only a few hours after a single intravenous or intramuscular administration in aqueous solution (e.g. sodium salt of benzylpenicillin). Their use requires repeated dosing at short intervals and is therefore impractical under clinical conditions. Hence, a common practice is to formulate antimicrobial preparations as aqueous or oily suspensions of poorly water-soluble salts (e.g. procaine benzylpenicillin) or as solutions in organic solvents (e.g. oxytetracycline), especially for use in farm animals. These depot products, when injected by a non-vascular route (usually intramuscularly but sometimes subcutaneously), are taken up slowly into solution at the injection site and provide more persistent concentrations in plasma

Table 6.5 Examples of species differences in elimination half-life

Drug	Half-life (h)			
	Cow	Horse	Dog	Man
Benzylpenicillin[a]	0.7	0.9	0.5	1.0
Ampicillin[a]	1.0	1.2	0.8	1.3
Gentamicin[a]	1.8	2.2	1.3	2.8
Trimethoprim[b]	1.3	3.2	4.6	10.6
Norfloxacin[b]	2.4	6.4	3.6	5.0
Sulfadiazine[b]	2.5	3.6	5.6	9.9
Metronidazole[b]	2.8	3.9	4.5	8.5
Sulfadimethoxine[b]	12.5	11.3	13.2	40.0

[a]For lipid-insoluble drugs eliminated mainly by renal excretion, half-life is relatively short, with little variation between species.
[b]For drugs of moderate or high lipid solubility, elimination is usually dictated mainly by biotransformation (most commonly but not exclusively) in the liver, but with some renal excretion of parent drug. Species variation in biotransformation rates are commonly considerable, being rapid in ruminants and horses and slower in humans.

and other biological fluids. The terminal half-life of antimicrobial drugs in depot formulations usually represents the absorption rather than elimination half-life (flip-flop pharmacokinetics). Another basis for prolonged duration of action is the recent introduction of cefovacin, a cephalosporin with a very high degree of binding to plasma protein, which is both slowly excreted in urine and not significantly metabolised in the liver. Therapeutic efficacy of long-acting formulations may therefore be obtained with single, or at most two, doses. This avoids the stress caused by repeated injections, minimises the risks of non-compliance and limits marked variations in drug plasma concentration during therapy. For drugs with time-dependent killing mechanisms, the presence of peaks and troughs may predispose to resistance development and this provides an additional advantage for depot formulation products.

6.4 Efficacy breakpoints based on concentration–time–effect relationships

6.4.1 Integrated pharmacokinetic and pharmacodynamic (PK–PD) indices

As a pharmacological basis for dosage to optimise the kill of pathogens and minimise the emergence of resistance, three PK–PD indices linking concentration (usually in serum or plasma) to MIC have been proposed (65–72): AUC/MIC, C_{max}/MIC ratios and T>MIC (expressed as a percentage of the inter-dose interval). AUC is the area under the plasma or blood concentration–time curve over 24 h, C_{max} is the maximum concentration, and T>MIC is the time for which concentration exceeds MIC (Figure 6.5). PK–PD indices are predictive parameters for treatment outcome based on empirical observations. This PK–PD integration approach utilises both of the pharmacological properties, pharmacokinetics and pharmacodynamics, which determine the outcome of therapy. Based on these surrogates, killing actions have been classified as time-dependent, concentration-dependent or co-dependent (Table 6.2). PK–PD indices should be derived from non-protein-bound drug concentrations in plasma, as only the free drug is microbiologically active.

For β-lactam agents, in general (1) increasing plasma concentrations above 4XMIC does not provide greater or more rapid bacterial killing and (2) maximum bactericidal activity may be achieved when T>MIC exceeds 40–50% of the dosage interval. For optimal antimicrobial effect, however, a dosage which provides T>MIC of 80–100% (72), particularly for Gram-negative pathogens, may be required. On the other hand, for concentration-dependent killing drugs of the fluoroquinolone group, it has been widely recommended that: (1) $AUC_{0-24\,h}$/MIC should exceed 125 h, that is, the average daily plasma concentration should be approximately five times greater than MIC: and (2) C_{max}/MIC should be at least 10 (73–75). An AUC/MIC of 125 h correlates well with bacteriological cure for fluoroquinolones in human clinical trials and in infection models in experimental animals. When comparing rapid intravenous injection of danofloxacin with slow intravenous infusion, similar

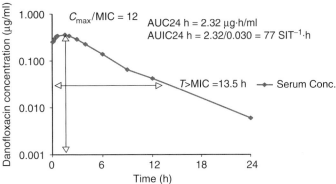

In vivo PK–PD integration in serum of goat 5 after single IM injection at a dose rate of 1.25 mg/kg danofloxacin

C_{max}/MIC = 12

AUC24 h = 2.32 µg·h/ml
AUIC24 h = 2.32/0.030 = 77 SIT^{-1}·h

T>MIC =13.5 h — Serum Conc.

Figure 6.5 An example of *ex vivo* PK–PD integration for danofloxacin administered intramuscularly in a goat, showing serum concentration–time relationship and derivation of C_{max}/MIC, AUC/MIC (AUIC24 h) and T>MIC (From Aliabadi and Lees (2001), *Am. J. Vet. Res.* 62: 1979–89).

AUC/MIC ratios but differing T>MIC and C_{max}/MIC ratios were achieved in a model of calf pneumonia (76). The bolus injection provided better bacteriological and clinical responses, confirming the concentration-dependent killing action of fluoroquinolones.

Different routes of administration may result in different pharmacokinetic profiles, which in turn may affect the intensity of selection for resistance. The impact of the administration route on the emergence of resistance has often been debated but few studies have addressed the question. A C_{max}/MIC of 10 has been proposed as a breakpoint value for minimising emergence of resistance to aminoglycosides and fluoroquinolones (74, 77, 78). Assuming that achieving a high plasma C_{max} is essential to prevent resistance development, pharmacokinetic studies of fluoroquinolone treatment in healthy animals indicate that the intramuscular route is superior to oral (and intragastric) administration routes (79–82). In pigs, experimentally infected with a 99:1 mixture of *Salmonella* Typhimurium susceptible and resistant to nalidixic acid, intramuscular administration of enrofloxacin resulted in reduced selection of the resistant variant compared to oral administration, and increased intramuscular doses were more efficient in preventing resistance development (83). When using intramuscular injection and designing dosage schedules, tissue tolerability must be assessed (84). Subcutaneous and intramuscular administration of danofloxacin in cattle has been shown to produce virtually identical plasma concentration profiles and AUCs following one, three or five consecutive daily doses (85). Oral administration given by continuous administration via drinking water (rather than via a nasogastric probe) further increases the risk of development of resistance since high peak concentrations cannot be achieved. Accordingly, reduced thirst in sick animals and hierarchy in a flock can potentially cause underdosing in some animals. For β-lactams and other time-dependent antimicrobial agents, a long half-life may provide the best treatment outcome. Subcutaneous administration of imipenem and meropenem to dogs results in extended half-lives in comparison with the intramuscular and intravenous routes (86, 87).

Numerical values of C_{max}/MIC, AUC/MIC and T>MIC cited in the scientific literature can provide useful guidelines to dosage determination. However, such values can be both drug- and bacterial species-specific, and may additionally depend on the experimental or clinical conditions of the study. For β-lactams, the longer PAE against Gram-positive than against Gram-negative bacteria is a potential cause of variability, and strain differences in the values of PK–PD indices have been reported. Veterinary data are especially sparse. However, in one study Guyonnet *et al.* (88) obtained AUC0–5 h/MIC values of 29.2, 7.9, 6.8 and 6.2 h against four strains of porcine *E. coli* for an *in vitro* bactericidal action of colistin. Thus, one strain was a clear outlier. For many antimicrobial breakpoint surrogate values, based on rate and extent of killing and resistance emergence, are not available. When breakpoints have been determined in experimental animals (usually mice or rats), infection models and/or in human clinical trials, the numerical values must be extrapolated to veterinary clinical circumstances with caution. There is an urgent need for further research to either validate breakpoint values determined in experimental animals and in humans for application in veterinary medicine, or yield alternative values.

Most authors have proposed MIC$_{90}$ as the relevant pharmacodynamic index for optimising dosage, but others have suggested MIC$_{50}$ (75) as less stringent and more readily determined than MIC$_{90}$. For fluoroquinolones there is evidence from many sources, based on *in vitro* data, animal disease models and clinical trials in humans, that the AUC/MIC ratio is the PK–PD surrogate that best correlates with efficacy. It is widely reported that daily dosage should provide a ratio of at least 125 h. However, doses yielding lower values are likely to be acceptable when the bacteriological burden is low, especially in immunocompetent animals.

6.4.2 Veterinary examples of PK–PD integration and modelling

An approach to designing optimal dosage schedules, based on PK–PD integration and PK–PD modelling, has been proposed (54–58, 89). This involves conducting bacterial time–kill studies sequentially *in vitro, ex vivo* and *in vivo*, followed by population PK–PD modelling in clinical trials (70, 71, 90) (see Sections 6.6 and 6.7). It is proposed that such studies are superior in many instances to the traditional approach based on dose titration studies. The latter will generally yield a clinically effective dose, whilst dosage based on

PK–PD modelling is designed to yield an optimal dose for bacteriological cure. Optimal dosage varies with the organism type and location. When applied to a given organism, PK–PD modelling allows for the two principal sources of inter- and intra-subject variability in treatment outcome, pharmacokinetics and pharmacodynamics. Veterinary examples of PK–PD integration and PK–PD modelling applied to dose schedule design studies are provided in Figures 6.5 and 6.6, respectively. Studies conducted *ex vivo* with danofloxacin in four ruminant species (calf, goat, sheep, camel) may be cited (54–58). Against pathogenic strains of *M.haemolytica* (calf, goat, sheep) and *E.coli* (camel), data describing the whole sweep of the AUC/MIC to bacterial count (CFU) relationship was obtained. Modelling the data to the sigmoidal E_{max} equation provided numerical values required for four parameters of activity, bacteriostasis, reduction in bacterial count of 50%,

reduction in bacterial count of 99.9% (bactericidal action) and eradication of organisms (Table 6.6). Subsequent calculations, based on MIC_{90} values for *M. haemolytica*, indicated, in the calf, for a bactericidal response or eradication of bacteria, respectively, doses of 4.1 and 7.5 mg/kg. If it is assumed that a bacteriological effect level intermediate between 99.9% kill and eradication of bacteria is appropriate, these values support the manufacturer's currently recommended dose of 6 mg/kg. This intermediate effect level is similar to that proposed by Mouton *et al.* (68) in humans. They suggested for fluoroquinolones a dosage based on an AUC/MIC ratio of 90% of E_{max}, whilst indicating that in immunocompetent subjects and when infections are not severe, the AUC/MIC ratio providing 50% of E_{max} may be acceptable. These considerations relate to efficacy but may not be applicable to resistance development (*vide infra*).

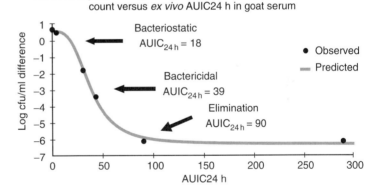

Figure 6.6 An example of PK–PD modeling for danofloxacin administered intramuscularly in a goat, illustrating the relationship between change in bacterial count from baseline and AUC/MIC (AUIC24 h) and derivation of values producing bacteriostasis, bactericidal action and eradication of bacteria (From Aliabadi and Lees (2001), *Am. J. Vet. Res.* 62: 1979–89).

Table 6.6 Critical *ex vivo* values of serum AUC24/MIC(h) for danofloxacin[a] in four ruminant species

Level of growth inhibition	Calf	Goat	Sheep	Camel
Bacteriostatic	15.9 ± 2.0	22.6 ± 1.7	17.8 ± 1.7	17.2 ± 3.6
Bactericidal	18.1 ± 1.9	29.6 ± 2.5	20.2 ± 1.7	21.2 ± 3.7
Eradication	33.5 ± 3.5	52.4 ± 8.1	28.7 ± 1.8	68.7 ± 15.6

[a]Intramuscular administration at a dose rate of 1.25 mg/kg. Antibacterial activity was evaluated by bacterial count *ex vivo* after 24 h incubation. The pathogens tested were strains of *Mannheimia haemolytica* (calf, goat, sheep) and *E. coli* (camel). The AUC24 h/MIC relationship to log_{10} change in bacterial count (CFU/ml) was modellised by a Hill model.
Values are mean ± SEM (*n*=6).
Data from Aliabadi and Lees (2001, 2003) and Aliabadi *et al.* (2003a,b).

6.4.3 Limitations and pitfalls in using PK–PD indices

One variable significantly affecting breakpoints is inoculum size (see Section 6.6). Moreover, numerical values of one or more of the surrogate PK–PD indices, C_{max}/MIC, AUC/MIC and T>MIC, required to provide a given level of efficacy for example a bactericidal response, will not necessarily be the ame as those which avoid or reduce selective pressure for resistance. Although research in this crucial area is limited, and in the veterinary field is virtually absent, some recent studies have investigated the potential optimal requirements for resistance avoidance.

Drusano (91) has defined the conditions for designing counterselective dosing schedules to avoid resistance emergence by mutations as follows: (a) the total organism burden should substantially exceed the inverse of the mutational frequency to resistance; (b) there should be a high probability of a resistant clone being present at baseline; and (c) the step size change in MIC of the mutated population should be relatively small, not more than 10-fold. Under these conditions, it is possible to select a dosage regimen suppressing both the wild-type susceptible population and more resistant sub-populations.

Mouton (92) has noted that AUC/MIC values of some fluoroquinolones are similar for a given magnitude of bacteriological effect. However, other studies have suggested differences between marbofloxacin and danofloxacin against a single strain of the calf pathogen *Mannheimia haemolytica* (55, 56). First, AUC/MIC values measured *ex vivo* in calf serum for the two drugs differed as the serum concentration multiples of MIC required to eradicate the selected strain of *M. haemolytica* were 1.40 for danofloxacin and 4.96 for marbofloxacin. This difference possibly reflects a difference in MPC for the two drugs. Second, slopes of the AUC/MIC–bacterial count relationship also differed, suggesting possible differences in potency and sensitivity for these two fluoroquinolones.

Macrolides and triamilides comprise drug classes that have proved less easy to categorise in terms of the PK–PD paradigm than agents of other classes. Generally, they are classified as time-dependent killing drugs, but some newer agents in human use, such as azithromycin, exert a significant PAE and the marker correlating best with outcome is AUC/MIC (93). For *P. multocida* of bovine origin, indices based on plasma concentration obtained using recommended doses of the triamilide tulathromycin are extremely low: AUC/MIC = 7.6 h, C_{max}/MIC = 0.04 and T>MIC = 0 h (94, 95). The explanation for these extraordinarily low values is unclear. Lung tissue concentrations greatly exceed those in plasma, and it has been postulated that concentrations in epithelial lining fluid (the biophase for bovine respiratory disease) may also exceed those in plasma. Certain macrolides are known to possess immunomodulatory and anti-inflammatory properties, so that non-antimicrobial actions in the host may contribute significantly to therapeutic response. In calves, tilmicosin induces neutrophil apoptosis, reduces pulmonary inflammation and controls *P. haemolytica* infection. A similar action has been reported for erythromycin. Reported anti-inflammatory and immunomodulatory actions of macrolides include increased airway epithelial cell ciliary motility, reduced leucocyte accumulation, decreased secretory functions of airway cells and reduced epithelial cell synthesis of pro-inflammatory cytokines, for example IL6 (96–102). Similar considerations apply to other macrolides used to treat respiratory infections in farm animals, such as tilmicosin, which is rapidly cleared from plasma but accumulates in lung tissue. Irrespective of the mechanism(s), macrolides and triamilides are effective *in vivo* at plasma concentrations markedly below those predicted from correlating plasma concentration obtained *in vivo* to MIC measured *in vitro*.

Another circumstance in which the conventional PK–PD paradigm may not be applicable in a simplistic manner comprises bacteria in biofilms. In biofilms bacteria exist as consortia rather than as planktonic or non-aggregated cells. The biofilm comprises biopolymers that provide a permeability barrier to drug penetration. Such organisms are less susceptible to antimicrobial agents than free-living cells. Infections associated with biofilms are increasingly recognised. In addition to protection against antimicrobial drugs, biofilms containing human clinical isolates contain more resistance phenotypes (103, 104). Organisms in biofilms have slow growth rates and most antimicrobial agents act only on dividing organisms. Another microbial protective mechanism of organisms in biofilms is reduced apoptosis (105), and a hyper-mutability state causing antimicrobial resistance has been reported in *P. aeruginosa* associated infection in human patients (106). Hence, several protective mechanisms result in the general inapplicability of the PK–PD approach to dosage determination for biofilm organisms.

6.5 Resistance breakpoints based on concentration–time–effect relationships

6.5.1 General considerations

Bacterial populations are heterogeneous, comprising sub-populations each with its own susceptibility to a given antimicrobial drug. Exposure to an antimicrobial drug exerts selective pressure, so that the most susceptible sub-populations are eradicated, leading to overgrowth of those sub-populations of least susceptibility. It is exposure, and especially repeated exposure, to sub-optimal drug concentrations that is the most important single factor in resistance emergence and its subsequent spread (12). As exposure is dose related, there is a direct link between administered dose and resistance development. These fundamental principles apply to commensal as well as pathogenic organisms, so that even with adequate exposure of pathogens, commensals may be underexposed. This situation may lead to development of resistance in the commensal flora and subsequent transfer of resistance genes both within and between pathogenic organisms and commensals at a later stage (13).

Numerical values of one or more of the surrogate PK–PD indices, C_{max}/MIC, AUC/MIC and T>MIC, required to provide a given level of efficacy for example a bactericidal response, will not necessarily be the same as those which avoid or reduce selective pressure for resistance. Although research in this crucial area is limited, and in the veterinary field is virtually absent, some recent studies have investigated examples that can be cited to illustrate the potential optimal requirements for resistance avoidance.

6.5.2 Concentration-dependent killing drugs

1. Preston *et al.* (107) reported that, for the fluoroquinolone levofloxacin, in human patients, a C_{max}/MIC $\geq$ 12.2 provided 100% microbiological kill. Other *in vitro* studies with ciprofloxacin and sparfloxacin have confirmed that high C_{max}/MIC ratios are required to avoid emergence of

resistance (108) and, in a murine peritonitis model, resistance to ciprofloxacin was lower for *P. aeruginosa* when C_{max}/MIC was 20 than for a value of 10 (109).

2. A classical study in human pneumococcal patients receiving fluoroquinolone therapy showed that resistance had emerged after 5 days in 50% of subjects when AUC/MIC values were <100 h. After 3 weeks of therapy this had increased to 93% of patients (110). However, when AUC/MIC was greater than 100 h the probability of organisms remaining susceptible exceeded 90%. In an earlier study, the same group (111) reported that resistance selection for fluoroquinolones was greater when C_{max}/MIC was less than 8. Both investigations were conducted in seriously ill and possibly immunocompromised human patients and the numerical values of AUC/MIC and C_{max}/MIC required to avoid resistance may be lower in animals and humans that are immunocompetent. Nevertheless, to avoid resistance with fluoroquinolones the value of AUC/MIC may need to be higher than that required to achieve bacteriological cure, as the next example illustrates.

3. In an *in vitro* study with *Staphylococcus aureus,* Firsov *et al.* (112) investigated the ability of the fluoroquinolones, gatifloxacin, ciprofloxacin, moxifloxacin and levofloxacin, to selectively enrich resistant mutants in a dynamic model, which reproduced *in vivo* pharmacokinetic patterns in man. A relationship for fluoroquinolones between AUC/MIC and resistance emergence at 72 h was established. When resistance frequency was plotted against the 24 h AUC/MIC ratio a bell-shaped curve was obtained, and for AUC/MIC values of less than 10 h or greater than 200 h there was no resistance. The maximum degree of resistance occurred with AUC/MIC values of 24–62 h. When AUC/MIC was in the range 201–244 h, concentrations exceeded MPC for 80% of the dosage interval. The AUC/MIC for fluoroquinolones generally accepted for optimal efficacy is 125 h, which is less than the 200 h value reported by Firsov *et al.* (112) for resistance avoidance.

4. In a hollow fibre infection model, and using a dense inoculum, Tam *et al.* (113) investigated resistance emergence of *P. aeruginosa* to garenoxacin; C_{max} was held constant and AUC/MIC ratios ranged from 0 to 200 h. With AUC/MIC values of

10, 48 and 89 h most susceptible organisms were replaced by resistant mutants; and all susceptible organisms were replaced by resistant mutants when AUC/MIC = 108 and 137 h, but resistant mutants did not emerge when AUC/MIC = 201 h.

5. Jumbe et al. (114) used *P. aeruginosa* in a mouse thigh infection model to study the effect of escalating doses of levofloxacin on the amplification of resistance. When AUC/MIC was 52 h resistant mutant amplification was maximal; when AUC/MIC = 157 h there was no amplification.

6. Based on the results of an *E. coli* model of septicaemia in chickens (115), Toutain et al. (72) determined for a fluoroquinolone, an ED_{50} of 8 mg/kg for reduction in mortality and an ED_{50} of 13 mg/kg for bacteriological cure. Although the higher dose compared to the lower dose does not ensure avoidance of emergence of resistance, it must be much less likely, as outcome is based on bacteriological cure.

7. For the aminoglycoside netilmicin acting on *E. coli* and *S. aureus*, Blaser et al. (77) reported a correlation between C_{max}/MIC and emergence of resistance. Organism regrowth was prevented when C_{max}/MIC was greater than 8. It has been found that for aminoglycosides in general, a C_{max}/MIC of 8–10 or higher is required to prevent resistance emergence (116).

8. In an *in vitro* bacterial time–kill study, using four strains of *E. coli* isolated from pigs, regrowth occurred when the concentration of colistin (a polypeptide belonging to the polymixin group) was less than 8 or 16 times MIC; growth inhibition with lower multiples of MICs was almost complete at 5 h but re-growth had occurred by 24 h. When the concentration was equal to or greater than 8 or 16 × MIC, re-growth at 24 h did not occur (90).

6.5.3   Time-dependent killing drugs

1. To investigate the time-dependent killing drug ceftizoxime, Stearne et al. (117) used a mixed infection murine model. Resistant clones were monitored and mutation frequency was shown to be related to the surrogate *T*>MIC, expressed as a percentage of dosing interval. When *T*>MIC values were either <40 or equal to 100% there

was no resistance, while peak mutation frequency occurred when *T*>MIC=70%. In fact, mutation to resistance was very low when *T*>MIC was 87% or greater. This contrasts with experimental animal and human clinical data, which have often reported that the optimal *T*>MIC for bacterial kill is of the order of 40–50% of the interdose interval for β-lactams. These findings suggest that a higher value of *T*>MIC, perhaps ideally 90 or even 100%, should be the objective for minimising resistance development for time-dependent killing cephalosporins.

2. Odenholt et al. (118) investigated whether certain concentrations of benzylpenicillin were critical for the selection of resistant subpopulations. They exposed a mixed culture of *Streptococcus pneumoniae* (containing susceptible, intermediate and resistant bacteria) *in vitro* to the antibiotic for different times above their respective MICs; they showed that selection of resistant bacteria occurred when concentrations were targeted only against fully susceptible strains.

3. Tam et al. (119) using an *in vitro* hollow fibre infection model, suggested an alternative PK–PD index for β-lactams of C_{min}/MIC, C_{min} being the minimum plasma concentration over the dosing interval required to prevent resistance emergence. Against a dense population of *P. aeruginosa* with drug concentrations up to 4 × MIC, resistant populations formed after exposure to piperacillin, ceftazidime and meropenem. Interestingly, meropenem was the most effective drug in reducing bacterial numbers at a concentration 4 × MIC but it also provided the greatest regrowth of resistant sub-populations. These workers found that, even when *T*>MIC = 100% and C_{min}/MIC ratios were less than 1.7, resistance emerged. They concluded that a C_{min} of 6 × MIC was required to suppress resistance emergence.

In summary, it seems likely that the PK–PD breakpoint commonly recommended for clinical and bacteriological efficacy (usually *T*>MIC of 40–80% of dosing interval) may be too low for avoidance of resistance emergence. Finally, it should be noted that optimal dosing strategies for minimising resistance may achieve this objective in two ways, first by eradicating all disease causing pathogenic bacteria and second by exerting minimal selection pressure on commensals. Of course, these two aims may often differ.

6.6 Pharmacodynamic and pharmacokinetic variability and the requirement for population studies: use of Monte Carlo simulations

At the first stage of dosage schedule design, it is usual to use mean values of integrated PK–PD surrogate markers to select dosage regimens for subsequent evaluation in the target species, initially in disease model studies and finally in confirmatory clinical trails. However, with a normal or near-normal distribution in such studies, approximately half the animal population will have an index below the mean value and the remainder will have a higher value. The final dosage, therefore, should not be based on mean or median values of PK–PD indices. To minimise resistance development, focus is required on those animals in the population that do not achieve the desired breakpoint. Toutain *et al.* (72) have therefore used an approach based on Monte Carlo simulations, integrating population pharmacokinetics and MIC values obtained from field cases. The objective is to allow for variability in both pharmacokinetics and pharmacodynamics in clinical subjects of the target species and thereby generate PK–PD indices appropriate for most animals and not only for the population mean (Figure 6.7).

Population pharmacokinetics and population PK–PD provide new and potentially improved means for establishing optimal dosage regimens, that is, those which provide bacteriological cure and minimise, prevent or delay resistance emergence. The necessity for the population approach lies in the differences that are likely to occur between PK–PD indices obtained in the early *in vitro* investigations and in studies using healthy animals on the one hand and those that are appropriate to 'field' circumstances on the other. The former may adequately or even precisely predict outcome when a drug is used in immunocompetent healthy animals, for example prophylactically, and when accurate per animal dosing is possible in individually treated companion animal subjects. However, such data are unlikely to apply in all instances when treating infectious disease. Therefore, the final and crucial step in dosage determination should, when possible, be taken using the population PK–PD approach within a clinical trial, using a sparse sampling strategy on a large number of animals. This provides the opportunity for minimising, at the population level, the selection and spread of resistant pathogens. Inadequate exposure of pathogens to the required drug concentration, in even a small minority of animals within a group, may result in establishment of a resistant sub-population that may transfer resistance genes both vertically and horizontally. This factor accounts for individual clinical failures as well as a stepwise loss of efficacy and development of resistance to a high level.

Inter-individual variability, resulting in under exposure of a significant proportion of treated animals, is an inevitable consequence when dose selection targets the population mean. There are also differences arising between healthy and diseased animals. A third source of variability arises in veterinary medicine for those animals, for example fish, pigs, poultry and calves,

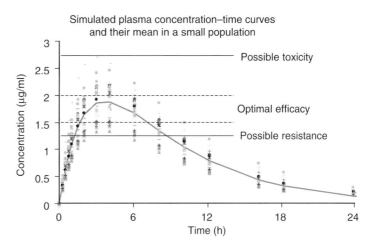

Figure 6.7 Hypothetical plasma concentration–time relationship for an antimicrobial drug, administered by a non-vascular route, illustrating the curve for mean concentration and each symbol representing an individual animal. Horizontal lines indicate concentrations above which host toxicity may occur, below which resistance is likely and the concentration window for optimal efficacy.

which normally or commonly receive drugs orally in feed or in drinking water with dosing on a group basis. The nominal mg/kg dose is not the dose actually received by any animal in the group. The competition between animals for access to medicated water or feed leads to variability in the ingested dose. The magnitude of the variability may also be increased when the drug is given metaphylactically to a group of animals, only some of which show clinical signs of infection. The latter animals may receive lower doses of drug than their more healthy companions. Hence, a reduced exposure of those animals carrying the largest bacterial load and most likely to have the highest pathogen mutational frequency is a likely additional factor predisposing to selection for resistance. The population PK–PD paradigm offers the opportunity of optimising dosage to minimise resistance based on the response of a given quantile of the target population, say 90% or even 95%, rather than the population mean.

Based on measured pharmacokinetic and pharmacodynamic variabilities in the target animal population, Monte Carlo simulations are used to establish the statistical distribution of the selected PK–PD index (82, 120). In these simulations, a hypothetical population of outcomes is generated, and this permits determination of the probability of attaining a preselected PK–PD breakpoint in a chosen proportion of the population. In veterinary medicine, Regnier et al. (121) and co-workers have used Monte Carlo simulations to establish, in the dog, a dosage regimen of marbofloxacin appropriate for treating infections in the anterior segment of the eye. The Toutain group also investigated the pharmacokinetic variability of doxycycline in the pig in a population field study (122). Pharmacokinetic and pharmacodynamic distributions were modelled to define the percentage of pigs attaining a given AUC/MIC value for several dosage rates of doxycycline. They concluded that a dose of 20 mg/kg or greater was required to attain a PK–PD breakpoint value of 24 h (based on total drug concentration) in 90% of pigs. This is equivalent to obtaining a mean total plasma concentration equal to the actual (but unknown) MIC over a 24 h dosage interval. The extent of protein binding of doxycycline in the pig is approximately 90% (123), indicating that the currently recommended dosage of 10 mg/kg daily does not attain an appropriate breakpoint for AUC/MIC for the free plasma concentration.

Monte Carlo simulations can be applied to the establishment of MIC resistance breakpoints for antibiograms, that is, to determine the MIC above which an organism can be classed as clinically resistant. This will be the MIC for which a defined dosage schedule fails to guarantee that 90% of the target animal population will be exposed to a mean plasma drug concentration equal to one of the *a priori* MICs of the MIC distribution.

6.7 Validation and extension of the population PK–PD approach to determination of optimal dosage regimens

At the present time, there is a lack of established PK–PD breakpoints derived from population studies in veterinary medicine. Ideally, these should be set separately for therapeutic, prophylactic and metaphylactic use of drugs, with the objective of preventing the emergence of resistance. Generally, the initial bacterial burden under prophylactic and metaphylactic conditions will be lower than that pertaining when therapy is required, and inter-animal variability is also less likely under the former conditions. Different breakpoint values and hence differing dosage requirements are therefore likely to apply. Jumbe et al. (114) showed that for levofloxacin the breakpoint AUC/MIC values against *P. aeruginosa* in mice inoculated in the thigh with 10^7 or 10^8 bacteria, were 31 and 161 h respectively. Thus a 10-fold increase in the pathogen burden increased five-fold the drug exposure required for the same antibacterial effect. The increase in the pathogen burden also increased the size of the resistant population. On the other hand, for time-dependent drugs, the value of *T*>MIC providing an optimal antibacterial effect was not affected by inoculum size or mechanism of resistance but was influenced by host immune status (124).

A further consideration for future research is the impact of population PK–PD approaches on zoonotic and commensal flora. Antimicrobial drugs are commonly administered orally in food-producing animals. Systemic bioavailability is sometimes low and this increases exposure of the gastrointestinal (GIT) flora. This might account for the shedding of zoonotic bacteria such as *Salmonellae* with resistance to drugs used in humans. In addition, the GIT flora might increase the gene pool of resistance, with possible transmission to humans in the food chain. Exposure of the GIT flora is not confined to orally administered drugs, but may also occur with parenterally administered drugs as a consequence of active efflux by enterocytes, as demonstrated for fluoroquinolones, or through active secretion into bile. The GIT ecosystem is complex and it is generally the local rather than plasma drug concentrations which must be used when applying the PK–PD paradigm to the GIT flora. Moreover, the pros and cons of long-acting versus short-acting products on commensal flora (as well as pathogenic organisms) is not well understood and data are lacking. On the one hand, maintained concentrations may assist bacterial kill of pathogens but, on the other, prolonged exposure may encourage resistance development by commensals. Also of significance in relation to resistance is the use of local therapy as an alternative to systemic administration. Although little data are available, it would seem likely (in general) that the former (a veterinary example is intramammary infusions) will expose pathogenic organisms to higher concentrations than can be achieved with systemic dosing, whilst sparing the exposure of commensals for example within the GIT. It will rarely, if ever, be the case that an optimal dosage regimen for target pathogens will also be optimal to spare the GIT flora from the emergence and spread of resistance.

References

1. Wright, G.D. (2005). Bacterial resistance to antibiotics: enzymatic degradation and modification. *Adv. Drug Deliv. Rev.* 57: 1451–70.
2. Kumar, A. and Schweizer, H.P. (2005). Bacterial resistance to antibiotics: active efflux and reduced uptake. *Adv. Drug Deliv. Rev.* 57: 1486–1513.
3. Piddock, L.J. (2006). Clinically relevant chromosomally encoded multidrug resistance efflux pumps in bacteria. *Clin. Microbiol. Rev.* 19: 382–402.
4. Martinez, J.L. and Baquero, F. (2000). Mutation frequencies and antibiotic resistance. *Antimicrob. Agents Chemother.* 44: 1771–7.
5. Baquero, F. (2001). Low-level antibiotic resistance. In Andersson, D.H.a.D.I. (ed.), *Antibiotic Development and Resistance.* Taylor and Francis Group, London, pp. 117–36.
6. Lipsitch, M. and Levin, B.R. (1997). The population dynamics of antimicrobial chemotherapy. *Antimicrob. Agents Chemother.* 41: 363–73.
7. Tenover, F.C. and McGowan, J.E., Jr. (1996). Reasons for the emergence of antibiotic resistance. *Am. J. Med. Sci.* 311: 9–16.
8. Baquero, F. and Negri, M.C. (1997). Strategies to minimize the development of antibiotic resistance. *J. Chemother.* 9 Suppl 3: 29–37.
9. Baquero, F., Negri, M.C., Morosini, M.I. and Blazquez, J. (1998). Antibiotic-selective environments. *Clin. Infect. Dis.* 27 Suppl 1: S5–S11.
10. Negri, M.C., Lipsitch, M., Blazquez, J., Levin, B.R. and Baquero, F. (2000). Concentration dependent selection of small phenotypic differences in TEM beta-lactamase-mediated antibiotic resistance. *Antimicrob. Agents Chemother.* 44: 2485–91.
11. Zhao, X. and Drlica, K. (2001). Restricting the selection of antibiotic-resistant mutants: a general strategy derived from fluoroquinolones studies. *Clin. Infect. Dis.* 33: S147–S156.
12. Burgess, D.S. (1999). Pharmacodynamic principles of antimicrobial therapy in the prevention of resistance. *Chest* 115: 195–233.
13. Baquero, F., Negri, M.C., Morosini, M.I. and Blazquez, J. (1997). The antibiotic selective process: concentration-specific amplification of low-level resistant populations. *CIBA Foundation Symposia,* 207: 93–111.
14. Lenski, R.E. (1997). The cost of antibiotic resistance–from the perspective of a bacterium. *Ciba Found Symp.* 207: 131–140; discussion 141–51.
15. Besier, S., Ludwig, A., Brade, V. and Wichelhaus, T.A. (2005). Compensatory adaptation to the loss of biological fitness associated with acquisition of fusidic acid resistance in *Staphylococcus aureus. Antimicrob. Agents Chemother.* 49: 1426–31.
16. Bjorkman, J., Nagaev, I., Berg, O.G., Hughes, D. and Andersson, D.I. (2000). Effects of environment on compensatory mutations to ameliorate costs of antibiotic resistance. *Science* 287: 1479–82.
17. Levin, B.R., Perrot, V. and Walker, N. (2000). Compensatory mutations, antibiotic resistance and the population genetics of adaptive evolution in bacteria. *Genetics* 154: 985–97.
18. Maisnier-Patin, S., Berg, O.G., Liljas, L. and Andersson, D.I. (2002). Compensatory adaptation to the deleterious effect of antibiotic resistance in *Salmonella typhimurium. Mol. Microbiol.* 46: 355–66.
19. Nagaev, I., Bjorkman, J., Andersson, D.I. and Hughes, D. (2001). Biological cost and compensatory evolution in fusidic acid resistant *Staphylococcus aureus. Mol. Microbiol.* 40: 433–9.
20. Nilsson, A.I., Kugelberg, E., Berg, O.G. and Andersson, D.I. (2004). Experimental adaptation of *Salmonella typhimurium* to mice. *Genetics* 168: 1119–30.
21. Reynolds, M.G. (2000). Compensatory evolution in rifampin-resistant *Escherichia coli. Genetics* 156: 1471–1481.
22. Schrag, S.J., Perrot, V. and Levin, B.R. (1997). Adaptation to the fitness costs of antibiotic resistance in *Escherichia coli. Proc. Biol. Sci.* 264: 1287–91.
23. Nilsson, A.I., Zorzet, A., Kanth, A., Dahlstrom, S., Berg, O.G. and Andersson, D.I. (2006). Reducing the fitness cost of antibiotic resistance by amplification of initiator tRNA genes. *Proc. Natl. Acad. Sci. USA* 103: 6976–81.

24. Andersson, D.I. (2006). The biological cost of mutational antibiotic resistance: any practical conclusions? *Curr. Opin. Microbiol.* 9: 461–5.

25. Criswell, D., Tobiason, V.L., Lodmell, J.S. and Samuels, D.S. (2006). Mutations conferring aminoglycoside and spectinomycin resistance in *Borrelia burgdorferi*. *Antimicrob. Agents Chemother.* 50: 445–52.

26. Enne, V.I., Delsol, A.A., Davis, G.R., Hayward, S.L., Roe, J.M. and Bennett, P.M. (2005). Assessment of the fitness impacts on E*scherichia coli* of acquisition of antibiotic resistance genes encoded by different types of genetic element. *J. Antimicrob. Chemother.* 56: 544–51.

27. Gillespie, S.H., Voelker, L.L. and Dickens, A. (2002). Evolutionary barriers to quinolone resistance in *Streptococcus pneumoniae*. *Microb. Drug Resist.* 8: 79–84.

28. Ramadhan, A.A. and Hegedus, E. (2005). Survivability of vancomycin resistant enterococci and fitness cost of vancomycin resistance acquisition. *J. Clin. Pathol.* 58: 744–6.

29. Sander, P., Springer, B., Prammananan, T., *et al.* (2002). Fitness cost of chromosomal drug resistance-conferring mutations. *Antimicrob. Agents Chemother.* 46: 1204–11.

30. Bjorkman, J., Hughes, D. and Andersson, D.I. (1998). Virulence of antibiotic-resistant *Salmonella typhimurium*. *Proc. Natl. Acad. Sci. USA* 95: 3949–53.

31. Cohen, S.P., McMurry, L.M., Hooper, D.C., Wolfson, J.S. and Levy, S.B. (1989). Cross resistance to fluoroquinolones in multiple antibiotic-resistant (Mar) *Escherichia coli* selected by tetracycline or chloramphenicol: decreased drug accumulation associated with membrane changes in addition to OmpF reduction. *Antimicrob. Agents Chemother.* 33: 1318–25.

32. Giraud, E., Cloeckaert, A., Kerboeuf, D. and Chaslus-Dancla, E. (2000). Evidence for active efflux as the primary mechanism of resistance to ciprofloxacin in *Salmonella enterica* serovar *typhimurium*. *Antimicrob. Agents Chemother.* 44: 1223–8.

33. Kern, W.V., Oethinger, M., Jellen-Ritter, A.S. and Levy, S.B. (2000). Non-target gene mutations in the development of fluoroquinolone resistance in *Escherichia coli*. *Antimicrob. Agents Chemother.* 44: 814–20.

34. Oethinger, M., Kern, W.V., Jellen-Ritter, A.S., McMurry, L.M. and Levy, S.B. (2000). Ineffectiveness of topoisomerase mutations in mediating clinically significant fluoroquinolone resistance in *Escherichia coli* in the absence of the AcrAB efflux pump. *Antimicrob. Agents Chemother.* 44: 10–13.

35. Corkill, J.E., Anson, J.J. and Hart, C.A. (2005). High prevalence of the plasmid-mediated quinolone resistance determinant qnrA in multidrug-resistant Enterobacteriaceae from blood cultures in Liverpool, UK. *J. Antimicrob. Chemother.* 56: 1115–7.

36. Mammeri, H., Van De Loo, M., Poirel, L., Martinez-Martinez, L. and Nordmann, P. (2005). Emergence of plasmid-mediated quinolone resistance in *Escherichia coli* in Europe. *Antimicrob. Agents Chemother.* 49: 71–6.

37. Robicsek, A., Strahilevitz, J., Sahm, D.F., Jacoby, G.A. and Hooper, D.C. (2006). qnr prevalence in ceftazidime-resistant *Enterobacteriaceae* isolates from the United States. *Antimicrob. Agents Chemother.* 50: 2872–4.

38. Wang, M., Sahm, D.F., Jacoby, G.A. and Hooper, D.C. (2004). Emerging plasmid-mediated quinolone resistance associated with the qnr gene in *Klebsiella pneumoniae* clinical isolates in the United States. *Antimicrob. Agents Chemother.* 48: 1295–9.

39. Bradford, P.A. (2001) Extended-spectrum beta-lactamases in the 21st century: characterization, epidemiology, and detection of this important resistance threat. *Clin. Microbiol. Rev.* 14: 933–51, table of contents.

40. Hasman, H. and Aarestrup, F.M. (2005). tcrB, a gene conferring transferable copper resistance in *Enterococcus faecium*: occurrence, transferability, and linkage to macrolide and glycopeptides resistance. *Antimicrob. Agents Chemother.* 46: 1410–6.

41. Liebana, E., Batchelor, M., Hopkins, K.L., *et al.* (2006). Longitudinal farm study of extended-spectrum beta-lactamase-mediated resistance. *J. Clin. Microbiol.* 44: 1630–4.

42. Riano, I., Moreno, M.A., Teshager, T., Saenz, Y., Dominguez, L. and Torres, C. (2006). Detection and characterization of extended-spectrum {beta}-lactamases in *Salmonella enterica* strains of healthy food animals in Spain. *J. Antimicrob. Chemother.* 58: 844–7.

43. Weill, F.X., Lailler, R., Praud, K., *et al.* (2004). Emergence of extended-spectrum-beta-lactamase (CTX-M-9)-producing multiresistant strains of *Salmonella enterica* serotype Virchow in poultry and humans in France. *J. Clin. Microbiol.* 42: 5767–73.

44. Carattoli, A. Lovari, S., Franco, A., Cordaro, G., Di Matteo, P. and Battisti, A. (2005). Extended-spectrum beta-lactamases in *Escherichia coli* isolated from dogs and cats in Rome, Italy, from 2001 to 2003. *Antimicrob. Agents Chemother.* 49(2): 833–5.

45. Feria, C., Ferreira, E., Correia, J.D., Goncalves, J. and Canica, M. (2002). Patterns and mechanisms of resistance to beta-lactams and beta-lactamase inhibitors in uropathogenic *Escherichia coli* isolated from dogs in Portugal. *J. Antimicrob. Chemother.* 49: 77–85.

46. Sidjabat, H.E., Hanson, N.D., Smith-Moland, E., *et al.* (2007). Identification of plasmamid-mediated extended-spectrum and AmpC beta-lactamases in *Enterobacter* spp. isolated from dogs. *J. Med. Medicrobiol.* 56: 426–34.

47. Blondeau, J.M., Zhao, X., Hanson, G. and Drlica, K. (2001). Mutant prevention concentrations of fluoroquinolones for clinical isolates of *Streptococcus pneumoniae*. *Antimicrob. Agents Chemother.* 45: 433–8.

48. Catry, B., Laevens, H., Devriese, L.A. Opsomer, G. and De Kruif, A. (2003). Antimicrobial resistance in livestock. *J. Vet. Pharmacol. Ther.* 26: 81–93.

49. Drlica, K., Zhao, X., Blondeau, J.M. and Hesje, C. (2006). Low correlation between MIC and mutant prevention concentration. *Antimicrob. Agents Chemother.* 50: 403–404.

50. Balaban, N.Q., Merrin, J., Chait, R., Kowalik, L. and Leibler, S. (2004). Bacterial persistence as a phenotypic switch. *Science* 305: 1622–5.

51. Keren, I., Kaldalu, N., Spoering, A., Wang, Y. and Lewis, K. (2004). Persister cells and tolerance to antimicrobials. *FEMS Microbiol. Lett.* 230: 13–18.

52. Levin, B.R. and Rozen, D.E. (2006). Non-inherited antibiotic resistance. *Nat. Rev. Microbiol.* 4: 556–62.

53. Wiuff, C., Zappala, R.M., Regoes, R.R., Garner, K.N., Baquero, F. and Levin, B.R. (2005). Phenotypic tolerance: antibiotic enrichment of noninherited resistance in bacterial populations. *Antimicrob. Agents Chemother.* 49: 1483–94.

54. AliAbadi, F.S. and Lees, P. (2001). Pharmacokinetics and pharmacodynamics of danofloxacin in serum and tissue fluids of goats following intravenous and intramuscular administration. *Am. J. Vet. Res.* 62: 1979–89.

55. AliAbadi, F.S. and Lees, P. (2002). Pharmacokinetics and pharmacokinetic/pharmacodynamic integration of marbofloxacin in calf serum, exudate and transudate. *J. Vet. Pharmacol. Ther.* 25: 161–174.

56. AliAbadi, F.S. and Lees, P. (2003). Pharmacokinetic–pharmacodynamic integration of danofloxacin in the calf. *Res. Vet. Sci.* 74: 247–59.

57. Aliabadi, F.S., Badrelin, H. Ali, Landoni, M.F. and Lees, P. (2003a). Pharmacokinetics and PK-PD modelling of danofloxacin in camel serum and tissue cage fluids. *Vet. J.* 165: 104–18.

58. AliAbadi, F.S., Landoni, M.F. and Lees, P. (2003b). Pharmacokinetics (PK) pharmacodynamics (PD) and PK–PD integration of danofloxacin in sheep biological fluids. *Antimicrob. Agents Chemother.* 47: 626–35.

59. Koritz, G.D., Kilroy, C.R. and Bevill, R.F. (1994). Pharmacokinetics–pharmacodynamic modelling of antibacterial therapy *in vitro*. In *Proceedings of the 6th International Congress of the European Association for Veterinary Pharmacology and Therapeutics*. Edinburgh, UK, Blackwell Scientific Publications.

60. Yancey, Jr., R.J., Evans, R.A., Kratzer, D.D. Paulissen, J.B. and Carmer, S.G. (1990). Efficacy of ceftiofur hydrochloride for treatment of experimentally induced colibacillosis in neonatal swine. *Am. J. Vet. Res.* 51: 831–47.

61. Dalhoff, A. and Shalit, I. (2003). Immunomodulatory effects of quinolones. *Lancet Infect. Dis.* 3: 359–71.

62. Hoyt, J.C. and Robbins, R.A. (2001).Macrolide antibiotics and pulmonary inflammation. *FEMS Microbiol. Lett.* 205: 1–7.

63. Ianaro, A., Ialenti, A., Maffia, P., *et al.* (2000). Anti-inflammatory activity of macrolide antibiotics. *J. Pharmacol. Exp. Ther.* 292: 156–63.

64. Lindecrona, R.H., Friis, C. and Nielsen, J.P. (2000). Pharmacokinetics and penetration of danofloxacin into the gastrointestinal tract in healthy and in*Salmonella typhimurium* infected pigs. *Res. Vet. Sci.* 68: 211–6.

65. Lees, P. and AliAbadi, F.S. (2000). Rationalising dosage regimens of antimicrobial drugs; a pharmacological perspective. *J. Med. Microbiol.* 49: 943–5.

66. Lees, P. and AliAbadi, F.S. (2002). Rational dosing of antimicrobial drugs; animals versus humans. *Int. J. Antimicrob. Agents* 19: 269–84.

67. McKellar, Q.A., Sanchez Bruni, S.F. and Jones, D.G. (2004). Pharmacokinetic/pharmacodynamic relationships of antimicrobial drugs used in veterinary medicine. *J. Vet. Pharmacol. Ther.* 27: 503–14.

68. Mouton, J.W., Dudley, M.N., Cars, O., Derendorf, H. and Drusano, G.L. (2002). Standardization of pharmacokinetic/pharmacodynamic (PK/PD) terminology for anti-infective drugs. *Int. J. Antimicrob. Agents* 19: 355–8.

69. Toutain, P.L. (2002). Pharmacokinetics/pharmacodynamics integration in drug development and dosage regimen optimisation for veterinary medicine. *AAPS Pharmaceuti. Sci.* 4: 1–25, article 38.

70. Toutain, P.L. (2003a). Pharmacokinetics/pharmacodynamics integration in dosage regimen optimisation for veterinary medicine. *J. Vet. Pharmacol. Ther.* 26 (Suppl 1): 1–8.

71. Toutain, P.L. (2003b). Antibiotic treatment of animals–a different approach to rational dosing. *Vet. J.* 165: 98–100.

72. Toutain, P.L., del Castillo, J.R. and Bousquet-Melou, A. (2002). The pharmacokinetic–pharmacodynamic approach to a rational dosage regimen for antibiotics. *Res. Vet. Sci.* 73: 105–14.

73. Craig, W.A. (1998). Pharmacokinetic/pharmacodynamic parameters: rationale for antibacterial dosing of mice and men. *Clin. Infect. Dis.* 26: 1–12.

74. Drusano, G.L., Johnson, D.E., Rosen, M. and Standiford, H.C. (1993). Pharmacodynamics of a fluoroquinolone antimicrobial agent in a neutropenic rat model of *Pseudomonas sepsis*. *Antimicrob. Agents Chemother.* 37: 483–90.

75. Schentag, J.J. (2000). Clinical pharmacology of the fluoroquinolones: studies in human dynamic/kinetic models. *Clin. Infect. Dis.* Suppl. 2: 540–544.

76. Sarasola, P., Lees, P., AliAbadi, F.S., *et al.* (2002). Pharmacokinetic and pharmacodynamic profiles of danofloxacin administered by two dosing regimens in calves infected with *Mannheimia (Pasteurella) haemolytica*. *Antimicrob. Agents Chemother.* 46: 3013–9.

77. Blaser, J., Stone, B.B., Groner, M.C. and Zinner, S.H. (1987). Comparative study with enoxacin and netilmicin in a pharmacodynamic model to determine importance of ratio of antibiotic peak concentrations to MIC for bacterial activity and emergence of resistance. *Antimicrob. Agents Chemother.* 31: 1054–60.

78. Marchbanks, C.R., McKiel, J.R., Gilbert, D.H., *et al.* (1993). Dose ranging and fractionation of intravenous ciprofloxacin against *Pseudomonas aeruginosa* and *Staphylococcus aureus* in an *in vitro* model of infection. *Antimicrob. Agents Chemother.* 37: 1756–63.

79. Bugyei, K., Black, W.D. and McEwen, S. (1999). Pharmacokinetics of enrofloxacin given by the oral, intravenous and intramuscular routes in broiler chickens. *Can. J. Vet. Res.* 63: 193–200.

80. Ding, H.Z., Zeng, Z.L., Fung, K.F., Chen, Z.L. and Qiao, G.L. (2001). Pharmacokinetics of sarafloxacin in pigs

and broilers following intravenous, intramuscular, and oral single-dose applications. *J. Vet. Pharmacol. Ther.* 24: 303–308.

81. Fernandez-Varon, E., Bovaira, M.J., Espuny, A., Escudero, E., Vancraeynest, D. and Carceles, C.M. (2005). Pharmacokinetic–pharmacodynamic integration of moxifloxacin in rabbits after intravenous, intramuscular and oral administration. *J. Vet. Pharmacol. Ther.* 28: 343–8.

82. Intorre, L., Mengozzi, G., Bertini, S., Bagliacca, M., Luchetti, E. and Soldani, G. (1997). The plasma kinetics and tissue distribution of enrofloxacin and its metabolite ciprofloxacin in the Muscovy duck. *Vet. Res. Commun.* 21: 127–36.

83. Wiuff, C., Lykkesfeldt, J., Svendsen, O. and Aarestrup, F.M. (2003). The effects of oral and intramuscular administration and dose escalation of enrofloxacin on the selection of quinolone resistance among *Salmonella* and coliforms in pigs. *Res. Vet. Sci.* 75: 185–93.

84. Fernandez-Varon, E., Ayala, I., Marin, P., *et al.* (2006). Pharmacokinetics of danofloxacin in horses after intravenous, intramuscular and intragastric administration. *Equine Vet. J.* 38: 342–6.

85. Giles, C.J., Magonigle, R.A., Grimshaw, W.T., *et al.* (1991). Clinical pharmacokinetics of parenterally administered danofloxacin in cattle. *J. Vet. Pharmacol. Ther.* 14: 400–10.

86. Barker, C.W., Zhang, W., Sanchez, S., Budsberg, S.C., Boudinot, F.D. and McCrackin Stevenson, M.A. (2003). Pharmacokinetics of imipenem in dogs. *Am. J. Vet. Res.* 64: 694–9.

87. Bidgood, T. and Papich, M.G. (2002). Plasma pharmacokinetics and tissue fluid concentrations of meropenem after intravenous and subcutaneous administration in dogs. *Am. J. Vet. Res.* 63: 1622–8.

88. Guyonnet, J., Monnoyer, S., Manco, B., Aliabadi, F.S. and Lees, P. (2003). *In vivo* pharmacokinetics and *in vitro* pharmacodynamics as a basis for predicting dosage of colistin in piglet g.i.t. disease. *J. Vet. Pharmacol. Ther.* 26 Suppl. 1: 148–9.

89. Lees, P., Aliabadi F.S. and Toutain, P-L. (2004). PK–PD modelling: an alternative to dose titration studies for antimicrobial drug dosage selection. *J. Reg. Affairs* 15: 175–80.

90. Toutain, P.L. and Lees, P. (2004). Integration and modelling of pharmacokinetic and pharmacodynamic data to optimise dosage regimens in veterinary medicine. *J. Vet. Pharmacol. Ther.* 27: 467–77.

91. Drusano, G.L. (2004). Antimicrobial pharmacodynamics: critical interactions of 'bug and drug'. *Nat. Rev. Microbiol.* 2: 289–300.

92. Mouton, J.W. (2005). Impact of pharmacodynamics on dosing schedules: optimising efficacy, reducing resistance, and detection of emergence of resistance. In *Antibiotic Policies Theory and Practice* (Eds. Gould, I.M. and van der Meer, J.W.M.). Kluwer Academic/Plenum Publishers, New York, pp. 387–407.

93. Mazzei, T. and Novelli, A. (1999). How macrolide pharmacodynamics affect bacterial killing. *Infect. Med.* 16: 22–8.

94. Benchaoui, H.A., Nowakowski, M., Sheripngton, J., Rowan, T.G. and Sunderland, S.J. (2004). Pharmacokinetics and lung tissue concentrations of tulathromycin in swine. *J. Vet. Pharmacol. Ther.* 27: 203–10.

95. Nowakowski, M.A., Inskeep, P.B., Risk, J.E., *et al.* (2004). Pharmacokinetics and lung tissue concentrations of tulathromycin, a new triamilide antibiotic, in cattle. *Vet. Ther.* 5: 60–74.

96. Goswami, S.K., Kivity, S. and Marom, Z. (1990). Erythromycin inhibits respiratory glycoconjugate secretion from human airways *in vitro. Am. Rev. Resp. Dis.* 141: 72–8.

97. Morikawa, K., Oseko, F., Morikawa, S. and Iwamoto, K. (1994). Immunomodulatory effects of three macrolides, midecamycin acetate, josamycin and clarithromycin, on human T-lymphocyte function *in vitro. Antimicrob. Agents Chemother.* 38: 2643–7.

98. Roche, Y., Gougerot-Pocidalo, M.A., Fay, M., Forest, N. and Pocidalo, J.J. (1986). Macrolides and immunity: effects of erythromycin and spiramycin on human mononuclear cell proliferation. *J. Antimicrob. Chemother.* 17: 195–203.

99. Takeyama, K., Tamaoki, J., Chiyotani, A., Tagaya, E. and Konno, K. (1993). Effect of macrolide antibiotics on ciliary motility in rabbit airway epithelium *in vitro. J. Pharm. Pharmacol.* 45: 756–8.

100. Takizawa, H., Desaki, M., Ohtoshi, T., *et al.* (1995). Erythromycin suppresses interleukin 6 expression by human bronchial epithelial cells: a potential mechanism of its anti-inflammatory action. *Biochem. Biophys. Res. Comm.* 210: 781–6.

101. Tamaoki, J., Noritaka, S., Tagaya, E. and Konno, K. (1994). Macrolide antibiotics protect against endotoxin-induced vascular leakage and neutrophil accumulation in rat trachea. *Antimicrob. Agents Chemother.* 38: 1641–3.

102. Umeki, S. (1993). Anti-inflammatory action of erythromycin: its inhibitory effect on neutrophil NADPH oxidase activity. *Chest* 104: 1191–1193.

103. Delissalde, F. and Amabile-Cuevas, C.F. (2004). Comparison of antibiotic susceptibility and plasmid content, between biofilm producing and non-producing clinical isolates of *Pseudomonas aeruginosa. Int. J. Antimicrob. Agents.* 24: 405–8.

104. Drenkard, E. and Ausubel, F.M. (2002). Pseudomonas biofilm formation and antibiotic resistance are linked to phenotypic variation. *Nature* 416: 740–3.

105. Gilbert, P., McBain, A. and Rickard, A.H. (2003). Biofilms and bacterial multi-resistance. In *Multiple Drug Resistant Bacteria* (ed. Amabile-Cuevas, C.F.). Horizon Scientific Press, Wymondham.

106. Oliver, A., Canton, R., Campo, P., Baquero, F. and Blazquez, J. (2000). High frequency of hypermutable *Pseudomonas aeruginosa* in cystic fibrosis lung infection. *Science* 288: 1251–3.

107. Preston, S.L., Drusano, G.L., Berman, A.L., *et al.* (1998). Pharmacodynamics of levofloxacin: a new paradigm for early clinical trials. *J. Am. Med. Assoc.* 279: 125–9.

108. Thorburn, C.E. and Edwards, D.I. (2001). The effect of pharmacokinetics on the bactericidal activity of ciprofloxacin and sparfloxacin against *Streptococcus pneumoniae* and the emergence of resistance. *J. Antimicrob. Chemother.* 48: 15–22.

109. Michae-Hamzehpour, M., Auckenthaler, R., Regamey, P. and Pechere, J.C. (1987). Resistance occurring after fluoroquinolone therapy of experimental *Pseudomonas aeruginosa* peritonitis. *Antimicrob. Agents Chemother.* 31: 1803–1808.

110. Thomas, J.K., Forrest, A., Bhaveni, S.M., *et al.* (1998). Pharmacodynamic evaluation of factors associated with the development of bacterial resistance in acutely ill patients during therapy. *Antimicrob. Agents Chemother.* 42: 521–7.

111. Forrest, A., Nix, D.E., Ballow, C.H., Goss, T.F., Birmingham, M.C. and Schentag, J.J. (1993). Pharmacodynamics of intravenous ciprofloxacin in seriously ill patients. *Antimicrob. Agents Chemother.* 37: 1073–81.

112. Firsov, A.A., Vostrov, S.N. Lubenko, I.Y., Drlica, K., Portnoy, Y.A. and Zinner, S.H. (2003). *In vitro* pharmacodynamic evaluation of the mutant selection window hypothesis using four fluoroquinolones against *Staphylococcus aureus*. *Antimicrob. Agents Chemother.* 47: 1604–13.

113. Tam, V.H., Louie, A., Deziel, M.R., Liu, W., Leary, R. and Drusano, G.L. (2005a). Bacterial-population responses to drug-selective pressure: examination of Garenoxacin's effect on *Pseudomonas aeruginosa*. *J. Infect. Dis.* 192: 420–8.

114. Jumbe, N., Louie, A., Leary, R., *et al.* (2003). Application of a mathematical model to prevent *in vivo* amplification of antibiotic-resistant bacterial populations during therapy. *J. Clin. Invest.* 112: 275–85.

115. Charleston, B., Gate, J.J., Aitken, I.A., Stephan, B. and Froyman, R. (1998). Comparison of the efficacies of three fluoroquinolone antimicrobial agents, given as continuous or polsed-water medication against *Escherichia coli* infection in chickens. *Antimicrob. Agents Chemother.* 42: 83–7.

116. Moore, R.D., Smith, C.R. and Lietman, P.S. (1984). Association of aminoglycoside plasma levels with therapeutic outcome in Gram-negative pneumonia. *Am. J. Med.* 77: 657–62.

117. Stearne, L.E., Lemmens, N., Goessens, W.H.F., Mouton, J.W. and Gyssens, I.C. (2002). In *European Conference Clinical Microbiology and Infectious Diseases*, Milan.

118. Odenholt, I., Gustafsson, I., Lowdin, E. and Cars, O. (2003). Suboptimal antibiotic dosage as a risk factor for selection of penicillin-resistant *Streptococcus pneumoniae*: *in vitro* kinetic model. *Antimicrob. Agents Chemother.* 47: 518–23.

119. Tam, V.H., Schilling, A.N., Neshat, S., Poole, K., Melnick, D.A. and Coyle, E.A. (2005b). Optimization of meropenem minimum concentration/MIC ratio to suppress *in vitro* resistance of *Pseudomonas aeruginosa*. *Antimicrob. Agents Chemother.* 49: 4920–7.

120. Lees, P., Concordet, D., Aliabadi, F.S. and Toutain, P.-L. (2006). Drug selection and optimization of dosage schedules to minimize antimicrobial resistance. In *Antimicrobial Resistance in Bacteria of Animal Origin* (ed. Frank, M.). Aerestrup, ASM Press, Washington, D.C. pp. 49–71.

121. Regnier, A., Concordet, D., Schneider, M., Boisrame, B. and Toutain, P.L. (2003). Population pharmacokinetics of marbofloxacin in the aqueous humour after intravenous administration in dogs. *Am. J. Vet. Res.* 64: 889–93.

122. del Castillo, J.R., Laroute, V., Pommier, P., *et al.* (2006). Interindividual variability in plasma concentrations after systemic exposure of swine to dietary doxycycline supplied with and without paracetamol: a population pharmacokinetic approach. *J. Anim. Sci.* 84: 3155–66.

123. Riond, J.L. and Riviere, J.E. (1989). Effects of tetracyclines on the kidney in cattle and dogs. *J. Am. Vet. Med. Assoc.* 195: 995–7.

124. MacGowan, A.P. (2004). Elements of design: the knowledge on which we build. *Clin. Microbiol. Infect.* 10 Suppl 2: 6–11.

Chapter 7

GUIDELINES FOR ANTIMICROBIAL USE IN SWINE

David G. S. Burch, C. Oliver Duran and Frank M. Aarestrup

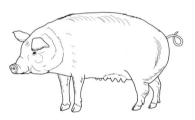

The demand for meat increased substantially during the post-war years and increased pig production was the main driver of the industry. The increased demand, coupled with a decrease in people engaged in agriculture, has led to intensified and more efficient production. Because of these socio-economic changes, over the last 30 years there has been a steady decline of small farms and an increase in the larger ones, particularly in the USA. In 2005, 53% of all hog inventories were in farms with more than 5000 pigs (1). More recently, the development of large corporate farms and production systems has led to further concentration in the ownership of pigs. Currently, three large companies produce 20% of pigs in the UK, while in the USA the 20 biggest companies own one-third of all the breeding sows (2). These changes have resulted in increased disease challenges due to larger units, increased population density and throughput and to a certain extent a reduction in the quality of stockmanship. As a result, they have frequently contributed to increased use of antimicrobials in pork production to compensate.

Antimicrobials have been widely used in swine production over several decades and are reported to be worth an estimated $1.7 billion dollars or 34% of the global animal health antimicrobial market, closely followed by poultry (33%) and cattle (26%) (3). A major exception is the USA where 50% of the $1.3 billion antimicrobial market was in cattle, primarily due to the feedlot system, and only 20% in pigs ($0.23 billion). Precise figures regarding tonnages of active ingredient and actual use in pigs are rarely published, but national bodies are starting to collate total antimicrobial usage in animals and some, like Denmark, can break them down by family class of antimicrobial (4, 5) and the species of animal in which they are used (6). The Danish antimicrobial market is not completely representative of the worldwide swine industry, as total antimicrobial usage is relatively low compared to other countries and usage in pigs accounts for over 80% of all animal consumption in terms of kg active compounds. However, tetracyclines dominate in most markets, followed by the macrolide/lincosamide/ pleuromutilin group of compounds. The use of penicillins, trimethoprim/sulfonamide combinations and aminoglycosides is also important (see Figure 7.1).

Total use of antimicrobials in Europe has probably been reduced following the ban on use of Antimicrobial Growth Promoters (AGPs) in 2006 (see Chapter 1). Recent Scandinavian data showed an overall reduction in total veterinary antimicrobial usage (7). In Denmark, an increase in the use of antimicrobials used for therapy in recently weaned and grower pigs due to *Escherichia coli* and *Lawsonia*

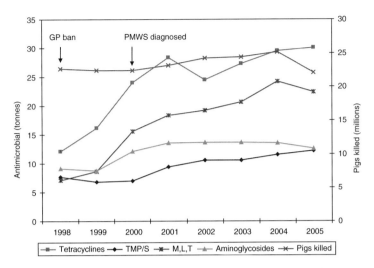

Figure 7.1 Therapeutic antimicrobial usage (tetracyclines, trimethoprim/sulfonamides, macrolides/lincosamides/pleuromutilins (MLT) and aminoglycosides) in Denmark after the withdrawal of growth promoters in 1999 (9) and number of pigs killed/year (millions).

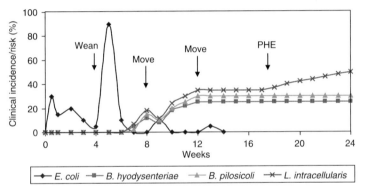

Figure 7.2 Enteric disease patterns in swine.

intracellularis respectively, was observed shortly after the ban of AGPs. However, the situation has stabilised following changes in management practices by farmers and veterinarians (8, 9). The appearance of severe clinical disease related to infections with Porcine Circovirus Associated Diseases (PCVAD) from 2000 has also resulted in increased antimicrobial use to combat secondary bacterial infections, and it is difficult to separate this effect from that of the AGPs ban.

The most common bacterial pathogens and diseases requiring antimicrobial use in swine are summarised in Table 7.1 and their disease patterns are highlighted in Figures 7.2 (enteric diseases), 7.3 (respiratory diseases) and 7.4 (septicaemic diseases). Any use of antimicrobial agents leads to development of bacterial resistance. Resistance development in swine pathogenic bacteria complicates treatment of infections and therefore has to be regarded as both an animal health problem and an economic burden. In addition, pigs are often colonised by bacteria capable of transferring

to, and causing infections in, humans, such as *Salmonella* and *Campylobacter*. Thus, the use of antimicrobials in pigs also leads to selection of resistance in these zoonotic bacteria and thereby potentially complicates treatment of human infections. This aspect has to be taken into account when choosing antimicrobials for treatment of bacterial infections in pigs and in other food animals. The purpose of this chapter is to describe the current use of antimicrobial agents in swine production and to suggest possible strategies to reduce their overall use and to use them more effectively, prudently and responsibly.

7.1 Antimicrobial usage in swine production

The antimicrobial compounds most commonly used in pig production are described in Table 7.2 together with their modes of administration, dosage rates and

Table 7.1 Common bacterial pathogens and diseases in swine

Bacterial species	Disease	Age
Enteric		
Escherichia coli	Neonatal scours.	1–3 days.
	Piglet scours.	7–14 days.
	Post-weaning diarrhoea.	5–14 days after weaning.
Clostridium perfringens	Type C – necrotic enteritis.	1–7 days.
	Type A – diarrhoea.	10–21 days, weaned pigs.
Clostridium difficile	Diarrhoea, ill thrift.	3–7 days.
Salmonella spp.	Typhimurium – occasional diarrhoea, septicaemia, death.	Grower pigs 6–16 weeks.
	Derby – occasional diarrhoea.	Grower pigs 6–16 weeks.
	Choleraesuis – septicaemia diarrhoea, death.	Finishing pigs 12–16 weeks.
Lawsonia intracellularis	Porcine proliferative enteropathy (ileitis).	Grower pigs.
	Regional/necrotic ileitis.	Grower pigs.
	Porcine haemorrhagic enteropathy.	Finishing pigs and young adults 16–40 weeks.
Brachyspira hyodysenteriae	Swine dysentery.	Growers and finishers, 6–26 weeks. All ages in primary breakdown.
Brachyspira pilosicoli	Intestinal spirochaetosis 'colitis'.	Grower pigs.
Respiratory		
Pasteurella multocida (D)	Atrophic rhinitis.	1–8 weeks.
Bordetella bronchiseptica		Nasal distortion, lasts for life.
Mycoplasma hyopneumoniae	Enzootic pneumonia.	Grower and finisher pig.
Pasteurella multocida	Mycoplasma-induced respiratory disease (MIRD).	Grower and finisher – secondary invader.
Actinobacillus pleuropneumoniae	Pleuro-pneumonia.	Grower and finisher – MDA last for 10 weeks.
Actinobacillus suis	Septicaemia.	5–28 days.
	Pleuro-pneumonia.	Weaning to slaughter.
Septicaemic/bacteraemic		
Streptococcus suis	Meningitis, endocarditis, arthritis, peritonitis.	2–10 weeks.
Haemophilus parasuis	Glässer's disease (arthritis, pericarditis, peritonitis).	2–10 weeks.
Mycoplasma hyosynoviae	Mycoplasmal arthritis.	16 weeks plus.
Erysipelothrix rhusiopathiae	Erysipelas (dermatitis, arthritis, endocarditis).	Growers, finishers and sows.

indications. Their relative activity against various porcine pathogens is highlighted in Tables 7.3–7.12. Antimicrobials are used in swine production for therapeutic, metaphylactic and prophylactic purposes as well as for growth promotion, although the latter use is banned in EU countries and in Australia (see Chapter 1 for definitions on therapy, metaphylaxis and prophylaxis). Prophylactic treatments coincide with defined times in the production cycle, occasionally at birth to reduce *Streptococcus* and *Haemophilus* transmission, frequently after weaning (say three to six weeks of age) to prevent post-weaning diarrhoea, or in the mid to late nursery phase (in the USA, six to ten weeks of age) or after moving and mixing of pigs. Only occasionally is prophylaxis used in the finishing stage after initial placement in the barn (10 or 12 weeks to slaughter), where medication becomes very costly, unless pigs from a number of sources are co-mingled. Feed traditionally lends itself well to prophylactic/metaphylactic medication of pigs, as it can be built easily into a medication programme for disease control, without having to physically handle the animal.

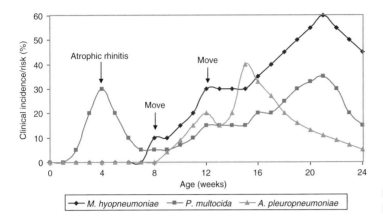

Figure 7.3 Respiratory disease patterns in swine.

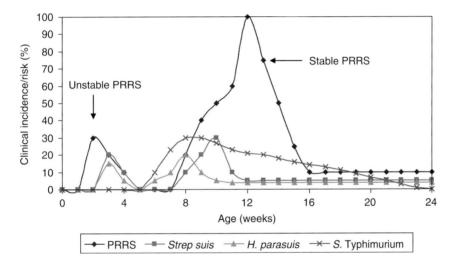

Figure 7.4 Septicaemic disease patterns in swine.

In growth promotion practice, antimicrobials are usually included in feed at low concentrations that preclude systemic disease-controlling effects. Particularly in the USA, antimicrobial feed premixes may be approved for treatment, prevention and growth promotion depending on the dose administered. For example, tiamulin was licensed for inclusion in feed at 220 ppm for treatment, 38.5 ppm for prevention and 11 ppm as a growth promoter respectively (10). Some products, like tylosin, are approved at 44–110 ppm for prevention and treatment, but also at 11–110 ppm for growth promotion depending on the diet. None of these dosages require a veterinary prescription, but the inclusion levels strictly follow Food and Drug Administration (FDA) label instructions. Nobody can deviate from the label, not even veterinarians. In Europe, since the banning of AGPs, antimicrobial premixes for medicated feeding stuffs (MFS) are supplied under a veterinary controlled MFS prescription for prevention or treatment purposes, although the mills generally purchase and include the premixes in the feed. In some countries, like Denmark, the medicines are supplied via the pharmacist, although this is changing as it was considered too restrictive and uncompetitive. Interestingly, in the USA, only one antimicrobial in feed, tilmicosin, currently requires the equivalent of a veterinary prescription or what is called a Veterinary Feed Directive (11). All others can be included in rations at the discretion of the farmer, nutritionist or mill manager.

Table 7.2 Routes of administration, dosages (mg/kg bodyweight) and target pathogens of antimicrobials used in swine

Antimicrobial class/ compound	Administration and dosage			Target pathogens
	Injection	In water	In feed	
Tetracyclines				*M. hyopneumoniae*
Oxytetracycline	10 (LA forms 20–30)	10–30	20	*P. multocida*
Chlortetracycline	—	20	10–20	*A. pleuropneumoniae*
Tetracycline	—	20–40	–	*H. parasuis*
Doxycycline	4–6	12.5	12.5	*L. intracellularis*
				E. coli (resistance)
				Salmonella spp. (resistance)
Trimethoprim/ sulfonamide	15	30	15	*P. multocida*
				B. bronchiseptica
				A. pleuropneumoniae
				S. suis
				S. hyicus
				H. parasuis
				E. coli
				Salmonella spp.
Penicillins				*S. suis*
Penicillin G	10 (LA form 15)	—	—	*P. multocida*
Penicillin V		10	10	*H. parasuis*
				A. pleuropneumoniae
				A. pyogenes
				C. perfringens
				E. rhusiopathiae
Synthetic penicillins				*S. suis*
Amoxicillin	7 (LA forms 15)	20	15–20	*P. multocida*
Ampicillin	7.5	—	—	*H. parasuis*
plus clavulanic acid	+1.75	—	—	*A. pleuropneumoniae*
				A. pyogenes
				C. perfringens
				E. rhusiopathiae
				E. coli
				Salmonella spp.
Cephalosporins				*S. suis*
Cefalexin	7	—	—	*P. multocida*
Ceftiofur	3 (LA forms 5)	—	—	*H. parasuis*
Cefquinome	1–2	—	—	*A. pleuropneumoniae*
				A. pyogenes
				C. perfringens
				E. rhusiopathiae
				E. coli
				Salmonella spp.
Fluoroquinolones				*M. hyopneumoniae*
Enrofloxacin	2.5	—	—	*P. multocida*
Danofloxacin	1.25	—	—	*A. pleuropneumoniae*
Marbofloxacin	2	—	—	*H. parasuis*
				E. coli
				Salmonella spp.
Thiamphenicols				*P. multocida*
Thiamphenicol	10–30	—	10	*A. pleuropneumoniae*
Florfenicol	15	15	15	*H. parasuis*
				S. suis
				B. bronchiseptica

Continued

Table 7.2 (Continued)

Antimicrobial class/ compound	Administration and dosage			Target pathogens
	Injection	In water	In feed	
Aminoglycosides				*E. coli*
Streptomycin	25	—	—	*Salmonella* spp.
Neomycin	– (NA)	11	11	
Apramycin	– (NA)	7.5–12.5	4–8	
Gentamicin	– (NA)	—	—	
Amikacin		—	—	
Aminocyclitol				
Spectinomycin (+ lincomycin)	– (NA)	10–50	1.1–2.2	
Polymixin				*E. coli*
Colistin	—	50 000 IU	50 000 IU	*Salmonella* spp.
Macrolides				*M. hyopneumoniae*
Tylosin	2–10	25	3–6 (T)	*L. intracellularis*
			1.2–2.4 (P)	*B. hyodysenteriae* (resistance tylosin)
				B. pilosicoli (resistance tylosin)
Acetyliso-valeryltylosin	—	—	2.5–5	
Tilmicosin	—	—	8–16	Plus *A. pleuropneumoniae*
Triamilide				*H. parasuis*
Tulathromycin	2.5 (LA form)	—	—	*P. multocida*
				S. suis (resistance)
Lincosamides				*M. hyopneumoniae*
Lincomycin	10	4.5	5.5–11 (T)	*M. hyosynoviae*
			2.2 (P)	*L. intracellularis*
				B. hyodysenteriae
				B. pilosicoli
Pleuromutilins				*M. hyopneumoniae*
Valnemulin	—	—	3.75–10 (T)	*M. hyosynoviae*
			1–1.5 (P)	*L. intracellularis*
				B. hyodysenteriae
Tiamulin	10–15	8.8	5–11 (T)	*B. pilosicoli*
			1.5–2 (P)	Plus *A. pleuropneumoniae*
Miscellaneous				
Growth promoters (not EU)				
Avoparcin	—	—	10–40 ppm	*C. perfringens*
Virginiamycin	—	—	5–100 ppm	*B. hyodysenteriae*
Bacitracin MD	—	—	10–250 ppm	
Flavophospholipol	—	—	2–4 ppm	
Avilamycin	—	—	10–40 ppm	
Carbadox	—	—	11–55 ppm	*B. hyodysenteriae*
				S. Choleraesuis
Anticoccidials				
Toltrazuril	—	20 (OD)	—	Isospora suis
Salinomycin	—	—	15–60 ppm	
Monensin	—	—	100 ppm (NA)	

NA – not approved; LA form – long-acting formulation; OD – oral doser; T – treatment; P – prevention; ppm – parts per million.

Table 7.3 Occurrence of antimicrobial resistance among *Salmonella enterica* serovar Typhimurium from swine in different European countries in year 2004

	Country, number and origin of isolates						
Origin and antimicrobial agent	The Netherlands	Belgium	Denmark	Germany	Poland	England/ Wales	Italy
	n=77	n=175	n=814	n=299	n=10	n=147	n=216
Amoxicillin	51.9						
Ampicillin	a	84	22.2	78.6	40	82	66.2
Amoxicillin + clavulanic acid			0	1.3	0	1	
Apramycin			1.4		0	4	
Ceftiofur		2	0	0	0		
Chloramphenicol	32.5	63	9.3	46.2	30	71	32.6
Ciprofloxacin	0		0.8	0	10	0	0.5
Enrofloxacin		0					0.9
Florfenicol	31.2	53	5.3	44.2	30		
Gentamicin	0	0	1.4	6.0	0	3	1.4
Kanamycin				14.1			0.5
Flumequin							
Nalidixic acid	1.3	4	0.9	1.7	20	4	10.2
Neomycin	0	2	7.8	14.1	0	10	2.5
Streptomycin		73	37.3	82.6	40	80	70.8
Sulfonamides	67.5	91	37.7	90.0	40	90	81.9
Doxycycline							
Tetracycline	72.7	89	39.9	77.9	40	93	80.6
Trimethoprim	29.9		6.3	26.8	0		20.3
Trimethoprim + sulfonamides		36		26.8		72	

[a] Indicates that this antimicrobial was not tested for in that country.

No extra-label usage of in feed antimicrobials is allowed by the FDA (12).

Therapeutic antimicrobials may also be given in feed, but because sick pigs have a reduced appetite and variable feed intake, and medicated feed may also take time to prepare and deliver, they are commonly given as *soluble formulations* in the drinking water to groups or houses of animals. This is becoming increasingly popular with the development of more reliable dosing/water-proportioner machines rather than using header tanks. *Injectables* and *piglet dosers* are widely used, but require individual handling of the animal. When they are small piglets are easy to handle, so metaphylactic injection programmes of antimicrobials are quite common to fight off piglet infections such as neonatal scours, navel infections or arthritis.

Injections of all pigs may also occur at weaning as part of a Medicated Early Weaning health protocol to eliminate certain bacterial infections from the growing population (13). Individual older pigs are injected when they are ill, but for therapy usually only after removal to a hospital pen. A sick pig is easier to inject in a pen but, as they recover, it becomes more difficult. Injecting unrestrained large sows or boars can be dangerous. Due to these risks and the reduced availability of labour, *long-acting injectable formulations* have been developed to facilitate administration and to reduce the need for repeated injections. While these preparations improve compliance by removing the need for repeated injections, if products are used that do not reach therapeutic concentrations for the target pathogens this may lead to therapy failure or encourage resistance development.

Table 7.4 Occurrence of antimicrobial resistance among *Escherichia coli* isolated from swine in different European countries in year 2004 (source www.arbao.org)

Origin and antimicrobial agent	Spain	Belgium	Denmark	Latvia	Latvia	Norway	Finland	Belgium	Sweden	England/Wales	France	Portugal	Switzerland
	169	137	177	19	11	45	61	105	386	313	758–1412	44	47
SWINE	Passive monitoring programme	Diseased animals	O149	Infected animals	Faeces	Enteritis/oedema disease	Infections	Diarrhoea (Young animals)	Intestinal, diagnostic mat	Disease outbreaks	Diagnostic laboratories/ pathogenic bacteria	Origin of the isolates infected animal	Intestine K88
Amoxicillin	33.7	a											4.2
Ampicillin		72.3	45.8	75	100	7	16	61.9	22	47	53.2		
Amoxicillin + Cl	1.8	0.7	0.6	15.8	0			1			2.0	36	0.0
Apramycin	13	13.1	13.6					1.9		8	3.3		
Ceftiofur		0.7	0			0	0	1.0	<1		0.6		
Chloramphenicol	40.8	38.7	41.8	0		4.0	7	29.5				45	38.3
Ciprofloxacin	14.2		0	0	0								
Enrofloxacin		2.9				0	0	13.3	6	2	5.5	30	0.0
Florfenicol	7.1	4.4	0			0	0	3.8			0.9		
Gentamicin	19.5	3.6	12	9	0	0	0	6.7	0		5.5	45	12.7
Kanamycin				33.3	63.6							27	
Flumequin											18.6	41	
Nalidixic acid	33.7	34.3	32	23	0	2	13	18.1					
Neomycin	20.1	1.5	35	39	16.7	2	7	1.0		11	10.9		
Streptomycin	74		77.4	50	100	47	54		4				
Sulfonamides	76.3		82			7	51		28			64	
Doxycycline	78.2				100								
Tetracycline	87	77.4	91	82	100	24	51	73.3	27	82	82.6	91	
Trimethoprim	66.9		48.6			7	44		27	55	66.4	98	57.4
Trimethoprim + sulfonamides		70.8						55.2					

a Indicates that this antimicrobial was not tested for in that country.

7 Swine

Table 7.5 Minimum inhibitory concentrations (MICs) of antimicrobial agents against *B. hyodysenteriae, B. pilosicoli, C. perfringens, C. difficile* and intracellular inhibitory concentrations (90% inhibition) for *L. intracellularis*

Organism/antimicrobial	MIC 50 (µg/ml)	MIC 90 (µg/ml)	Range (µg/ml)
B. hyodysenteriae – Australia (76 isolates) (63)			
Valnemulin	0.031	0.5	≤0.016–2.0
Tiamulin	0.125	1.0	≤0.016–2.0
Lincomycin	16	64	≤1.0–64
Tylosin	>256	>256	≤2.0>256
B. hyodysenteriae – Czech Republic (100 isolates) (64)			
Valnemulin	0.125	4.0	—
Tiamulin	0.25	2.0	—
Lincomycin	32	64	—
Tylosin	>128	>128	—
Acetylisovaleryltylosin	25	50	—
Chlortetracycline	4	8	—
B. pilosicoli – N. America (25 isolates) (65)			
Valnemulin	0.06	0.5	0.03–2.0
Tiamulin	0.125	1.0	0.06–8.0
Lincomycin	32	64	4.0–>128
Tylosin	>512	>512	<16–>512
Carbadox	0.06	0.06	0.03–0.125
L. intracellularis – UK (1–3 isolates) (55)[a]			
Valnemulin	—	—	<1.0–<4.0
Tiamulin	—	—	<2.0–<8.0
Lincomycin	—	—	<0.25
Tylosin	—	—	<2.0–<100
Tilmicosin	—	—	<0.125–<0.5
Chlortetracycline	—	—	<1.0–<16
Spectinomycin	—	—	<64
L. intracellularis – USA (4 isolates) EU (4 isolates) (56)[a]			
Carbadox	—	—	0.125–0.25
Chlortetracycline	—	—	0.25–64
Lincomycin	—	—	8–>128
Tiamulin	—	—	0.125–0.5
Tylosin	—	—	0.25–32
Valnemulin	—	—	0.125
C. perfringens – Belgium (58 isolates) (66)			
Tiamulin	—	–	0.25–4.0
Lincomycin	2.0	256	0.12–>512
Penicillin G	0.12	0.5	0.06–1.0
Tetracycline	16	32	0.06–>64
C. perfringens - Belgium (95 isolates) (ref 67)			
Tylosin	≤0.12	≤0.25	≤0.12–>64
C. difficile – USA (80 isolates) (57)			
Bacitracin	>256	>256	NR
Ceftiofur	256	>256	NR
Erythromycin	0.5	>256	NR
Tetracycline	8	32	NR
Tiamulin	4	8	NR
Tilmicosin	0.5	>256	NR
Tylosin	0.25	64	NR
Virginiamycin	0.25	2	NR

[a] Based on determination of intracellular MICs.

Table 7.6 Minimum inhibitory concentrations (MICs) of antimicrobial agents against *M. hyopneumoniae* and *M. hyosynoviae*

	MIC 50 (µg/ml)	MIC 90 (µg/ml)	Range (µg/ml)
M. hyopneumoniae – Hannan *et al.*, 1997 (68) – Global (20 isolates)			
Enrofloxacin	0.025	0.05	0.01–0.1
Tiamulin	0.05	0.05	0.01–0.1
Tylosin	0.1	0.25	0.025–0.25
Oxytetracycline	0.25	1.0	0.025–1.0
M. hyopneumoniae – Vicca *et al.*, 2004 (69) – Belgium (21 isolates)			
Enrofloxacin	0.03	0.5	0.015–>1.0
Tiamulin	≤0.015	0.12	≤0.015–0.12
Tylosin	0.03	0.06	≤0.015–>1.0
Tilmicosin	0.25	0.5	≤0..25–>16
Lincomycin	≤0.06	≤0.06	≤0.06–>8.0
Spectinomycin	0.25	0.5	≤0.12–0.5
Oxytetracycline	0.12	1.0	0.03–2.0
Doxycycline	0.12	0.5	0.03–1.0
Florfenicol	≤0.12	0.25	≤0.12–0.5
M. hyosynoviae – Hannan *et al.*, 1997 (68) – Global (18 isolates)			
Enrofloxacin	0.1	0.25	0.05–0.25
Tiamulin	0.005	0.025	0.0025–0.01
Tylosin	0.25	1.0	0.025–>10
Oxytetracycline	0.5	5.0	0.25–10

Table 7.7 Antimicrobial resistance in porcine bacterial pathogens in the UK (59)

Antimicrobial	*P. multocida*	*A. pleuropneumoniae*	*S. suis*	*E. rhusiopathiae*	*A. pyogenes*
No. of isolates	573	201	92	44	69
Ampicillin	3	6	0	0	0
Penicillin	–	–	0	0	0
Tetracycline	12	31	75	33	1
Trimethoprim/sulfonamide	8	14	9	59	6
Enrofloxacin	0	1	0	–	0
Ceftiofur	–	1	0	0	0

The pharmacokinetics of antimicrobials is discussed in Chapter 6. However, there are a number of key aspects to swine medicine that are both important and specific. The bulk of antimicrobials used in swine are via the feed, approximately 80% of the total consumption. Dose intake is linked directly to feed intake and inclusion level. One of the common problems veterinarians encounter regarding efficacy is underdosing. If the animal is sick with a high temperature, it will stop eating. It is essential to treat pigs with no appetite by injection to get them to start eating the medicated feed. The age of the pig is also important. Most dose rates are based upon a 20 kg pig eating 1 kg of feed/day or 5% of bodyweight. Finishing pigs are often given restricted feed to control fat deposition,

in male castrates especially, and there can be a halving of relative feed intake to 2.5% from 80 kg and above. Lactating sows are usually fed to about 2.5% and dry sows can be fed at a rate of 1% of bodyweight. To achieve a target dose of chlortetracycline to treat a uterine infection, five times the normal weaner inclusion rate is required. This is also important in eradication programmes to ensure the correct dose is administered to the various age groups. Many in-feed administration products give relatively lower plasma levels and bioavailability (14), especially products that are mainly metabolised in the liver (e.g. macrolides, pleuromutilins and lincosamides), due to the slower passage down the gut. Products excreted via the kidney (e.g. tetracyclines, trimethoprim/sulfonamides

Table 7.8 Minimum inhibitory concentrations (MICs) of antimicrobial agents used against *A. pleuropneumoniae*, *P. multocida* and *S. suis* (60)

Antimicrobial (NCCLS resistance breakpoints – µg/ml)	MIC 50 (µg/ml)	MIC 90 (µg/ml)	Range (µg/ml)
A. pleuropneumoniae – N. America (89 isolates)			
Penicillin (≥0.25)	0.5	32	≤0.12–64
Tetracycline (≥8)	16	32	≤0.12–64
Trimethoprim/sulfonamide (≥4/76)	≤0.06	≤0.06	≤0.06–0.12
Tilmicosin (≥32)	2.0	4.0	≤0.12–4.0
Florfenicol (≥8)	0.25	0.5	≤0.06–0.5
Enrofloxacin (≥2)	≤0.03	≤0.03	≤0.03–0.06
Ceftiofur (≥8)	≤0.03	≤0.03	≤0.03–0.06
P. multocida – N. America (186 isolates)			
Penicillin (≥0.25)	≤0.12	≤0.12	≤0.12–>64
Tetracycline (≥8)	2.0	24	0.25–>64
Trimethoprim/sulfonamide (≥4/76)	≤0.06	0.25	≤0.06–>8.0
Tilmicosin (≥32)	4.0	8.0	≤0.12–>64
Florfenicol (≥8)	0.25	0.5	≤0.06–4.0
Enrofloxacin (≥2)	≤0.03	≤0.03	≤0.03–0.5
Ceftiofur (≥8)	≤0.03	≤0.03	≤0.03–4.0
S. suis – N. America (167 isolates)			
Penicillin (≥0.25)	≤0.12	0.25	≤0.12–32
Tetracycline (≥8)	64	64	0.25–>64
Trimethoprim/sulfonamide (≥4/76)	≤0.06	0.12	≤0.06–1.0
Tilmicosin (≥32)	>64	>64	≤0.12–>64
Florfenicol (≥8)	1.0	2.0	0.12–4.0
Enrofloxacin (≥2)	0.25	0.5	≤0.03–1.0
Ceftiofur (≥8)	≤0.03	0.06	≤0.03–4.0

Table 7.9 MICs 50, MICs 90, ranges (µg/ml) and antimicrobial resistance (%) among 229 Spanish isolates of *A. pleuropneumoniae* (61)

Antimicrobial	MIC 50	MIC 90	Range	Breakpoint	Resistance
Penicillin	1.0	64	0.12–128	≥4.0	15
				≤0.25	99
Amoxicillin	0.5	64	0.25–64	≥8.0	15
Cefalothin	0.5	2.0	0.5–32	≥16	0.4
Tetracycline	32	64	0.25–128	≥16	74
Gentamicin	8.0	8.0	4.0–8.0	≥16	9.2
Trimethoprim	≤1.0	≤1.0	≤1.0–32	NR	NR
Sulfisoxazole	64	>512	32–>512	≤512	17
Florfenicol	0.25	0.5	0.12–1.0	≤8.0	0
Nalidixic acid	2.0	4.0	1.0–32	NR	NR

NR – not recorded.

and penicillins) are not normally affected. It must also be remembered that some products given orally are hardly absorbed from the gut, such as the aminoglycosides (e.g. neomycin, apramycin) and aminocyclitols (e.g. spectinomycin). Thus, it is of little use to give them orally for systemic or respiratory infections.

Soluble products given via the drinking water or in liquid feed pass through the stomach more quickly and are therefore more rapidly absorbed. Therapeutic levels of soluble products (e.g. tiamulin) can be achieved in the lung to treat respiratory pathogens such as *Actinobacillus pleuropneumoniae*, but these

Table 7.10 Recent data on the occurrence of antimicrobial resistance among *S. suis* isolated from swine in different countries (62)

Antimicrobial agent	Belgium	Canada	Canada	Canada	Croatia	Denmark	Denmark	England/Wales	France	Finland	Japan	Netherlands	Norway	Poland	Poland	Portugal	Spain	USA	USA
Country, year of isolation and number of isolates	1999–2000	1986–1988	1988	Prior to 1991	Prior to 1995	1995–1996	2003	2003	2003	1984–1987	1987–1996	2003	1986	2002	2003	2003	1992	1999–2001	Prior to 1992
	87	59ᵃ	135	80	33ᵃ	180	557	34	Differs	35	689	762	21	150	151	14	65	151	48
Fluoroquinolones	1	—	—	—	9.1	2.2	0	0	2.9	—	0.3	—	—	8.6	9.9	64	—	2.0	—
Macrolides	71	33.9	60.7	66.3	0	41.7	29.1	36	52.9	0	—	35	28.6	28.0	—	93/71	63	90.7	58
Gentamicin	—	66.1	0.0	2.5	—	—	—	—	0.0	—	—	—	—	—	0.0	100	—	4.6	9
Penicillin	—	0	3.0	2.5	51.1	1.1	0.9	0	—	0	0.9	0	—	10.6	7.9	21	7	4.0	—
Sulfonamides	—	—	—	47.5	—	—	0.9	—	—	—	—	—	—	—	—	—	—	96.0	44
Tetracycline	85	83.0	78.5	95.0	72.2	32.2	52.2	68	69.9	42.8	86.9	48	66.7	73.3	55.0	93/79	61	95.4	63
Co-trimoxazole	—	39.0	1.5	—	—	1.7	51.5	3	15.5	31.4	0.0	8	—	30.0	16.6	100	61	0.0	—

ᵃOnly serotype 2.

7 Swine

Table 7.11 Antimicrobial resistance of 124 US isolates of *H. parasuis* (70) and MIC 50, MIC 90 and Range (µg/ml) of Danish isolates (71)

Antimicrobial agent (disc conc)	Resistance (%)	MIC 50	MIC 90	Range
Penicillin (10 IU)	2.1	0.015	0.25	0.015–0.25
Ampicillin (10 µg)	0.0	1.0	1.0	1.0
Cefalothin (30 µg)	0.0	—	—	—
Ceftiofur (30 µg)	2.1	0.03	0.03	0.03
Tetracycline (30 µg)	14.9	1.0	2.0	0.06–2.0
Trimethoprim/sulfonamide (5 µg)	6.4	0.03	2.0	0.015–8.0
Gentamicin (10 µg)	4.3	—	—	—
Amikacin (30 µg)	6.4	—	—	—
Enrofloxacin (5 µg)	0.0	—	—	—
Ciprofloxacin	—	0.015	0.125	0.015–0.5
Florfenicol	—	0.25	0.5	0.125–0.5
Tilmicosin	—	2.0	2.0	2.0–4.0
Tiamulin	—	4.0	8.0	1.0–16

Table 7.12 Occurrence of antimicrobial resistance in *S. hyicus* from different countries (62)

	Country, year, (number of isolates) and percentage of resistance				
	Belgium	Denmark	Germany	Japan	United Kingdom
Antimicrobial agent	1974–1976 (46)	2003 (68)	1989 (32)	1979–1984 (124)[a]	1988 (37)
Chloramphenicol	—	0	9	0	0
Florfenicol	—	0	—	—	—
Fluoroquinolones	—	4	—	—	—
Gentamicin	—	0	—	0	0
Macrolides	74	21	3	41	11
Penicillin	60	84	25	38	32
Streptomycin	72	44	43	23	51
Sulfonamides	—	2	100	—	—
Tetracycline	60	35	66	54	41
Trimethoprim	—	24	—	—	—

[a]Both healthy and diseased.

levels are not reached when the same drug is given in the feed.

7.2 Zoonotic infections transmitted by pigs

The two main food-borne pathogens associated with swine are *Salmonella* (especially *S.* Typhimurium and *S.* Derby) and *Campylobacter* (primarily *C. coli*), both causing mainly enteric disease in humans, but occasionally more severe infections. While these zoonotic agents are mainly transmitted to humans by consumption of contaminated pork, infection with less known zoonotic agents like *Streptococcus suis* and methicillin-resistant *Staphylococcus aureus* (MRSA) usually occurs in people working closely with pigs, such as farmers, slaughterhouse workers, butchers or veterinarians. These zoonotic infections are reviewed in further detail below.

7.2.1 *Salmonella*

The main serovar found in pigs is *S.* Typhimurium, which accounts for about 65% of isolations from pigs in the UK (VLA *Salmonella* 2004, 2005), while *S.* Derby accounts for about 17%. Among human cases in the UK in 2004, 64% were due to *S.* Enteritidis, which is found predominantly in poultry, 11% was due to *S.* Typhimurium, which can be found in most animal species, and <1.0% due to *S.* Derby (15). Some cases of *S.* Typhimurium are more commonly associated with phage types from pigs (such as U288 and 193) so a definite link to pigs as a source has been established (15). However, many phage types can be found in a variety of animal and poultry species, and it is therefore difficult to apportion the number of cases directly due to pigs/pork. Danish and imported pork was estimated to account for approximately 29% of all attributed human *Salmonella* infections acquired in Denmark (16). However, the question is controversial. If *S.* Derby is used as an indicator, on a proportional basis, the percentage of all UK human cases due to pork consumption could be under 5% (D.G.S. Burch – unpubl. obs.).

The resistance patterns of *S.* Typhimurium, from a number of EU countries, are highlighted in Table 7.3, with high susceptibility being recorded for amoxicillin/clavulanic acid, ceftiofur (third-generation cephalosporin), ciprofloxacin (fluoroquinolone) and gentamicin (aminoglycoside). In Poland, slightly higher resistance levels have been reported on the basis of a low number of isolates (Table 7.3). It can be concluded that pork does pose a potential zoonotic hazard in relation to *Salmonella*, but that it is a relatively small risk in comparison with poultry meat and products, especially if handled and cooked properly. The likelihood of treatment failure due to antimicrobial resistance, on those rare occasions when antimicrobial therapy should be required, is generally considered to be low. However, antimicrobial resistant *Salmonella* such as *S.* Typhimurium DT104 can have serious human health consequences both due to the occurrence of infections that would otherwise not have occurred and due to treatment failures and increased severity of infections. The use of antimicrobial agents in humans disturbs the intestinal microflora. Individuals taking an antimicrobial agent for respiratory infections, for example, are therefore at an increased risk of becoming infected with intestinal pathogens resistant to that agent. Barza and Travers (17) estimated that in the USA resistance to antimicrobial agents results annually in an additional 29 379 *Salmonella* infections, leading to 342 hospitalisations and 12 deaths. Several studies have examined the severity of infections with antimicrobial resistant

Salmonella and found that infections with resistant *Salmonella* were associated with a higher death rate, increased hospitalisation rate and longer illness than infections with susceptible isolates (18–21). In particular, infections with quinolone-resistant *Salmonella* are associated with increased mortality and morbidity compared to infections with quinolone-susceptible *Salmonella* (22,23). Not all types of resistance are of equal importance. Fluoroquinolones are in many countries the drug of choice for treatment of salmonellosis in humans. Cephalosporins are the drugs of choice for the treatment of salmonellosis in children, as fluoroquinolones cannot be administered due to toxic effects on children. Accordingly, the use of fluorquinolones and cephalosporins in pigs should be avoided unless the pathogen is resistant to any other antimicrobial agent available in the veterinary arsenal.

7.2.2 Campylobacter

The majority of *Campylobacter* infections in man are due to *Campylobacter jejuni*. Burch (24), in a literature review, estimated that 92% of human infections are caused by *C. jejuni* and only 8% by *C. coli*. The dominant *Campylobacter* species isolated from pigs is *C. coli* (96%). The prevalence of *C. jejuni* is higher in chickens (90%) and in cattle (99%), which is similar to the incidence of human Campylobacteriosis associated with these species. Conversely to chickens, turkeys can have quite a high prevalence of *C. coli*, although *C. jejuni* tend to be the dominant species (25). Several studies have indicated that poultry is the most important reservoir of *Campylobacter* infections in man (26, 27).

Macrolides and fluoroquinolones are the drugs of choice for treatment of severe campylobacteriosis in humans. There is only limited information on the importance of antimicrobial resistance in *Campylobacter* for human health. In the only available study, Helms *et al.* (28) found that patients infected with quinolone or macrolide-resistant strains of *C. jejuni* had an increased risk for an adverse event compared to patients infected with susceptible strains. This finding still needs to be verified in other studies. Macrolide (erythromycin) resistance in *C. coli* isolated from pigs can be quite high, up to 85% in the UK (29) and it cannot be discounted that this could have some human health implications. However, since most infections in man are caused by *C. jejuni*, the importance of macrolide resistance in *C. coli* should not be overestimated.

7.2.3 *Streptococcus suis*

Human infections with *S. suis* serotypes 2 and 14 have been reportedly associated with people producing or processing pigs in the UK (30). Among the 41 laboratory confirmed cases between 1981 and 2000 (approximately 2 per year), 27% were pig farmers or stockmen, 22% retail butchers, 12% abattoir workers, 12% no apparent risk and 27% no epidemiological data. Recently, a large *S. suis* outbreak in China was related to slaughterhouse employees working in poor health and safety conditions (31,32). Although the risk of infection is low, it can cause fatalities in man. Penicillin still remains highly active against *S. suis* (>90% of isolates are susceptible).

7.2.4 Methicillin-resistant *Staphylococcus aureus*

MRSA colonisation in animals has been implicated in infections in humans in several cases, and MRSA should today be considered as a zoonosis. Conversely to pets, which are usually infected or colonised with classical human variants of MRSA (33), a new clone (multi-locus sequence type ST398) appears to have emerged in pigs. This MRSA clone was first reported in a family of pig farmers in the Netherlands (34). Subsequently, in a survey, MRSA was found in 23% of Dutch farmers and in 4.6% of veterinarians and veterinary students in the Netherlands (34, 35). In the same country, a recent study of the pig population has revealed a colonisation rate of 39% of all slaughter pigs and 80% of pig slaughter batches (36). All isolates belonged to clone ST398, which seems to have established itself in the pig population in the Netherlands. In the autumn of 2006, the same clone was detected in patients in Denmark, most of which had close contacts to production animals, mainly swine. A retrospective study has shown that MRSA ST398 had already occurred in Danish slaughter pigs in 2005 (37). The same sequence type has also described in *S. aureus* strains isolated from pigs and farmers in France, though the isolates were not methicillin resistant (38). MRSA ST 398 has also been described in Germany, including in veterinarians (nasal carriage), human patients, companion animals and a single pig (39).

With our current knowledge, it seems quite evident that ST398 is a MRSA clone transmitted from pigs to humans; its origin is unknown, though it – or its antecedents – could have originated in humans. Further studies are underway in several countries, but it seems that MRSA ST398 is widespread in the pig populations, at least in the Netherlands and Denmark, but most likely in all European countries with intensive swine production. ST398 mainly colonises animals, but has been found to cause infections, in a few cases. The limited number of reports is probably due to the difficulties of isolating this bacterium from animals, because it is necessary to use selective enrichment. It must be expected that several new reports will be published in the near future. The reason for the colonisation of MRSA ST398 in pigs and the epidemiology of this clone is currently not known. It possibly first emerged in 2003, as it was not detected in 2002 in the human monitoring being done in the Netherlands nor in monitoring from 1992 to 2003 of human isolates in Germany. It can be speculated that the use of cephalosporins and other antimicrobials has provided a niche for this clone, but until further studies are carried out this is merely speculation. The importance for human health and the possibilities for infection control are currently unclear. In the Netherlands, the advice is to keep pig breeders in isolation when they are admitted to a hospital, until surveillance cultures are proven negative. This also applies to veterinarians and slaughterhouse personnel. For cattle breeders, screening without isolation on admission to a hospital is sufficient.

7.3 Prudent antimicrobial use in pigs

7.3.1 Principles of disease control in swine medicine

Disease control is not only about using medicines. Frequently, what has gone wrong is the production system. Hence, the challenge is to correct the underlying management problems. Post-weaning diarrhoea is the classic example. If the temperature of the weaning accommodation is kept high and constant (26–29°C), and drafts are avoided, there is normally little trouble. Pigs can be weaned into deep straw in barns at four weeks of age, in the middle of a UK winter, with no clinical problems. The 'right' environment is very important to the pig and to disease prevention. In general, various approaches can be used to avoid or eliminate the infectious agents and to avoid the clinical disease.

Avoid or eliminate the infectious agent

The health status of a herd is critical in relation to antimicrobial use. A herd can be started up free of specific infectious agents. Alternatively, the infectious agent can be eliminated by carrying out depopulation and repopulation with clean stock or by using herd closure and antimicrobial medication. Having sources of *high-health or Specific Pathogen Free (SPF) stock* is essential to prevent introduction of common bacterial pathogens such as *Mycoplasma hyopneumoniae*, toxigenic *Pasteurella multocida* type D, *A. pleuropneumoniae* and *Brachyspira hyodysenteriae*. Ideally, this list should be extended to include several viruses such as those causing Porcine Reproductive and Respiratory Syndrome (PRRS), Aujeszky's disease and Transmissible Gastroenteritis. Many countries have eradicated Classical Swine Fever and Foot and Mouth Disease, but such diseases are still endemic in certain areas of Asia and South America. It is difficult for producers to obtain stock free of Parvovirus, *L. intracellularis*, *S. suis* or *Haemophilus parasuis*, unless they use caesarean-derived pigs and extreme isolation and biosecurity measures. Breeding stock companies and large production systems operate health pyramids to flow high health pigs in linear fashion. The top of the pyramid is usually the genetic nucleus. This way the highest health pigs always flow down the pyramid towards the lowest health status pigs, and crossing over of pyramids is avoided in order to reduce transmission of infectious agents.

Sourcing of new genetic stock is important, and stricter protocols for diagnosis should possibly be imposed to ensure absence of specified infections. Often herd veterinarians will only certify 'no clinical disease is observed', but the pigs may still be carriers or even test positive for a disease-causing organism by polymerase chain reaction (PCR). In some cases, unwanted antimicrobial resistance may be introduced by this route into a herd or country. *Matching the health status of a herd with a supplier* is also important. Supplying enzootic pneumonia-free gilts or boars to an infected farm is not recommended, as the replacements and their offspring will come down with the acute form of the disease when exposed to the causative agent.

Veterinarians have established protocols and economic justification for depopulation of pig herds affected by certain costly infections (40). Sometimes, it is more cost effective or easier to eradicate using herd closure and mass medication. Many different protocols have been developed for eradication of enzootic pneumonia, *A. pleuropneumoniae*, swine dysentery and atrophic rhinitis (41). Basically, the herd is closed to new pig introductions, growing pigs are moved off site to clean accommodation, and the breeding herd immunity is usually well developed, either by natural infection or vaccination if suitable, while disease transmission is eliminated by antimicrobial prophylaxis and metaphylaxis. Once a high-health herd is established, it is essential to keep diseases out. Ideally, there should be no other pig farm within three miles (5 km). There are *strict biosecurity protocols* to keep infections out, so there is no direct access for feed deliveries, pig loading or animal entry. Ideally, *the site should be closed to new pig replacements*, as they still remain the most common cause of herd breakdown, in spite of separate *quarantine* or isolation facilities (41). *Semen* can also be a carrier of viral infections, as demonstrated by the Swine Fever outbreak in Holland (42) and by well-documented PRRS breakdowns following introduction of PRRSv contaminated semen into naive herds (43). However, import of live animals for breeding and finishing remains the more common means of bringing diseases onto a farm. Persons can carry infectious agents on their skin and clothes and pig farms should not be entered by external visitors without them going through a shower, a clothes changing system, and a one to three-day down time without pig contact.

Avoid clinical disease

There are a variety of production systems in every pig-producing region of the world and almost every farm is different with respect to structure and management problems. Working within the farm system and improving it to reduce infectious challenge is the key to being a successful swine veterinarian. However, some basic principles still apply. Various key areas need to be addressed to avoid clinical disease: herd management and size, population density, parity segregated production, weaning age, pig housing environment and immunity.

Herd management and size

Attention to detail is critical. Small closed breeding finisher herds, which are family owned, usually do well when compared with farms where employees look after pigs.

Mixing pigs from different sources should be avoided. The old cooperative farm system, where grower pigs from many breeding farms were mixed together for finishing, usually had severe disease problems. The more mixing that took place, especially from different farms, the greater the stress to the pigs, and the greater the risk of introducing new diseases to which they had little or no immunity. In the past, finishing units would mix pigs from 20 different sources and, basically, the lowest common disease denominator applied. In smaller single-site or farrow-to-finish farms, *all-in-all-out housing/room systems* coupled with good hygiene have very successfully reduced the spread of disease from one group of pigs to another. Eventually, following the principles developed for disease elimination, without depopulation, the *three-site production system* was developed in the USA, to try to halt or limit the spread of disease from one production stage to another (13). The three-site system consists of having the breeder sites, the nursery sites and finishing sites not just in separate houses, but on separate farms. Larger sow farms (site 1) allow for more cost effective use of growing pig buildings. Specialised labour can be employed on the different sites. Often pigs are weaned at between 14 and 18 days to the nursery site to prevent the spread of a number of infections, but the usefulness of early weaning in preventing disease is still under debate. In the EU, for welfare reasons, piglets are required to be weaned at 28 days. Initially, nursery sites (also known as site 2) consisted of 7 or 8 rooms to accommodate 1 week of production. As a consequence, a large number of sows were required to efficiently fill a nursery in one week, hence the development during the 1990s of the large integrated systems in the USA. Following the increase of PRRS infections, it was determined that even the age variation from weaning to 10 weeks on one site was detrimental to pig health, so *multi-site production systems* were developed. In these systems, the entire site is filled with pigs of the same age and moved *all-in-all-out.* Generally, age varies by 7–14 days maximum. This in turn has fuelled a further increase in the sow herd size to allow for efficient filling of large nurseries. The closer the farms follow the multi-site production system, the fewer disease problems occur,

although ileitis, *S. suis* meningitis and Glässer's disease still occur. However, this is not a system that can be easily adopted, especially in Europe where herd sizes are usually smaller and land is not readily available.

Stress is reduced by avoiding movement and mixing of pigs during the production cycle. Many larger systems are adopting wean-to-finish production (C.O. Duran, pers. comm.). This production system consists of weaning pigs offsite, into accommodation where they remain until slaughter. These systems incorporate the benefits of all-in-all-out and no mixing of different ages and reduces the need for transport between phases. The weaned piglet thermal requirements are met with temporary provision of supplemental heat in the form of heat lamps or brooder heaters. Disease challenges are much reduced by this system, particularly enzootic pneumonia.

Population density

For respiratory diseases particularly, a reduction in pigs per airspace has resulted in less severe infections, although some of these benefits have been reached with correct ventilation and management. Increased pig density in pens or barn has also been linked to increased stress and disease transmission resulting in higher mortality and reduced growth. Ideal space per head recommendations will vary depending on the housing type and production system (44).

Production based on segregated sow parities

Recently, the benefits of raising pigs segregated by the parity of the sows have been applied in Canada and the USA (45). This system reduces disease challenges by reducing variation in the immune status of the piglets by grouping them with piglets of like maternally derived antibody (MDA) and disease carrier status. Generally, this system raises the gilt offspring separate from offspring of sows of parity one and above. These systems reduce antimicrobial and vaccine use by allowing finely tuned interventions due to a very predictable time of disease challenge.

Weaning age

One of the other key elements to disease elimination without depopulation was early weaning below 21 days of age, sometimes below 10 days (13). This was found to reduce the transfer of infections from the sow to the piglets, utilising the transfer of MDAs to protect the piglets and preventing colonisation. This was effective for several viral infections, notably pseudorabies virus (PRV), porcine parvovirus (PPV), TGE and also *A. pleuropneumoniae*, atrophic rhinitis, *M. hyopneumoniae*, although it was less effective against some bacterial infections, where transmission from sow to piglet occurs around the time of parturition (e.g. *S. suis* and *H. parasuis*). In the EU, welfare legislation encourages weaning no earlier than 28 days of age. This has been helpful in reducing the effects of post-weaning diarrhoea and has been found to mitigate the severity of PMWS/PCVAD, but could increase the risk of infection transfer from sows to piglets. Recent studies in the USA investigating the profitability of weaning pigs below 21 days have further encouraged moves away from early weaning (46).

Housing environment

It is beyond the scope of this chapter to detail all the ideal conditions for pig environments at different ages, but it is essential to avoid conditions that increase pathogen exposure and challenge. Most important are providing the correct temperature to maintain pigs in their thermo-neutral zone, and avoiding drafts while removing moisture, gases and pathogens with adequate ventilation. Removal of manure and soiled bedding, plus sanitation processes, are also critical to the reduction of build-up of microbes in the environment. Disease prevention by appropriate housing and environmental management has been reviewed elsewhere (47).

Herd/population immunity

Disease control relies heavily on the protection of the pigs via natural or induced immunity. Early exposure to herd pathogens for replacement breeding stock can result in solid protection of their offspring (acclimatisation) (48, 49). This is often achieved by exposure to manure, mature cull sows or sick pigs, supplemented by vaccines. Stimulation of immunity by vaccination also plays a major role in pig production. Vaccination of the breeding herd to protect against infections in the sow is essential for good production and helps to build up herd immunity. These include viral infections such as PPV, PRRSV, PRV and in some countries porcine circovirus type 2 PCV2 as well as erysipelas (*Erysipelothrix rhusiopathiae*). Vaccination of the sow in late gestation is also used for stimulating MDA protection in the baby piglet against *E. coli*, *Clostridium perfringens* type C and type A, atrophic rhinitis in the farrowing house and erysipelas in the grower. Early intake of sow colostrum in the first 24 h of life

is essential for the piglets to absorb sufficient IgG antibodies and acquire circulating immunity. Continued production of IgA antibodies during lactation provides mucosal protection in the piglet gut.

Vaccine use in growing pigs was geared towards prevention of acute respiratory or systemic infections like *A. pleuropneumoniae* or erysipelas. These vaccines were traditionally whole cell, killed and adjuvanted, requiring two injections in growing pigs. The vaccination of piglets was revolutionised with the introduction of the *M. hyopneumoniae* vaccines, where piglets as young as a week old were shown to develop immunity against this endemic infection. The piglet's immune system appears to be sufficiently well developed to respond to vaccination at this age, although it is not fully matured until four weeks of age. However, it has been shown that high levels of MDA can reduce the vaccinal response in some cases (50,51). Some mycoplasmal vaccines were coupled with *H. parasuis* to give early protection against Glässer's disease. Other common vaccines, against viral infections like PRV, PRRSV and SIV, can help reduce secondary bacterial challenges in growing pigs (52). A recent development is the availability of live oral vaccines for *Salmonella choleraesuis*, *Lawsonia intracellularis*, *E. rhusiopathiae* and F18 *E. coli*. These improve protection against these costly diseases and it is expected that they will reduce antimicrobial usage for treatment and control. Excitingly, new PCV2 vaccines have been developed for young pigs in North America and it is hoped that this scourge will be successfully controlled worldwide in the future.

There appears to be a need for new vaccines, as well as improving old vaccines, particularly in the areas of mucosal immunity, improved practical delivery and application of needle-less technology. Recent work on development of sub-unit vaccines, which permit poly-vaccination to cover a spectrum of common pig diseases in one shot, provides hope for the future (53).

7.3.2 Choice of antimicrobials for swine diseases

Besides using approaches to avoid infectious agents and clinical disease and the use of vaccines where possible, there are definite cases where antimicrobial therapy is required. In such cases, the authors advise that an accurate diagnosis is made, and that cultures and antimicrobial susceptibility data are used to support the therapy of choice. Once the most appropriate antimicrobial is chosen, then a suitable route of administration and dosage should be used to reach the organism and to ensure clinical efficacy. The following sections provide pathogen- and disease-specific guidelines for efficacious antimicrobial use in swine practice. In addition to clinical efficacy, an important additional factor is to try to limit the use of antimicrobials that are critical in human medicine, such as fluoroquinolones and the cephalosporins (see Chapter 4). In the USA, prudent use guidelines would also include trimethoprim/sulfonamide combinations. They may be

used under certain extreme conditions, but prudent use guidelines recommend their use only as a last resort (see Table 7.13).

Diarrhoea/enteritis

Data on the occurrence of antimicrobial resistance among *E. coli* from enteric infections in pigs in different countries are given in Table 7.4. Major differences in the occurrence of resistance are obvious. In general, there is a frequent occurrence of resistance to

Table 7.13 First, second and last resort choices for antimicrobial therapy of common porcine infections

Infection/disease	First choice	Second choice	Last resort
E. coli: Neonatal scours	Trimethoprim/S* (OD**, Inj) Colistin (Sow vaccination)	Neomycin, Apramycin (OD)	Amoxicillin (OD, Inj) Amoxicillin/clavulanate (Inj) Cephalosporins*** (Inj), Fluoroquinolone (OD, Inj)***
Piglet scours	Colistin (OD)	Neomycin, Trimethoprim/S* (OD; Inj)	As above
Post-weaning diarrhoea	Zinc oxide (IF)	Colistin (IF, IW), Neomycin (IF, IW) Trimethoprim/S* (IF, IW)	As above
MMA syndrome	Trimethoprim/S*(Inj)	Amoxicillin (Inj) Ampicillin (Inj)	As above
Salmonella spp: Diarrhoea	Colistin (IW, IF)	Neomycin (IF, IW) Trimethoprim/S* (IF, IW) Spectinomycin (IF, IW)	As above
Septicaemia	Trimethoprim/S (Inj)	Amoxicillin (Inj)	As above
C. perfringens: Necrotic enteritis	Penicillin (Inj) (Sow vaccination)	Amoxicillin (Inj)	Amoxicillin/clavulanate (Inj) Tylosin (Inj)
L. intracellularis: Ileitis	Pleuromutilins (Inj, IW, IF) (Pig vaccination)	Tetracyclines (IW, IF)	Tylosin (Inj), Macrolides (IW, IF) Lincomycin (IW, IF)
PHE	Tiamulin (Inj)	Tylosin (Inj)	
B. hyodysenteriae: Swine dysentery	Pleuromutilins (Inj, IW, IF)	Lincomycin (Inj, IW, IF)	Macrolides (Inj, IW, IF)
B. pilosicoli: Colitis	Pleuromutilins (Inj, IW, IF)	Lincomycin (Inj, IW, IF)	Macrolides (Inj, IW, IF)
M. hyopneumoniae: Enzootic pneumonia	Pleuromutilins (Inj, IW, IF) (Pig vaccination)	Tetracyclines (Inj, IW, IF) Lincomycin (Inj, IW, IF)	Macrolides (Inj, IW, IF)

Continued

Table 7.13 (Continued)

Infection/disease	First choice	Second choice	Last resort
P. multocida:			
Pneumonia	Penicillin (Inj)	Florfenicol (Inj)	Amoxicillin (Inj, IW, IF)
	Penethamate (Inj)	Tulathromycin (Inj)	
		Trimethoprim/S* (Inj, IW, IF)	
		Tetracyclines (Inj, IW, IF)	
A. pleuropneumoniae:			
Pleuropneumonia	Penicillin (Inj)	Florfenicol (Inj)	Amoxicillin (Inj, IW, IF)
	Penethamate (Inj)	Tulathromycin (Inj)	Cephalosporins***,
		Tetracycline (Inj, IW, IF)	Fluoroquinolone (Inj)***
	(Pig vaccination)	Trimethoprim/S* (Inj, IW, IF)	Tilmicosin (IF)
H. parasuis:			
Glässer's disease	Penicillin (Inj)	Florfenicol (Inj)	Amoxicillin
	(Pig vaccination)	Tetracycline (Inj, IW, IF)	Amoxicillin/
		Trimethoprim/S* (Inj, IW, IF)	clavulanate, Florfenicol
S. suis:			
Meningitis	Penicillin (Inj, IW, IF)	Amoxicillin, (Inj, IW, IF)	
		Trimethoprim/S* (Inj, IW, IF)	
E. rhusiopathiae:			
Erysipelas	Penicillin (Inj)	Amoxicillin (Inj, IW, IF)	
	(Sow/pig vaccination)		
M. hyosynoviae:			
Arthritis	Tiamulin (Inj, IW, IF)	Lincomycin (Inj, IW, IF)	

*Trimethoprim/sulfonamides on US critical antimicrobial list, but widely used in the rest of the world in pig medicine.
**Inj – injectable; OD – oral dosing; IW – in water; IF – in feed.
***Wherever possible, the use of fluoroquinolones and cephalosporins should be reserved for human use.

ampicillin, streptomycin, sulfonamides and tetracyclines. However, it is not possible to predict for *E. coli* whether an isolate is susceptible or resistant, and choice of empiric treatment has to be made on the basis of knowledge of the individual herd and local data on resistance patterns. This is why routine submission of samples to a microbiological laboratory is important to generate records on susceptibility data.

The MICs for *B. hyodysenteriae* and *B. pilosicoli* are very low for pleuromutilins (valnemulin and tiamulin), and although resistance has now been reported in a number of EU countries to a few strains (see Table 7.5), one would expect over 90% of isolates to be susceptible. Pleuromutilins are not used in human medicine and apparently do not cross-select for resistance to critically important antimicrobials. Accordingly, these antimicrobials should be regarded as the first choice for treatment of swine dysentery colitis enteritis associated with *Brachyspira* spp. Lincomycin achieves much higher levels in the colon, so much higher MICs are found, but most isolates (>70%) would be resistant to tylosin. Some authors

(54) consider that both organisms are so commonly resistant to tylosin and lincomycin that these antimicrobials cannot be recommended.

Pleuromutilins are also the drugs of choice for treatment of *L. intracellularis* infections (Table 7.13). This bacterium grows inside the cell and MIC testing requires growth in cell cultures. This is not an easy or possibly sensitive procedure. Mackie (55) looked at the effects of antimicrobial concentrations in the culture fluid and their effects on inhibition of growth of the organism inside the cell. Not all were titrated to their lowest concentration. A recent study (56), which titrated eight US and EU isolates down to 0.125 μg/ml, showed that tiamulin, valnemulin and carbadox were highly active, and that lincomycin, tylosin and chlortetracycline had a more variable activity.

Clostridium perfringens is very susceptible to penicillin (first choice) and tylosin (second choice), whereas there is a variable degree of susceptibility to tiamulin, lincomycin and tetracycline. *Clostridium difficile* seems to show some susceptibility to macrolides and virginiamycin (57).

Respiratory/systemic diseases

The variability in susceptibility/resistance patterns of the various respiratory and systemic bacterial pathogens is shown in Tables 7.6–7.12. Culture and susceptibility testing of *Mycoplasma* species is difficult and only carried out at a few reference laboratories (see Table 7.6). However, *M. hyopneumoniae*, *M. hyosynoviae* and *M. hyorhinis* are generally susceptible to tiamulin, whereas low levels of resistance have been reported towards tylosin, tilmicosin, lincomycin, tetracycline and fluoroquinolones (58).

A. pleuropneumoniae is generally susceptible to all commonly used antimicrobials, including the penicillins, which should therefore be considered as the first choice antimicrobial for treating this pathogen. Teale *et al.* (59) reported on porcine isolates submitted for diagnostic investigation to the Veterinary Laboratories Agency in the UK between 1999 and 2002 (see Table 7.7). Resistance was measured by the Kirby-Bauer disc method using a 13 mm-diameter as the breakpoint for ceftiofur resistance. This differs from the CLSI (formerly NCCLS) definition of resistance, which is based on a higher zone interpretive breakpoint ($R \leq 17$ mm).

Penicillins also remain very active against *S. suis*, *E. rhusiopathiae* and *A. pyogenes*. Some resistance to ampicillin, trimethoprim/sulfonamide and tetracycline is shown by *A. pleuropneumoniae* and, in uncontrollable resistance situations, the fluoroquinolones or cephalosporins have been effectively used by injection. However, these antimicrobials should be used as last resorts, limited to the hypothetical situations in which the target strain is resistant to all first, second and third choice drugs listed in Table 7.13. High MICs of penicillins and tetracyclines have been reported among *A. pleuropneumoniae* isolates in North America (60), but there does not appear to be any resistance to trimethoprim/sulfonamide, tilmicosin, florfenicol, enrofloxacin and ceftiofur. *P. multocida* can also be resistant to penicillin, tetracyclines or tilmicosin, but is generally susceptible to trimethoprim/sulfonamide, florfenicol, enrofloxacin or ceftiofur (Table 7.8). Trimethoprim/sulfonamide is not available as a feed premix or water soluble in the USA for use in pigs, which may account for its high activity, in contrast to tetracyclines, which are also commonly used in the EU. Fluoroquinolones are also not licensed for use in swine in the USA, which may account for their lack of resistance, but ceftiofur is widely available and no resistance is displayed.

When evaluating data on antimicrobial susceptibility, it is very important to take into consideration the methods and breakpoints used to measure resistance. Guttierez-Martin *et al.* (61) reported on the susceptibility of 229 Spanish isolates of *A. pleuropneumoniae*, which had been isolated between 1997 and 2004. They used a microdilution doubling-dilution technique and resistance was based on CLSI interpretation. The levels of penicillin resistance differed substantially depending on the interpretive breakpoint used. High prevalence (99%) of resistance to penicillin was recorded according to the lower MIC breakpoint (Table 7.9), suggesting that penicillin was likely to be ineffective if given by the oral route. However, the higher breakpoint indicated that possibly only 15% of the strains would be resistant if penicillin was given by injection, as much higher blood levels are achieved by this administration route. There would appear to be a very high level of resistance to the tetracyclines in Spain, similar to the USA.

Penicillin is active against most strains (>90%) of *S. suis*, (60) and resistance to trimethoprim/sulfonamide, florfenicol and ceftiofur has never been reported. In Europe, *S. suis* often shows MICs of fluoroquinolones close to the breakpoint and thus these antimicrobials cannot be recommended (62). Similarly, tetracyclines and macrolides are scarcely active against this Gram-positive pathogen (Table 7.10).

H. parasuis is generally susceptible even to the more commonly used antimicrobials such as penicillin, although low-level resistance to tetracycline has been reported (Table 7.10). Altogether, parenteral administration of penicillin is particularly useful for treating respiratory and systemic bacterial pathogens in pigs as it results in markedly higher serum concentrations compared with oral administration. However, unfortunately, in the USA no injectable formulations of penicillins are labelled for use in pigs and this factor limits the use of these antibiotics.

Others

Staphylococcus hyicus can be quite a difficult condition to treat on some farms (Table 7.12) and the occurrence of resistance varies considerably between countries (62). Resistances to macrolides, tetracyclines, penicillin, streptomycin or sulfonamides are frequently observed in most countries. Thus, like for *E. coli*, resistance in *S. hyicus* is difficult to predict and choice of the most appropriate antimicrobial drug for empiric treatment has to be done on the basis of knowledge of the individual herd and data on susceptibility at the farm level.

7.4 Conclusions

Antimicrobials are, and will be, essential to maintain the health, welfare and productivity of pigs. It is critical to retain the use and maintain the effectiveness of the antimicrobials that are currently available to combat current and future disease problems as they arise. There is therefore a responsibility on behalf of the users of these medicines to preserve their efficacy. If antimicrobials are withdrawn, as has been seen in the USA with fluoroquinolones for poultry, they will never be restored and important last resort drugs will be lost for future use in veterinary medicine. The responsibility lies with the veterinarians or the farmers, depending on the national legislation, to use antimicrobials in a responsible way, to minimise their use and seek alternatives without compromising the health of the animal.

References

1. Anonymous (2006). Farms, land in farms and livestock operations, 2005 Summary, Agriculture Statistics Board, National Agricultural Statistical Service, USDA, 34–5. Available at: http://usda.mannlib.cornell.edu/usda/nass/FarmLandIn//2000s/2006/FarmLandIn-01-31-2006.pdf2 Accessed on: May 2007.
2. Anonymous (2005). Pork Powerhouses, 2005. Successful farming, http://www.agriculture.com/ag/pdf/2005-pork-powerhouses.pdf, 16 October. Accessed on: May 2007.
3. Vivash-Jones, B. (2000). COMISA report. The year in review. COMISA, Brussels, Belgium.
4. Veterinary Medicines Directorate (2005). Sales of antimicrobial products authorised for use as veterinary medicines, antiprotozoals, antifungals, growth promoters and coccidiostats, in the UK in 2004 (ed. Goodyear, K.). Veterinary Medicines Directorate, New Haw, Surrey, UK.
5. SVARM, 2005 (2006). Use of antimicrobials. In *Swedish veterinary resistance monitoring* (eds. Bengtsson, B., Greko, C. and Grönlund-Andersson, U.). National Veterinary Institute, Uppsala, Sweden, pp. 8–12.
6. Danmap 2004 (2005). Antimicrobial consumption. In *Use of Antimicrobial Agents and Occurrence of Antimicrobial Resistance in Bacteria from Food Animals, Foods and Humans in Denmark* (eds. Emborg, H.-D., Heuer, O.E. and Larsen, P.B.). Danish Zoonosis Centre and Danish Institute for Food and Veterinary Research, Søborg, Denmark, pp. 15–22.
7. Grave, K., Jensen V.F., Odensvik, K. Wierup, M. and Bangen, M. (2006). Usage of veterinary therapeutic antimicrobials in Denmark, Norway and Sweden following termination of antimicrobial growth promoter use. *Prev. Veter. Med.* 75 (1–2): 123–32.
8. Nielsen, J.P. and Stege, H.S. (2006). Consumption of prescribed antimicrobials after the growth promoter termination in Denmark. *Proceedings of the 19th International Pig Veterinary Society Congress.* Copenhagen, Denmark, 1: 191.
9. Danmap 2005 (2006). Antimicrobial consumption. In *Use of Antimicrobial Agents and Occurrence of Antimicrobial Resistance in Bacteria from Food Animals, Foods and Humans in Denmark* (eds. Heuer, O.E. and Hammerum, A.E.). Danish Institute for Food and Veterinary Research and Danish Zoonosis Centre, Søborg, Denmark, pp. 15–16.
10. Animal Health Institute (1995). *Feed Additive Compendium.* The Miller Publishing Company, Minnetonka, Minnesota, USA.
11. Anonymous (1999). Proposed rules. *US Federal Register* 64 (127): 35966–72.
12. Anonymous (2002). Extralabel drug use in animals. *21 Code of Federal Register*, Chapter 1, part 530.II. 4/1/2002 Edition. US Federal Government, Washington DC.
13. Harris, D.L. (2000). Exclusion and elimination of microbes. In *Multi-site Pig Production* (ed. Harris, D.L.). Iowa State University Press, Ames, Iowa, USA, pp. 57–78.
14. Nielsen, P. (1997). The influence of feed on the oral bioavailability of antibiotics/chemotherapeutics in pigs. *J. Vet. Pharmacol. Ther.* 20 (Supplement 1): 30–1.
15. Veterinary Laboratories Agency (VLA) (2005). Antimicrobial sensitivity in Salmonella. In *Salmonella in Livestock Production in GB – 2004* (eds. Davies, R. and Kidd, S.A.). VLA, Weybridge, UK, pp. 144–55.
16. Annual report on zoonoses – http://www.dfvdk/Default.aspx?ID=9202#74145, Accessed on: May 2007.
17. Barza, M. and Travers, K. (2002). Excess infections due to antimicrobial resistance: the 'Attributable Fraction'. *Clin. Infect. Dis.* 34 (Suppl 3): S126–30.
18. Holmberg, S.D., Wells, J.G. and Cohen, M.L. (1984). Animal-to-man transmission of antimicrobial-resistant *Salmonella*: investigations of U.S. outbreaks, 1971–1983. *Science* 225: 833–5.
19. Lee, L.A., Puhr, N.D., Maloney, E.K., Bean, N.H. and Tauxe, R.V. (1994). Increase in antimicrobial-resistant Salmonella infections in the United States, 1989–1990. *J. Infect. Dis.* 170: 128–34.
20. Martin, L.J., Fyfe, M., Dore, K., *et al.* (2004). Multiprovincial *Salmonella typhimurium* case–control study steering committee. Increased burden of illness associated with antimicrobial-resistant *Salmonella enterica* serotype *typhimurium* infections. *J. Infect. Dis.* 189: 377–84.
21. Varma, J.K., Mølbak, K., Barrett, T.J., *et al.* (2005). Antimicrobial-resistant nontyphoidal *Salmonella* is associated with excess bloodstream infections and hospitalizations. *J. Infect. Dis.* 191: 554–61.

22. Helms, M., Vastrup, P., Gerner-Smidt, P. and Mølbak, K. (2002). Excess mortality associated with antimicrobial drug-resistant *Salmonella typhimurium*. *Emerg. Infect. Dis.* 8: 490–5.

23. Helms, M., Simonsen, J. and Mølbak, K. (2004). Quinolone resistance is associated with increased risk of invasive illness or death during infection with *Salmonella* serotype Typhimurium. *J. Infect. Dis.* 190: 1652–4.

24. Burch, D.G.S. (2002). Risk assessment – Campylobacter infection transmission from pigs to man using erythromycin resistance as a marker. *Pig J.* 50: 53–8.

25. Wesley, I.V., Muraoka, W.T., Trampel, D.W. and Hurd, H.S. (2005). Effect of preslaughter events on prevalence of *Campylobacter jejuni* and *Campylobacter coli* in market-weight turkeys. *Appl. Environ. Microbiol.* 71 (6): 2824–33.

26. Kramer, J.M., Frost, J.A., Bolton, F.J. and Wareing, D.R.A. (2000). Campylobacter contamination of raw meat and poultry at retail sale: identification of multiple types and comparison with isolates from human infection. *J. Food Prod.* 63 (12): 1654–59.

27. Hopkins, K.L., Desai, M., Frost, J.A., Stanley, J and Logan, J.M.L. (2004). Fluorescent amplified fragment length polymorphism genotyping of *Campylobacter jejuni* and *Campylobacter coli* strains and its relationship with host specificity, serotyping and phage typing. *J. Clin. Microbiol.* 42 (1): 229–35.

28. Helms, M., Simonsen, J., Olsen, K.E. and Molbak K. (2005). A study of adverse health events associated with antimicrobial drug resistance in *Campylobacter* species: a registry-based cohort study. *J. Infect. Dis.* 191 (7): 1050–5.

29. Teale, C. (2002). Antimicrobial resistance in porcine bacteria. *Pig J.* 49: 52–69.

30. Barlow, A.M., Hunt, B.W., Heath, P.J. and Smith, R.M.M. (2003). The prevalence and clinical diseases caused in pigs by different serotypes of *Streptococcus suis* (June 2000 to September 2002) and human infection (1981 to October 2002) in England and Wales. *Pig J.* 51: 164–76.

31. Yu, H., Jing, H., Chen, Z., *et al.* (2006). *Streptococcus suis* study groups. Human *Streptococcus suis* outbreak, Sichuan, China. *Emerg. Infect. Dis.* 12 (6): 914–20.

32. Ye, C., Zhu, X., Jing, H., *et al.* (2006). *Streptococcus suis* sequence type 7 outbreak, Sichuan, China. *Emerg. Infect. Dis.* 12 (8): 1203–8.

33. Moodley, A., Stegger, M., Bagcigil, A. F., *et al.* (2006). PFGE and *spa* typing of methicillin-resistant *Staphylococcus aureus* isolated from domestic animals and veterinary staff in the UK and Ireland. *J. Antimicrob. Chemother.* 58: 1118–23.

34. Voss, A., Loeffen, F., Bakker, J., Klaassen, C. and Wulf, M. (2005). Methicillin-resistant *Staphylococcus aureus* in pig farming. *Emerg. Infect. Dis.* 11 (12): 1965–6.

35. Wulf, M.W.H., Van Nes, A., Eiklenboom-Boskamp, A., *et al.* (2006). MRSA-prevalence in Dutch veterinarians and veterinary students. *Proceedings 19th International Pig Veterinary Society Congress.* Copenhagen, Denmark, 1: 193.

36. de Neeling, A.J., van den Broek, M.J.M., Spalburg, E.C., *et al.* (2007). High prevalence of methicillin resistant *Staphylococcus aureus* in pigs. *Vet. Microbiol.* 122 (3–4): 366–72.

37. Guardabassi, L., Stegger, M. and Skov, R. (2007). Retrospective detection of methicillin resistant and susceptible *Staphylococcus aureus* ST398 in Danish slaughter pigs. *Vet. Microbiol.* 122 (3–4): 384–6.

38. Armand-Lefevre, L., Ruimy, R. and Andremont, A. (2005). Links clonal comparison of *Staphylococcus aureus* isolates from healthy pig farmers, human controls and pigs. *Emerg. Infect. Dis.* 11 (5): 711–4.

39. Witte, W., Strommenger, B., Stanek, S. and Cuny, C. (2007). Methicillin-resistant *Staphylococcus aureus* ST398 in humans and animals, Central Europe. *Emerg. Infect. Dis.* 13: 255–8.

40. Baker, R.B. (2005). Strategies and techniques for disease eradication: eradication of multiple diseases from herds. *Proceedings of the 4th International Swine Disease Eradication Symposium, Allen D. Leman Conference,* Saint Paul, Minnesota, 17–20 September 2005, 1–5.

41. Harris, D.L. and Alexander, T.J.L. (1999). Methods of disease control. In *Diseases of Swine, 8th edn* (eds. Straw, D'Allaire, Mengeling and Taylor). Iowa State University Press, Ames Iowa, pp. 1077–110.

42. Hennecken, M., Stegeman, J.A., Elbers, A.R., van Nes. A., Smak, J.A. and Verheijden, J.H. (2000). Transmission of classical swine fever virus by artificial insemination during the 1997–1998 epidemic in The Netherlands: a descriptive epidemiological study. *Vet. Quart.* 22 (4): 228–33.

43. Guerin, B. and Pozzi, N. (2005). Viruses in boar semen: detection and clinical as well as epidemiological consequences regarding disease transmission by artificial insemination. *Theriogenology* 63 (2): 556–72.

44. Brumm, M. (2004). Housing decisions for the growing pig. *Proceedings of the London Swine Conference – Building Blocks for the Future 1–2 April, 2004,* 31–44.

45. Moore, C. (2003). Parity segregations, successes and pitfalls. *Proceedings of the A.D.Leman Conference,* Minneapolis, MN, USA, 36–42.

46. Main, R.G., Dritz, S.S., Tokach, M.D., Goodband, R.D. and Nelssen, J.L. (2004). Increasing weaning age improves pig performance in a multisite production system. *J. Anim. Sci.* 82 (5): 1499–1507.

47. Wathes, C and Whitehouse, C. (2006). Environmental management of pigs. In *Whittemore's Science and Practice of Pig Production* (eds. Kyriazakis, I. and Whittemore, C.T.). Blackwell Publishing, Oxford, UK, pp. 533–90, Chapter 17.

48. Muirhead, M.R. and Alexander, T.J.L. (eds.) (1997). Reproduction non-infectious infertility. In *Managing Pig Health and the Treatment of Disease: A Reference for the Farm.* 5M Enterprises, Sheffield, UK, pp. 140–1.

49. Pesente, P., Rebonato, V., Sandri, G., Giovanardi, D., Ruffoni, L.S. and Torriani, S. (2006). Phylogenetic analysis of ORF5 and ORF7 sequences of porcine reproductive and respiratory syndrome virus (PRRSV) from PRRS-positive Italian farms: a showcase for PRRSV epidemiology and

its consequences on farm management. *Vet. Microbiol.* 114 (3–4): 214–24.

50. Thacker, E. and Thacker, B. (2000). Factors affecting *Mycoplasma hyopneumoniae* vaccine efficacy. *Proceedings of the 16th International Pig Veterinary Society Congress.* Melbourne 17–20 September 2000, 164.

51. Jayappa, H., Davis, R., Rapp-Gabrielson, V., Wasmoen, T., Thacker, E.L. and Thacker, B. (2001). Evaluation of efficacy of *M. hyopneumoniae* bacterin following vaccination of young pigs in the presence of varying levels of maternal antibodies. *Proceedings of the American Association of Swine Veterinarians,* March 2001, pp. 237–41.

52. Brockmeier S.L., Halbur, P.G. and Thacker, E.L. (2002). Porcine respiratory disease complex. In *Polymicrobial Diseases* (eds. Kim A. Brogden and Janet M. Guthmiller). ASM Press, Washington, DC, USA, pp. 231–59.

53. Desrosiers, R., Clark, E., Tremblay, D. and Tremblay, R. (2007). *Proceedings 38th American Association of Swine Veterinarians annual Meeting,* March 2007. Orlando, USA, pp. 143–5.

54. Franklin, A., Pringle, M. and Hampson, D.J. (2006). Antimicrobial resistance in *Clostridium* and *Brachyspira* spp. and other anaerobes. In *Antimicrobial Resistance in Bacteria of Animal Origin* (ed. Aarestrup, F.M.). ASM Press, Washington, DC, pp. 127–44.

55. Mackie, R.A. (1996). Masters by Research Thesis: 'An *in vitro* study of antimicrobial agents against the obligately intracellular bacterium *Lawsonia intracellularis*.' University of Edinburgh, Scotland.

56. Wattanaphansak, S., Gebhart, C., Singer, R. and Dau, D. (2007). *In-vitro* testing of antimicrobial agents for *Lawsonia intracellularis*. *Proceedings 38th American Association of Swine Veterinarians Meeting,* Orlando, USA, 255–6.

57. Post, K.W. and Songer, J.G. (2002). Antimicrobial susceptibility of *Clostridium difficile* isolated from neonatal pigs. *Proceedings 17th International Pig Veterinary Society Congress,* Ames, Iowa, USA, 2, 62.

58. Aarestrup, F.M. and Kempf, I. (2006). Mycoplasma. In *Antimicrobial Resistance in Bacteria of Animal Origin* (ed. Aarestrup, F.M.). ASM Press, Washington, DC, pp. 239–48.

59. Teale, C.J., Martin, P.K. and Watkins, G.H. (2004). *VLA Antimicrobial Sensitivity Report 2003.* Crown Copyright Unit, Norwich, UK.

60. Salmon, S., Portis, E. and Lindeman, C. (2003). Minimum inhibitory concentrations for Ceftiofur and comparator antimicrobial agents against bacterial pathogens of swine. *Proceedings of the American Association of Swine Veterinarians Congress,* Orlando, Florida, USA, pp. 235–9.

61. Gutierrez-Martin, C.B., del Blanco, N.G., Blanco, M., Navas, J. and Rodríguez-Ferri, F.E. (2006). Changes in antimicrobial susceptibility of *Actinobacillus pleuropneumoniae* isolated from pigs in Spain during the last decade. *Vet. Microbiol.* 115: 218–22.

62. Aarestrup, F.M. and Schwarz, S. (2006). Staphylococci and streptococci. In *Antimicrobial Resistance in Bacteria of Animal Origin* (ed. Aarestrup, F.M.). ASM Press, Washington, DC, pp. 187–206.

63. Karlsson, M., Oxberry, S.L. and Hampson, D.J. (2002). Antimicrobial susceptibility testing of Australian isolates of *Brachyspira hyodysenteriae* using a new broth dilution method. *Vet. Microbiol.* 84: 123–33.

64. Cizek, A., Lobova, D. and Smola, J. (2002). *In vitro* susceptibility of *Brachyspira hyodysenteriae* strains isolated in the Czech Republic from 1996–2001. *Proceedings 17th International Pig Veterinary Society Congress.* Ames, Iowa, USA, 2, 191.

65. Kinyon, J.M., Murphy, D., Stryker, C., Turner, V., Holck, J.T. and Duhamel, G. (2002). Minimum inhibitory concentration for US swine isolates of *Brachyspira pilosicoli* to valnemulin and four other antimicrobials. *Proceedings 17th International Pig Veterinary Society Congress.* Ames, Iowa, USA, **2,** 50.

66. Dutta, G.N. and Devriese, L.A. (1980). Susceptibility of *Clostridium perfringens* of animal origin to fifteen antimicrobial agents. *J. Vet. Pharmacol. Therap.* 3: 227–36.

67. Devriese, L.A., Daube, G., Hommez, J. and Haesebrouck, F. (1993). *In vitro* susceptibility of *Clostridium perfringens* isolated from farm animals to growth-enhancing antibiotics. *J. Appl. Bacteriol.* 75: 55–7.

68. Hannan, P.C.T., Windsor, G.D., de Jong, A., Schmeer, N. and Stegeman, M. (1997). Comparative susceptibilities of various animal-pathogenic mycoplasmas to fluoroquinolones. *Antimicrob. Agents Chemother.* 41 (9): 2037–40.

69. Vicca, J., Stakenborg, T., Maes, D., *et al.* (2004). *In-vitro* susceptibilities of *Mycoplasma hyopneumoniae* field isolates. *Antimicrob. Agents Chemother.* 48 (11): 4470–2.

70. Trigo, E., Mendez-Trigo, A.V. and Simonson, R. (1996). Antimicrobial susceptibility profiles of *Haemophilus parasuis*. A retrospective study from clinical cases submitted during 1994 and 1995 to a veterinary diagnostic laboratory. *Proceedings of the 14th International Pig Veterinary Society Congress.* Bologna, Italy, 313.

71. Aarestrup, F.A., Seyfarth, A.M. and Angen, O. (2004). Antimicrobial susceptibility of *Haemophilus parasuis*, and *Histophilus somni* from pigs and cattle in Denmark. *Vet. Microbiol.* 101: 143–6.

Chapter 8

Guidelines for antimicrobial use in poultry

Ulrich Löhren, Antonia Ricci and Timothy S. Cummings

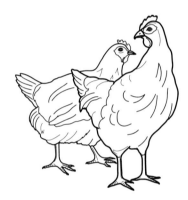

8.1 Antimicrobial use in poultry

Antimicrobial agents used in poultry include growth promoters, coccidiostats and antimicrobials for therapeutic or prophylactic use. All these forms of antimicrobial treatment are briefly described in the following sections.

8.1.1 Growth promoters

Antimicrobials were first used for growth promotion purposes as early as the late 1940s when it was discovered that chickens grew faster when fed tetracycline fermentation by-products. Subsequently, other antimicrobials were approved for growth promotion and performance enhancement over the years. Initially, antimicrobials like tetracyclines, tylosin and bacitracin could be used in poultry at low concentrations as feed additives for 'growth promotion', whereas higher dosages were restricted to veterinary use.

The Swann report (1) that was published in 1969 recommended that therapeutic antimicrobials should not be used as growth promoters. This resulted in most countries adapting their legislation over time, so that certain antimicrobial products were either banned or had to be used either as feed additives (without veterinarian prescription) or as therapeutic products under veterinarian prescription only. This attitude was more or less strictly applied by all food animal producing countries of Western Europe and North America.

In the mid-1990s, certain poultry integrators in Europe made significant efforts to improve hygiene, disinfection and biosecurity to reduce bacterial loads as a precursor to reducing the use of antimicrobial growth promoters. In 1997, avoparcin was banned from use in the EU, followed by the ban of other antimicrobial growth promoters (virginiamycin, bacitracin, spiramycin and tylocin) in 1999. Following the precautionary principle, the use of growth promoters was prohibited in the EU because it was liable to induce resistance to antimicrobial drugs used in human medicine. In 2006, all remaining growth promoters were banned from use in animal feeds in the EU, but the USA and other Third Countries have not introduced similar restrictions. These actions have been strenuously debated due to the lack of conclusive scientific evidence to support all the bans, but the overall worldwide usage of antimicrobial use as growth promoters is a downwards trend (2).

8.1.2   Coccidiostats

Intensive production of commercial poultry over the past 60 years has been largely due to the introduction of coccidiostats in the feed. These products interfere with various stage(s) of intestinal development of the coccidia. In the early days, sulfonamides were primarily used as coccidiostats, and they are still registered for veterinary prescription for therapy of coccidiosis. The vast majority of coccidiostats are regulated by feed legislation as feed additives. In the 1980s, a new group of coccidiostats was added: the polyether ionophores. The main target and purpose of ionophores is coccidiosis control, but this group also has limited antibacterial activity, especially against *Clostridium*. For this reason, ionophores were and are used almost exclusively as coccidiostats. Their significance has increased in the EU since antimicrobial growth promoters were banned. Worldwide, ionophores are still the mainstay of most programmes for the control of coccidiosis. Ionophores are not perceived as antimicrobials by most public health authorities, as these agents are not used in human medicine.

Live vaccines have been developed to prevent coccidiosis. These vaccines are a valuable tool for combating the loss of efficacy by coccidiostats against resistant *Eimeria* strains, and could eventually replace coccidiostats if the ionophores are banned as feed additives. There is circumstantial evidence that non-specific enteritis occurs more frequently in flocks vaccinated with live vaccines, as compared to flocks reared on ionophore coccidiostats, which has been associated with the cycling of the coccidial vaccine strains in the bird's intestine. For this reason, specific antimicrobial treatment can be needed if the enteritis becomes significant. Further steps into changing distribution and legislation on the use of coccidiostats should be carefully considered, as their removal could have significant implications for the poultry industries of the world.

8.1.3   Therapeutic antimicrobials

Antimicrobials for therapeutic use are, in most countries, regulated by specific veterinarian or pharmaceutical legislation. Their use in most countries is restricted to veterinarian prescription. Misuse and overuse of antimicrobials occurs more easily in countries where the farmer has easy access to antimicrobials not requiring veterinary prescription. In these cases, antimicrobials tend to be used on a trial and error basis (Donoghue, 2006; personal communication), in an effort to elicit a favourable response, which can be difficult to obtain or interpret depending upon the characteristics of the bacterial pathogen being treated (see Section 8.4).

In avian medicine, antimicrobials can be applied to the target animal by individual injection or oral application (to pet birds or valuable stocks only), or by mass application to the whole flock via drinking water (major way of administration) or feed (used on a limited basis). Individual injection or application (e.g. by oral gavage) will rarely be an option due to the sheer numbers of birds involved. The most practical method of application of therapeutic substances (including antimicrobials) is by oral administration, either via drinking water or feed. Whereas individual therapy in large animals is often done by the farmer himself, the owners of large poultry flocks are typically fully integrated, commercial poultry companies in industrialized nations. These companies often have veterinarians on staff or have access to qualified veterinary poultry expertise and diagnostic facilities to help make prudent therapeutic decisions. In these instances, therapeutic choices are made with economic, as well as efficacy and welfare, issues factoring into the decision, because medication of large groups of animals can be very costly.

In contrast to large animal practice, poultry veterinarians or the farmer can easily justify sacrificing a few sick birds or taking some fresh dead carcasses from the flock to a specialized diagnostic laboratory. There, a necropsy is typically performed with individual samples taken for cultivation and identification of the causative organism. Antimicrobial susceptibility patterns on any resultant isolate are routinely performed as well. Hence, the modern poultry veterinarian bases his diagnosis and resultant therapy on the clinical picture of the flock, bird pathology, bacteriology and history of the problem at hand. This is standard procedure for poultry medicine in large poultry producing regions of the world.

8 Poultry

It should be noted that actual treatment of poultry flocks has never been an extensive practice due to the relatively good health status of poultry flocks, the relatively few efficacious antimicrobials available for use and the prohibitive expense of medicating flocks. As a result, antimicrobial therapy of chicken flocks in the USA and Europe has been decreasing in recent years and a shift in the use of therapeutic antimicrobials has been observed in Europe (3). A small increase in the use of therapeutic antimicrobials coincided with the growth promoter ban, which was suggested as an undesirable side effect of the ban (4).

The issue of antimicrobial residues became more of a concern in the 1980s, so withdrawal times (different durations for the same product in different countries) for antimicrobials were introduced. From the beginning of antimicrobial residue testing, the poultry industry has always exercised responsible use of antimicrobials to allow for proper withdrawal times, as residues in edible tissues would have an impact on the use of all meat (or eggs) from the whole flock (instead of an individual animal) for human consumption. As a result, antimicrobial residues in poultry flocks at time of slaughter or in poultry meat (or eggs) have rarely been a problem.

In Europe, only those antimicrobials for which a MRL value (maximum residue level) according to the procedure laid down in regulation 2377/90 is set may be used in food delivering poultry flocks. Table 8.1 lists those antimicrobials for which a MRL value is set and therefore may be used in Europe. The withdrawal times are based on the MRL and on the different pharmacology of the antimicrobial molecules.

Although not a new debate, the concern about the rise of antimicrobial resistance in certain human pathogens began to surface again in the 1990s. Despite the general consensus that the increase in bacterial resistance in human medicine has been strongly associated with overuse by physicians (5), the legislative emphasis continues to focus on what extent the use of therapeutic antimicrobials in food animals has contributed to the increasing antimicrobial resistance issue in human medicine (6). Currently in the USA, legislation is routinely proposed to ban or limit antimicrobial use. The use of fluoroquinolones in poultry was banned in 2004. Many poultry companies are reducing antimicrobial use at the request of their customers or to meet export requirements.

There are a few other issues to be considered concerning the use of antimicrobials in poultry. There is a concern about the effectiveness of alternative approaches for therapy of diseased poultry flocks. These approaches are often less effective, and animal welfare considerations should also be respected. Although the commercial aspect of treating diseased flocks with antimicrobials should never compromise public health, neither should their removal be allowed without proper scientific evidence or carefully designed and interpreted risk assessments. On the other hand, antimicrobials should never be used for prophylactic purposes to substitute for poor hygiene or management.

8.1.4 Guidelines and codes of practice

With respect to the necessary therapeutic use of antimicrobials in food animals, codes of practice have been agreed upon by various national veterinary associations (7). Although such codes of practice are not as binding as legislation and are largely voluntary, they have made a big impact on the veterinary therapeutic use of antimicrobials in veterinary medicine (8). Most of these guidelines share common principles. A good example is the 'Guidelines for prudent use of antimicrobials in animals', which was published by the German Federal Veterinarians Association (BTK) and a Working Group of Senior Veterinarians (ArgeVet) in 2000 (9). The scope of these guidelines is to minimize the impact of antimicrobial usage on development of resistance in animals, and they should be regarded as the minimum requirement that must always be followed by veterinarians when administering antimicrobials to animals. The guidelines constitute the rules of veterinary science (good veterinary practice), which are to be complied with during any use of antimicrobials in animals, and which must be observed each and every time an animal (or a poultry flock) is treated properly in accordance with the national drug legislation. Antimicrobials should only be prescribed by veterinarians. They may be used by the animal (or poultry flock) owner only according to written instructions under veterinary supervision. The prescribing veterinarian must check this at suitable intervals by monitoring the success of treatment.

The use of antimicrobials is only justified for therapy if it has been proven by appropriate

Table 8.1 Major antimicrobial classes used in avian medicine

Antimicrobial class	Drug name	Type of activity	Intestine absorption	Spectrum of activity
Sulfonamides	Several compounds are available in this class	Bacteriostatic	Good	Gram + Gram −
Potentiated sulfonamides	Trimethoprim and sulfonamides	Bactericidal	Good	Gram + Gram −
Aminoglycosides	Apramycin	Bactericidal	Poor	Mainly Gram −
	Gentamicin	Bactericidal	None	Mainly Gram −
	Neomycin	Bactericidal	Poor	Mainly Gram −
	Spectinomycin	Bactericidal	Intermediate	Mainly Gram −
	Streptomycin	Bactericidal	Poor	Mainly Gram −
	Dihydrostrepto-mycin	Bactericidal	Poor	Mainly Gram −
β-Lactames	Benzylpenicillin Potassium Pen. G	Bactericidal	Good	Gram +
	Ampicillin	Bactericidal	Intermediate	Gram + (Gram −)
	Amoxicillin	Bactericidal	Good	Gram + (Gram −)
	Ceftiofur	Bactericidal	Cannot be given orally	Gram + Gram −
Fluoroquinolones	Enrofloxacin	Bactericidal	Very good	Gram ±
	Difloxacin	Bactericidal	Good	Gram ±
	Flumequin	Bactericidal	Good	Gram ±
Lincosamides	Lincomycin	Bacteriostatic	Good	Gram + *Mycoplasma*
Macrolides	Erythromycin	Bacteriostatic	Good	Gram − *Mycoplasma*
	Spiramycin	Bacteriostatic	Good	Gram − *Mycoplasma*
	Tylosin	Bacteriostatic	Good	Gram − Mycoplasma
	Timicosin	Bacteriostatic	Good	Gram − *Mycoplasma*
Pleuromutilines	Tiamulin	Bacteriostatic	Good	*Mycoplasma*
Polypeptides	Colistin sulfate	Bacteriocidal	None	Gram −
Tetracyclines	Tetracycline	Bacteriostatic	Intermediate	Gram ±
	Chlortetracycline	Bacteriostatic	Good	Gram ±
	Oxytetracycline	Bacteriostatic	Good	Gram ±
	Doxycycline	Bacteriostatic	Good	Gram ±

8 Poultry

diagnostic measures that the animals are infected by a pathogen susceptible to the antimicrobial that is to be administered. In veterinary practice, prophylaxis is only admissible in substantiated exceptional cases (immunosuppressed animals, long and/or elective surgery, etc.), which are *not* applicable to commercial poultry flocks. The diagnosis shall generally be based on identification of the pathogen and therapeutic options should be guided by susceptibility testing, knowledge of local resistance patterns, history of antimicrobial efficacy in the field, expense and relative importance of any antimicrobial options to human medicine. Diagnosis and susceptibility testing are always required when switching the therapy to another antimicrobial agent, when considering compounding (mixing of drugs for use in combination), or when using the antimicrobial in an extra-label manner (not used in compliance with the label instructions).

With respect to national legislation procedures, a solution needs to be found that enables the pharmaceutical producers to get easier registration of new claims for existing antimicrobials or new antimicrobials for food animals. This is especially true for species like chickens, which have been restricted in usage of many feed and/or water antimicrobials in some countries in recent years. Certain opportunities exist in some regions, where some poultry species (like turkeys and ducks) are considered a minor animal species. But a dilemma can present itself at times with regard to label claims. For example, enrofloxacin is one of the very few, highly efficacious, registered antimicrobials for specific diseases in turkeys in certain countries. However, this is also one of the critically important antimicrobial classes in human medicine (see Chapter 4) and according to most judicious guidelines one should first consider the use of antimicrobial products according to their label indications.

As alluded to earlier, previous guidelines on prudent use of antimicrobials are widely accepted in avian medicine. The development of these guidelines are timely and beneficial to the veterinary and medical professions as a whole, in addition to helping fulfil portions of the veterinarian's obligation to use scientific knowledge to promote public health and relieve animal suffering. Poultry veterinarians as a group are highly specialized, and have typically striven for a more precise clinical and microbiological diagnosis. Whereas in the past, in some countries, the use of antimicrobials has been regarded as a tool to control zoonotic bacterial infections like *Salmonella* in poultry, it is generally accepted that other measures should be used to control foodborne pathogens. EU Decision 1177/06 clearly states that antimicrobials may never be used as a control method within a specific *Salmonella* control programme. The EU poultry industry takes the lead and unanimously supports this legislation: no use of antimicrobials to control *Salmonella*. This has been the course of action in the USA as well, with Hazard Analysis Critical Control Point (HACCP) principles being implemented at the processing plants to reduce pathogen loads.

8.2   Major antimicrobials used in avian medicine

The most important antimicrobials used in avian medicine are listed in Table 8.1.

Sulfonamides are the oldest antimicrobials with minimal application significance in human medicine, and are therefore regarded as first choice products. Due to their toxicity, their small therapeutic scale and their longer withdrawal times, they are not used to a great extent. Potentiated sulfonamides (combinations with trimethoprim) are much more suitable for the same indications. They possess anticoccidial activity and should not be used within the first three weeks after live vaccination against coccidiosis.

Penicillins have been used for decades in human medicine. Some penicillins are inactivated by the presence of hydrochloric acid in the proventriculus. Only benzylpenicillin and penicillin V potassium can be given orally. Penicillins are first choice products against *Clostridium* infections in poultry. Ampicillin and amoxicillin belong to the group of aminopenicillins. Both are regarded as first choice antimicrobials in avian medicine, although they still have some impact in human medical usage. Their choice in avian medicine should be based on registration, withdrawal times and the degree of systematic efficacy, which is needed under the actual therapeutic situation. Both have limited solubility in higher concentrations (like that needed for dosatrons) and their stability in drinking water is limited. Solutions should be renewed every 8 h.

Polypeptides (like colistinsulfate or polymixin E) are used in human medicine mainly for topical application (too toxic for systemic use). They can therefore be considered in avian medicine as a first or second choice product. Their *in vitro* activity against Gram-positive bacteria remains excellent. Although not very well absorbed, some efficacy is seen in the field after a prolonged oral administration (minimum 1 week) against systematic *E. coli*. This may help to avoid the usage of third choice products like quinolones.

Lincosamides (available in combination with spectinomycin or as the sole antimicrobial) are used as a starter medication for broiler chicks in some countries, like the UK. This practice should not be encouraged.

Cephalosporins have a high importance in human medicine. They are therefore considered as third choice antimicrobial in avian medicine (product of last reserve). Their activity against both Gram-positive and Gram-negative bacteria is excellent. Because cephalosporins have to be injected, they are very rarely used with poultry and then only under very limited conditions and only with very valuable poultry stocks.

Among the *quinolones,* the first-generation product is flumequine and the second-generation products are enrofloxacin, difloxacin and norfloxacin. Flumequine is only registered in a few countries. Within the second-generation quinolones, enrofloxacin has by far the greatest significance in avian medicine. Because a closely related product (ciprofloxacin) is still considered as the drug of choice for many human bacterial diseases, these antimicrobial agents should be considered as product of last reserve (third choice product) in avian medicine. Quinolones are highly water soluble and can reach high tissue levels after oral application. If used in a rational way (10 mg/kg/body weight for minimum 3 days), the prevalence of resistance against these antimicrobials usually remains low.

8.3 Registration of antimicrobials for use in poultry

It is the intention of this book, as well as of the various national guidelines and Codes of practice, to encourage veterinarian use of 'first choice' products initially. These are products with an antibacterial spectrum as narrow as possible and/or with limited importance in human medicine. Many of these antimicrobials are older products, which often require re-registration in the light of higher registration standards. For this reason, some older products have lost their old general registration for poultry in some countries. Pharmaceutical producers will have to submit separate registration data for chicken (broilers, rearing pullets and layers) and for minor avian species like turkeys, ducks, geese and guineafowl. Unfortunately, many antimicrobials (especially those of first choice) are not registered for use in poultry in many countries. For example, in the Netherlands, there was until recently no oral penicillin (like benzylpenicillin or penicillin G) registered for any avian species. Hence, the poultry veterinarians have to go for a second choice product with broader spectrum like ampicillin or amoxicillin.

With regard to turkeys and ducks, these cannot be regarded as minor species. However, in most countries, older narrow-spectrum products are not registered for these species and only newer products with broader spectrum are available according to label claims. For example, in Germany, two fluoroquinolones (enrofloxacin and difloxacin) are registered for use in turkeys, while a first or second choice product should only be used in the framework of the guideline cascade. This is also true for ampicillin, amoxicillin, colistin, potentiated sulfonamides, tetracyclines and chlortetracycline, which all have no registration for turkeys. The situation is even worse for ducks. To safeguard the option of treating flocks of the so-called minor species (turkeys, ducks) with products of first or second choice, it would be highly beneficial if some type of international standard was adopted to provide a practical, streamlined process for registration of older antimicrobials or to obtain new label claims. This type of activity should most likely arise from an international agency such as European Medicines Agency (EMEA) or Codex Alimentarius (see Chapter 5).

With the relatively short lifespan of the meat-producing poultry species (broilers, turkeys and ducks), the withdrawal time is of importance for choosing the best antimicrobial. Many times, a health problem will develop just prior to processing, which significantly limits available therapeutic options. As a safety precaution, current legislation typically overestimates the importance of antimicrobial residues in meat products, but does not take into account the safeguard of critically important antimicrobial agents in human medicine. There is concern about the varying withdrawal times in different EU Member States for the same antimicrobial with the same EU MRL meat value, whereas the final poultry meat products can be traded globally in many countries without major restrictions. Certain anti-inflammatory substances, like acetylsalicylic acid, may be indicated under certain circumstances instead of an antimicrobial, but these are not registered for poultry in most countries.

8.4 Resistance trends in poultry pathogens and zoonotic bacteria

Antimicrobial resistance has been extensively studied in certain poultry pathogens and zoonotic bacteria. As far as *Salmonella* is concerned, the occurrence of resistance seems to have increased over the years, and is associated with the selective pressure exerted by the use of antimicrobials in poultry. There are large variations among regions, sectors and sources, and the ability to acquire resistance seems to vary between different serovars. Antimicrobial-resistant *Salmonella* are commonly isolated from different food animal species and food products throughout Europe (10). Over the last decade, clones of *Salmonella* with multiple drug resistance have been distributed widely in many European countries; in particular multiresistant *S.* Typhimurium definitive phage types (DTs) 204b and 104.

Data from the EU in 2005 (10), indicate that resistance to tetracycline is common in *Salmonella* strains from food animals. Resistance to streptomycin, sulfonamides and ampicillin were also often observed. Although fluoroquinolone resistance in many countries remains infrequent, resistance to nalidixic acid, which is an indicator of developing resistance to fluoroquinolones, was observed by most reporting countries. As regards *Salmonella* isolates from poultry in 2005, the highest proportions of isolates resistant to chloramphenicol, sulfonamides and tetracyclines were reported by the Netherlands and the UK. For *S.* Typhimurium, the highest levels of resistance among isolates from chickens were reported for ampicillin (up to 73.9%), sulfonamide (up to 69.6%) and tetracycline (up to 73.9%) (10).

Resistance to different types of antimicrobials, including quinolones, has become quite common among *S.* Typhimurium and many strains are multi-resistant (10). In several European countries as well as North America, a multi-resistant clone of *S.* Typhimurium DT 104 (MR-DT 104) became epidemic during the 1990s. MR-DT 104 has been isolated from many different food animals including poultry. It typically exhibits resistance to ampicillin, chloramphenicol, streptomycin, sulfonamides and tetracyclines (ACSSuT). Since the mid-1990s, the occurrence of resistance to quinolones has increased in MR-DT104 isolates. In the UK, the emergence of quinolone-resistant MR-DT104 in poultry, cattle, pigs and humans followed soon after the licensing of enrofloxacin for use in food-production animals.

In contrast to *S.* Typhimurium, *S.* Enteritidis isolates are, in general, susceptible to most antimicrobials. In poultry isolates of *S.* Enteritidis, in 2005, the highest level of resistance was reported for nalidixic acid (up to 51.2%). Resistance to tetracycline was generally low (from 0% to 10.5%). Italy was the only country to report resistance to ciprofloxacin and enrofloxacin. The proportions of resistant isolates were

0.2% and 0.8% respectively, in *Salmonella* spp. MS generally reported high proportions of fully sensitive *S.* Enteritidis isolates from chickens, ranging from 48.8% to 95.9%.

It should be noted that resistance to quinolones in *S.* Enteritidis from cases of human infection is emerging in many EU countries, and in poultry (11). In 2005, detection of nalidixic acid-resistant *S.* Enteritidis isolates from poultry was reported in Austria (3.9%), Germany (4.9%), Italy (34.3%) and the Netherlands (51.2%), in Denmark, resistance to nalidixic acid in *S.* Enteritidis increased from 0% in 2001 to 23% in 2002. Use of fluoroquinolones in food animals in Denmark decreased markedly in 2002 after several initiatives by the authorities (11). The increase in resistance was most likely a result of clonal spread caused by trade in day-old chicks carrying nalidixic acid-resistant *S.* Enteritidis. This illustrates how the association between usage of antimicrobials and occurrence of resistance may be confounded by other factors, such as transmission of resistant bacterial strains between premises. In 2002, fluoroquinolone resistance was detected in 1% of poultry *S.* Enteritidis isolates from Italy, 5% from Spain and 13% from Portugal.

In several EU countries since the 1990s, a significant increase in the prevalence of resistance to macrolides and fluoroquinolones among *Campylobacter* has been reported. This has been recognized as an emerging public health problem due to the ability of these bacteria to enter the food chain (13). In Norway in 2001, the prevalence of quinolone resistance among *Campylobacter* isolates from domestic poultry and from domestically acquired cases of campylobacteriosis in humans was low (2.7% versus 7%), as opposed to a high prevalence of quinolone resistance in isolates from imported human cases (60%) (12). In Australia, where fluoroquinolones have not been authorized for use in animals, indigenous fluoroquinolone resistant *Campylobacter* are not seen in human (15). In the USA, fluoroquinolone resistance in human *Campylobacter* isolates fluctuated between 13% and 18% (16). After an initial rise in resistance during the 1990s (14), the fluoroquinolone approval for use in poultry was withdrawn in 2004. Van Boven *et al.* (17) compared the selection of quinolone resistance in *C. jejuni* and *E. coli* in individually housed broilers, and demonstrated that treatment with enrofloxacin at doses routinely prescribed (50 ppm) rapidly reduced the faecal counts of *E.coli* below the detection limit, and did not induce resistance in this bacterial species.

However, the same treatment quickly selected for high frequencies of fluroquinolone-resistant strains of *C. jejuni*.

Resistance among clinical isolates of poultry *E. coli* can be high and multiple resistance is common, as demonstrated in studies from Spain and the USA (18, 19). In a collection of strains isolated from various types of poultry in the USA, 63% of the strains were found to harbour class 1 type integrons, mostly located in a transposon related to Tn*21* (19). In the USA, an increase in resistance to fluoroquinolones among avian pathogenic *E. coli* has been reported (21). In 2005, Zhao *et al.* (20) reported, in the USA, the presence of multiple antimicrobial-resistant phenotypes (≥3 antimicrobials) in 92% of *E. coli* isolated from diagnosed cases of avian colibacillosis. The majority of isolates displayed resistance to sulfamethoxazole (93%), tetracycline (87%), streptomycin (86%), gentamicin (69%) and nalidixic acid (59%). Fifty-six *E. coli* isolates displaying resistance to nalidixic acid were co-resistant to difloxacin (57%), enrofloxacin (16%), gatifloxacin (2%) and levofloxacin (2%). Similar data were previously reported by Bass *et al.* (19), who observed how the resistance to specific antimicrobials, like streptomycin, continued to be prevalent among avian *E. coli* isolate, despite the discontinuance of a given antimicrobial as a therapeutic agent. In this study, the presence of integrons among clinical isolates was demonstrated and linked to the presence of multiple-antimicrobial resistance with continued resistance to antimicrobials that have been withdrawn from use in poultry medicine. In Ireland, Cormican *et al.* (22) compared levels of antimicrobial resistance in pathogenic *E. coli* isolated from hens and from turkeys, and observed higher levels of resistance in turkeys, where antimicrobial use is more common. Resistance to sulfonamides, potentiated sulfonamides and nalidixic acid were more common in *E. coli* originating from turkeys. Ciprofloxacin resistance, at a level of 2.9%, was observed only in *E. coli* isolates from turkeys.

As far as *Staphylococcus* is concerned, Aarestrup *et al.* (23) tested 118 isolates from infections of poultry in Denmark for their susceptibility to 19 antimicrobial agents. All isolates were found susceptible to avoparcin, flavophospholipol, gentamicin, kanamycin, monensin, nitrofurantoin, oxacillin, salinomycin, trimethoprim and vancomycin. Seven per cent of *S. aureus* isolates and 35% of the novobiocin-resistant coagulase-negative staphylococci (CNoS) were

classified as resistant to bacitracin. A surprisingly high percentage of *S. aureus* (30%) were resistant to ciprofloxacin, whereas 24% were resistant to erythromycin and 19% to sulfamethoxazole.

Johansson *et al.* (24) performed a study to determine the *in vivo* susceptibility of *Clostridium perfringens* isolated from poultry to antimicrobials used in poultry production, including the ionophore coccidiostat narasin. Isolates were obtained from broilers, laying hens and turkeys in Sweden, Denmark and Norway. Tetracycline-resistance was the most common antimicrobial resistance trait found in *C. perfringens* in this study despite marked differences among the three countries, whereas all isolates proved to be susceptible to narasin. Three per cent of the Swedish isolates and 15% of the Danish isolates were resistant to bacitracin, and 13% of the Norwegian isolates were resistant to virginiamycin (a streptogramin). All isolates were susceptible to avilamycin, erythromycin, ampicillin and vancomycin, where negligible use of these substances occurred in poultry production in the investigated countries. Similarly, in the USA, avilamycin, avoparcin, penicillin and narasin were found to exhibit the most potent *in vitro* anti-clostridial activity on *C. perfringens* strains of avian origin (25).

Poultry products and farms have been implicated as a source of vancomycin-resistant *Enterococcus* (VRE) in humans (26). The role that non-human sources and reservoirs, other than hospitalized patients, may play in the spread of *Enterococcus* is controversial and poorly understood (27). In the USA, where glycopeptides have not been used for production animals, among *E. faecium* and *E. faecalis* isolated from 13 chicken and 8 turkey farms, none was resistant to vancomycin, whereas quinupristin/dalfopristin, gentamicin and ciprofloxacin resistance rates in *E. faecium* were 85%, 12% and 23% in chicken, and 52%, 13% and 24% in turkey isolates. Quinupristin/dalfopristin (streptogramin) resistance in *E. faecium* was more common on chicken and turkey farms using virginiamycin compared with farms not using a streptogramin. Ciprofloxacin resistance was more common on turkey farms using enrofloxacin compared with those with no enrofloxacin use (27). Conversely, it should be noted that one large, clinical study involving 28 000 human clinical isolates from 200 medical centres in the USA and Canada revealed streptogramin resistance to be 0.2% in *E. faecium* isolates despite decades of use of virginiamycin in the poultry industry (28). In Spain, no resistance to vancomycin, teicoplanin, penicillin or ampicillin was detected in *Enterococcus* isolated from poultry (29), but strains showed high-level aminoglycoside resistance for streptomycin (34.5%), kanamycin (27.3%) and gentamicin (7.3%).

Considering the fact that resistance trends in poultry pathogens may differ greatly from country to country, it is extremely interesting to compare data concerning resistance in different European countries with different patterns of antimicrobial use. When comparing data, different methods used (microdilution versus agar diffusion test), variances in susceptibility among different bacterial species of the same genus and various other factors must be taken into account. For example, antimicrobial susceptibility of *Ornithobacterium rhinotracheale* (ORT) shows great differences between geographical regions (30, 31). ORT is a respiratory pathogen in chicken and turkeys, and causes more problems in turkeys where it is regarded as primary pathogen. In chicken, ORT is often involved in respiratory problems as a secondary organism. Lister (31) reported susceptibility in *E. coli* (APEC) and *Pseudomonas* isolates from turkey in the UK. Data from 1996 and 2003–2005 did not show differences in susceptibility for *E. coli* (Table 8.2).

Bywater (32), when reviewing published literature, reported susceptibility patterns in zoonotic (*Salmonella, Campylobacter*) and indicator bacteria (*E. coli*) from poultry flocks in Sweden, France, the UK and the Netherlands. He concluded that the variation seen between countries could have resulted from differences in prescribing practices, in the disease distribution (resulting in differences in antimicrobial demand), or in clonal distribution of particular strains (e.g. *Salmonella*). Easy access to antimicrobials of third choice (like enrofloxacin) may lead to overuse with serious consequences on resistance development. Comparison over time between France (only original enrofloxacin product registered) and Spain (cheaper generic enrofloxacin products on the market) suggests that market dynamics can influence antimicrobial usage patterns and thus impact on antimicrobial resistance development (Table 8.3).

8.5 Good veterinary practices for antimicrobial use in poultry

Rational choice of antimicrobial agents should be based on clinical judgement and laboratory

Table 8.2 Antimicrobial susceptibility in *E. coli* and *Pseudomonas* isolates from poultry in the UK (31)

Antimicrobial drug	E. coli 1996 (%)	E. coli 2003–2005 (%)	Pseudomonas 2000–2005 (%)
Enrofloxacin	95	95	98
Ampicillin	58	62	4
Tetracyclin	21	32	35
Spectinomycin	95	95	72
Tylosin	3	0	0
Potentiated sulfonamides	55	80	12
Apramycin	96	98	100
Neomycin	89	95	84

Table 8.3 Enrofloxacin resistance in clinical *E. coli* isolates from poultry in Spain and France (35)

Spain		France	
1991–1995 $n = 338$	1996–2000 $n = 198$	1991–1995 $n = 154$	1996–2000 $n = 248$
10.3%	41.9%	7.1%	2.5%

diagnosis, including bacterial isolation and sensitivity testing (wherever possible), medical knowledge and experience, economic considerations, epidemiological background and information at the flock level. Antimicrobials should never replace fundamental shortcomings in poultry production such as biosecurity measures and proper hygiene. The administration of antimicrobials in disease situations is supportive of good farm management and properly designed immunization programmes (see Section 8.7).

The use of antimicrobials should meet the requirements of a valid veterinarian–client–patient relationship.

- The veterinarian assumes the responsibility for initiation of antimicrobial therapy and the farmer agrees to follow his instructions.
- The veterinarian is acquainted to the farm by regular visits.
- The veterinarian is available for follow-up evaluation and emergency visits.

Unless the clinical picture (signs, gross lesions) is pathognomonic, a flock diagnosis should be confirmed by laboratory testing. In urgent situations, a lab confirmation cannot be waited for before an antimicrobial treatment is initiated. In this case, the veterinarian will be guided by his professional knowledge and experience in similar situations. Susceptibility testing of the causative microorganism(s) in a representative bird sample (typically ill subjects, recent deaths), prior to or concurrently with the onset of medication, is common practice in avian medicine.

In contrast to antimicrobial use in individual human patients and in large animal practice, the avian medicine practitioner has to make use of antimicrobials in some instances for total flock medication, where often only a small percentage of birds may be showing clinical symptoms. Individual birds are not treated in the modern poultry industry. Although a diseased flock consists partially of sick and lethargic birds with varying degrees of symptoms, it is important to treat the flock as a whole to lower the infection pressure for flock mates.

Certain other principles pertaining to responsible antimicrobial usage include:

- The use of antimicrobials as soon as premonitory disease signs appear. The earlier in the disease process therapy is initiated, the better the chance of a favourable response. For intensively kept poultry, it is also vital to minimize the further spread of the disease to adjacent flocks and neighbouring farms.
- By minimizing bird morbidity and mortality with properly selected and timed antimicrobial therapy, the veterinarian also sustains improved animal welfare. Medication in anticipation of rising mortality and major disease damage is justifiable to minimize bird suffering as well as to improve performance.
- In addition to group medication, very sick birds, which will not drink enough of the medicated water, may be culled (broilers, rearing pullets) or individually treated (valuable breeder and turkey stocks) in some cases.
- The careful use of antimicrobials to anticipate developing disease in a flock should never be confused with, or serve as an excuse for, the injudicious use of antimicrobials in healthy flocks to cover shortcomings in hygiene and management.

Antimicrobial products should be administered according to the label directions established by the manufacturer and approved by the regulatory authority. Label directions encompass indications (claims) and dosage (dose, duration of application). The antimicrobial should always be used at full dose and never reduced in an attempt to save money. It is best for the antimicrobial dosage to be calculated on the basis of mg of active ingredient per kg bodyweight. In most broiler flocks, actual live weight can be seen on the display of automatic scales, which are today standard in modern broiler houses. For turkeys, the actual weight can be taken from the age and the growth profile of the breed. Replacement pullets and breeders are normally weighed every week. Modern poultry houses have water meters, so the amount of water to be consumed can be taken from the day before. Consideration needs to be made for the effect of temperature swings on water consumption patterns in poultry flocks:

- When choosing the appropriate antimicrobial, the veterinarian has to take into account: susceptibility results, withdrawal times, pharmacodynamic and pharmacokinetic properties.
- When different products come into consideration, the veterinarian should choose as first choice a narrow-spectrum antimicrobial or an antimicrobial with limited importance in human medicine.
- Treatment failures may occur if a low dosage or short duration of treatment is attempted.
- An unsatisfactory clinical outcome can also be triggered by concurrent immune suppressive viral diseases (Chicken Infectious Anemia, Gumboro, Reo, Marek), metabolic diseases, or too high infection pressure (overwhelming infections).

8.6 Disease-specific guidelines for antimicrobial use

The following sections provide guidelines for specific pathogens and diseases in poultry. As a rule, guidelines tend to be generic in nature, although they emphasize important use principals that are effective. Obviously, the guidelines do not take into consideration national differences regarding registration and withdrawal times, which are regulated by national legislation. Antimicrobial agents are categorized into first, second and last choice: (i) first choice antimicrobials are products with no or minimal use in human medicine; second choice antimicrobials are products which are used in human medicine, but which are not first choice products in the human medical community (see Chapter 4); and third choice products are important antimicrobials in human medicine, which should therefore be regarded as reserve antimicrobials for treatment of poultry flocks.

8.6.1 Unspecific enteritis (Dysbacteriosis)

After the withdrawal of growth promoters in the EU, the incidences of unspecific enteritis in turkeys and broilers have increased. The ban of growth promoters coincided in some countries with the ban of highly digestible animal protein in the feed due to the BSE crisis. As a consequence of this ban of meat and bone meal, animal proteins had to be replaced by plant protein sources with a higher content of NSP (non starch polysaccharides) and of potassium, namely soy bean meal which is rich in potassium. NSPs are not digestible to the avian gut, but may lead to a bacterial overgrowth in the intestine. Primarily Gram-positive bacteria, particularly *Clostridium* in the upper part of the jejunum and the duodenum, are thought to be involved in this form of unspecific enteritis (dysbacteriosis). If untreated, the disease may lead to caked and wet litter with increased food pad dermatitis and hock burns (animal welfare problems). If the birds live longer (turkeys) this may lead to ascending *Staphylococcus aureus* infections from the litter into the hock and knee joints with very serious uniformity and welfare problems. Medication may be warranted under these circumstances. Dysbacteriosis should not be confused with wet litter caused by poor ventilation or leaking water supply (spillage of water). Before medication is considered for cases of suspected dysbacteriosis, any potential nutritional influences should be assessed, such as use of NSP enzymes and control of sodium in the diet. If management and nutritional inputs are not felt to be contributing factors, then antimicrobial medication for dysbacteriosis needs to be considered. Antimicrobials of choice are those effective against *Clostridium* spp., although these bacteria may not be isolated in many instances. In most countries, benzylpenicillin is the drug of choice. If not registered for usage in poultry, macrolides (tylosin) or aminopenicillins (ampicillin or amoxicillin) represent valid alternatives. Antimicrobial susceptibility testing is not needed, as bacterial intestine overgrowth is in most cases of unspecific nature. There is circumstantial evidence that in broiler flocks vaccinated against coccidiosis, dysbacteriosis is more likely to occur. Cycling of the vaccine strains has been suggested to promote selection of clostridia in the intestinal flora. Ionophores can be used if feed additive antimicrobials to prevent unspecific enteritis are banned for this purpose.

8.6.2 Clostridial infections (*C. perfringens* and *C. colinum*)

Clostridium are opportunistic, spore-forming bacteria that can survive heat treatment of the feed. They cause sudden mortality in a broiler flock (necrotic enteritis) or may lead to higher condemnation rates at slaughter (cholangiohepatitis). Chronic forms of necrotic enteritis have also been described. In contrast to dysbacteriosis, these *Clostridium* infections typically present a clear clinical picture, which can be recognized at post-mortem examination and the causative microorganism isolated. Again, in flocks vaccinated with a live coccidiosis vaccine, the likelihood of *Clostridium* infections may increase compared to flocks using coccidiostats as feed additives. *C. perfringens* is the main causative organism of necrotic enteritis. A new breeder vaccine is under registration in Europe, which should help protect the offspring in the first weeks of life. If this product works under field conditions, its use should be considered to avoid antimicrobial treatment against necrotic enteritis. In acute outbreaks, flocks are routinely treated to reduce mortality and economical losses. The antimicrobials of choice are similar to dysbacteriosis (Table 8.4). Where registered for oral application, streptomycin or dihydrostreptomycin can be used as possible alternatives. Antimicrobial susceptibility of *C. perfringens* and other clostridia causing avian disease is predictable, thus susceptibility tests can be excluded.

8.6.3 Colibacillosis

Colibacillosis is the most common bacterial infection in chickens or turkeys, and can be involved in a number of syndromes affecting multiple ages. It is part of the yolk sac omphalitis syndrome during the first week of life, when colibacillosis is transmitted by dirty eggs or induced by poor hatchery hygiene. In adult layers, colibacillosis may lead to salpingitis and egg peritonitis. Colibacillosis is typically a secondary pathogen in respiratory infections resulting in pericarditis, perihepatitis and/or airsacculitis. Following systemic infections, *E. coli* can also result in synovitis and osteomyelitis. Some *E. coli* are primarily pathogenic to chicken (APEC, avian pathogenic *E. coli*). APEC strains are *E. coli* O:1, O:2 and O:78 K 80. Colicin and type 1 fimbriae seem to correlate with virulence, but non-APEC strains can sometimes also cause

Table 8.4 Antimicrobial agents for treatment of common bacterial diseases in poultry

Disease/pathogen	1st choice	2nd choice	Last choice
Dysbacteriosis	Benzylpenicillin	Aminopenicillins	Tylosin
Necrotic enteritis and other clostridial infections	Benzylpenicillin	Aminopenicillins or tylosin	Tylosin
Clostridium perfringens and others			
Colibacillosis	Potentiated sulfonamides	Aminopenicillins, tetracyclines, colistin, spectinomycin, aminoglycosides	Enrofloxacin
Escherichia coli			
Mycoplasmosis	Tiamulin[a]	Tetracyclines, lincomycin, (macrolides)	Enrofloxacin
Ornithobacterium rhinotracheale	Tiamulin[a] Aminopenicillins	Tetracyclines	
Staphylococcus or *Streptococcus*	Benzylpenicillin or potentiated sulfonamides	Aminopenicillins, tetracyclines	Macrolides
Fowl cholera	Potentiated sulfonamides	Tetracyclines, spectinomycin	Enrofloxacin
Pasteurella multocida	Aminopenicillins		
Riemerella anatipestifer	Aminopenicillins	Tetracyclines	Enrofloxacin
Infectious Coryza	Sulfonamides, potentiated sulfonamides or streptomycin	Tetracyclines, lincomycin, spectinomycin, macrolides	Enrofloxacin
Haemophilus paragallinarum			
Bordetella avium	No antimicrobials	Aminopenicillins, tetracyclines	Enrofloxacin
Erysipelothrix rhusiopathiae	Benzylpenicillin	Aminopenicillins	Enrofloxacin
Salmonellosis	No antimicrobials[c]	BAST	Unnecessary[b]

Aminoglycosides: streptomycin, apramycin, neomycin; aminopenicillins: amoxicillin, ampicillin; macrolides: erythromycin, spiramycin, tylosin, tilmicosin; tetracyclines: tetracycline, oxytetracycline, doxycycline; fluoroquinolones: enrofloxacin.

BAST, based on antimicrobial susceptibility testing.

[a] Tiamulin has neurotoxic effects when combined with ionophores and sulfonamides.

[b] *Erysipelotrix rhusiopathiae* infections can normally be treated successfully with penicillin or aminopenicillins. It is therefore unnecessary to mention a last choice product.

[c] A *Salmonella* infection should only be treated on the bases of a clinical outbreak for welfare reasons. In this case a first choice antimicrobial cannot be suggested. Therapy should always be based on antimicrobial testing. Zoonotic *Salmonella* infections should be eradicated by other means than antimicrobial treatment.

8 Poultry

Box 8.1 Predisposing factors involved in colibacillosis in poultry.

- Viral infections
  - Avian Pneumovirus
  - Infectious Bronchitis virus
  - Newcastle Disease virus
  - Low pathogenic Avian Influenza (LPAI) virus such as H9
- Other bacterial infections
  - *Mycoplasma*
  - *Ornithobacterium rhinotracheale* (ORT)
  - *Bordetella avium*
- Management conditions
  - Dry dusty conditions
  - High ammonia concentrations
  - Poor litter conditions

ity test. Wherever feasible, treatment should be on the basis of a susceptibility testing. First choice antimicrobials are potentiated sulfonamides. Tetracyclines and aminopenicillins (ampicillin, amoxicillin) should be used on the basis of antimicrobial susceptibility testing. After termination of treatment, relapses can occur depending on the nature of secondary bacterial infections. Colistin, neomycin or apramycin should be used in less severe cases and if time allows longer treatment (minimum 1 week). Spectinomycin has reasonable efficacy but is often only registered as a combination with lincomycin. Because of the combination, this has to be regarded as a third choice product. In some cases using a fluoroquinolone as first product is inevitable because of resistance to first and second choice antimicrobials.

8.6.4 Mycoplasmosis (*M. gallisepticum, M. synoviae* and *M. meleagridis*)

Primary breeding stock have eliminated the mycoplasmas of concern in the birds they provide to the industry, hence the ideal way to control *Mycoplasma* infections is by eradication. Unfortunately, this is not always possible because lateral spread plays a significant role in some areas where operations have multiage groups, and this renders stamping out more difficult. Vaccination reduces clinical symptoms but does not eliminate *Mycoplasma* shedding (neither vertical nor horizontal). Diagnosis is primarily based on serology (serum plate agglutination, ELISA, HAR) and on PCR. Because the organism is fastidious and requires specialized media for growth, isolation can be difficult and time consuming. Susceptibility testing of *Mycoplasma* isolates is even more difficult and can therefore only be conducted at specialized laboratories. Fortunately, the susceptibility patterns of *Mycoplasma* are predictable. Susceptibility testing should, however, be initiated on a geographical basis (if horizontal transmission of a *Mycoplasma* clone is assumed in a given area) if for whatever reason an infected breeder flock will be kept in production.

Most antimicrobials used to treat mycoplasmosis have a narrow spectrum of activity, while severe field infections are often complicated by secondary infections (mostly *E. coli*). In any case, a susceptibility test is required for the secondary infections. Based on the clinical picture (single *Mycoplasma* infection or complicated by secondary infections), the following

colibacillosis. In these cases various predisposing factors may be responsible for colibacillosis in poultry (see Box 8.1).

Mild Colibacillosis is often present in young chicken and in adult layers and breeders. Low-level colibacillosis does not prompt treatment. If mortality and/or morbidity increase to the point that treatment is to be considered, it is advisable to do a post mortem and take a swab for bacterial cultivation and susceptibility testing. *E. coli* is easy to grow and to identify. Isolates should be serotyped and further classified to see if the strain belongs to APEC or not. It may also be advisable to save *E. coli* isolates from flocks for potential production of an autogenous vaccine, if appropriate. It has been often observed that in one flock, different *E. coli* strains have been involved in mortality and clinical symptoms; hence it is best to have at least two different *E. coli* isolates from the same flock classified, including a susceptibility testing. Other factors to consider when selecting an antimicrobial treatment include whether the colibacillosis is systemic and the stage of the disease process.

Unfortunately, some products to which avian *E. coli* is usually susceptible, like colistinsulfate or aminoglycosides (neomycin, apramycin, spectinomycin), are not well absorbed and therefore do not reach sufficient blood and tissue levels. There is, however, circumstantial evidence that these products can be efficiently used in treating certain less severe *E. coli* infections if given for a longer time (at least seven days), especially when potentiated sulfonamides or tetracyclines are contraindicated by the susceptibil-

antimicrobial agents can be used: tiamulin (has neurotoxic effects when combined with ionophores and sulfonamides due to interference with drug degradation by the kidneys), tetracyclines or macrolides (tylosin or tilmicosin). Tetracyclines may be active against secondary bacterial infections, whereas tiamulin and macrolides are only active against *Mycoplasma*. In the case of non-complicated *Mycoplasma* infections, treatment with tylosin or tilmicosin is preferred. In complicated cases, a macrolide should be combined with a product against the secondary infection involved, in most cases *E. coli*. Lincomycin–spectinomycin combinations have limited efficacy against *Mycoplasma*, but most secondary bacteria involved are susceptible. Fluroquinolones (enrofloxacin) have good efficacy against *Mycoplasma* as well as against all major complicating secondary agents.

8.6.5 *Ornithobacterium rhinotracheale* (ORT)

Ornithobacterium rhinotracheale (ORT) infections are difficult to diagnose. The organism requires some skill for cultivation and sensitivity testing. A sensitivity test at the beginning or concurrently to the onset of medication is not practical in many cases. As resistance patterns often change in the field, cultivation and susceptibility testing should be routinely performed. Treatment on a trial and error basis should not be accepted. As with *Mycoplasma*, secondary infections have to be taken into consideration when choosing the product in a responsible way. ORT infections should be treated with tiamulin if incompatibilities with ionophores in the feed can be completely excluded. Second choice antimicrobials are amoxicillin, ampicillin and tetracyclines.

8.6.6 *Staphylococcus* and *Streptococcus* infections

The treatment strategies against infections associated with *Staphylococcus* and *Streptococcus* are similar. Infections with these organisms result in chronic diseases in poultry. Both bacterial species are mainly involved in chronic leg lesions, such as arthritis and femur head necrosis. Medication can usually wait until susceptibility testing is performed. *S. aureus* infections causing joint infections in replacement pullets and in turkeys are difficult to treat since most antimicrobials do not reach the needed MIC values in the joint and/

or bone tissues. Benzylpenicillin can be a good first empiric choice, especially for streptococcal infections. Other possible options are tetracyclines, aminopenicillins and macrolides (erythromycin, spiramycin).

8.6.7 Fowl cholera (Pasteurellosis)

Pasteurellosis is caused by the Gram-negative bacterium, *P. multocida*. *P. gallinarum* falls into the same group, but is of much less clinical importance. Susceptibility testing prior to or concurrent to the onset of medication is always indicated, as this pathogen can cause significant, acute mortality in turkeys. It tends to be more chronic in chickens, as they are less susceptible. First choice antimicrobials are potentiated sulfonamides and aminopenicillins.

8.6.8 *Riemerella anatipestifer* infections

R. anatipestifer causes major disease in the duck industry. Early infections can be controlled by maternal vaccination or by vaccination of the ducklings with autogenous vaccines. *R. anatipestifer* infections may also occur in turkeys, but the postmortem picture can be easily confused with colibacillosis. Susceptibility testing prior to or concurrent to the onset of medication should be conducted for *R. anatipestifer* infections. In emergency cases, tetracyclines or aminopenicillins are the drugs of choice.

8.6.9 Infectious coryza

Infectious coryza (*Haemophilus paragallinarum*) rarely occurs north of the equator. Most infections south of the equator are associated with *Mycoplasma* infections, which have to be taken into consideration when treating for this disease. Because of the more chronic nature of infectious coryza, susceptibility testing should be performed before the onset of medication. First choice antimicrobials are sulfonamides, potentiated sulfonamides and streptomycin (where registered) (Table 8.4).

8.6.10 Bordetella avium infections

Bordetella avium infections often act as secondary pathogens to other respiratory diseases of viral or bacterial origin. *B. avium* infections are likely underdiagnosed because the organism is easily overgrown by other complicating bacteria. *B. avium* can also be isolated from apparently healthy flocks. *B. avium* infections are difficult to treat via drinking water as blood concentrations of the antimicrobial do not readily get to the site of infection. In textbooks (33), contradictory results of antimicrobial treatments are reported even when the isolate was sensitive to the applied drug. Vaccination approaches and/or water line sanitation are recommended on farms with a history of this problem. When antimicrobial treatment is required, tetracyclines should be regarded as first choice agents.

8.6.11 Erysipelas

Erysipelothrix rhusiopathiae infections are infrequent in commercial layers, turkeys and rarely broilers. In most outbreaks, the flock had contact with pigs or open ranges. Penicillins are the antimicrobials of choice for treatment of avian erysipelas.

8.6.12 Salmonellosis

Antimicrobial treatments of *Salmonella* infected flocks as a mean of control are not allowed according to EU Regulation 1177/06. In case of severe welfare implications, flocks may be treated in accordance with the local government veterinarian authority. In this case, the same treatment restrictions for antimicrobials of first, second and last choice for colibacillosis will also be applicable to a salmonellosis treatment. Upon approval for treatment, an antimicrobial susceptibility testing is a prerequisite of any salmonellosis therapy.

8.7 Options to avoid antimicrobial treatment by biological approaches

Besides good management, proper hygiene and proper application of biosecurity practices, antimicrobial treatment can be avoided by other biological approaches such as registered vaccines, autogenous vaccines, probiotics and competitive exclusion flora.

8.7.1 Registered vaccines

There are only few bacterial vaccines registered for poultry. With *Mycoplasma gallisepticum* (MG) there are some inactivated and live vaccines available on the market which protect the target species (chicken), for which they are registered. These MG vaccines do not sufficiently protect turkeys and they do not stop vertical shedding in breeder flocks, so they cannot be used as an alternative for eradication in breeders. Some bacterial vaccines aim at preventing the disease in the breeders and protecting the offspring by maternal antibodies. This is the concept behind certain commercially available vaccines such as for fowl cholera, *E. coli* and ORT. Obviously, there are too many fowl cholera, *E. coli* and ORT serotypes that do not confer cross protection, so that the one vaccine concept does not fit for all circumstances.

Vaccines for many common viral diseases are available for use in poultry, which work quite effectively if properly applied. The modern poultry industry takes full advantage of this option and designs vaccination programmes appropriate for the pathogens in the region. This helps minimize and even prevent treatment against secondary bacterial infections (*E. coli*, ORT and Mycoplasmas), which often complicate respiratory challenges with ubiquitous viral pathogens (Avian Pneumovirus, Infectious Bronchitis, Newcastle Disease). It is highly desirable to encourage quicker registration procedures for vaccine approvals, so that vaccine manufacturer's can adapt their vaccines in a timely fashion to the changing requirements of the market.

8.7.2 Autogenous vaccines

Some bacterial diseases are of such significant local importance that autogenous vaccines may be a worthwhile approach, especially with infections associated with *E. coli*, ORT, *Pasteurella*, *B. avium* and *R. anatipestifer*. According to definition, autogenous vaccines may only be used on the farm where the isolate comes from. This may be a regulation that the large animal practitioner can live with, but it poses a unique problem for the poultry industry where a strict separation between rearing farms and growing or production farms is standard. Rearing farms are ideally located in a less poultry populated area, and the birds are transported after rearing to a more dense area where a high infection pressure is present. It is important to vaccinate the birds on the rearing farm with the antigen they will be exposed to on the grower or production farm. For this reason, it is highly desirable to adapt this regulation to the needs of the modern poultry industry.

8.7.3 Probiotics and competitive exclusion flora

It is well documented that Competitive Exclusion (CE) microflora products (undefined gut flora from healthy – SPF – chicken) like Aviguard and Broilact can prevent or minimize colonization with a low-level *Salmonella* challenge. This concept has been used primarily in Finland for many years. Recently, Hofacre (34) has demonstrated that it possible to use this concept to also replace multi-resistant *E. coli* from the chicken intestine. Because CE products are undefined, registration authorities had problems licensing the product in many countries. These products are also costly to use. In many operations, trials with probiotics (single defined products) are under way. These products may also prove helpful in replacing the performance and gut health benefits that growth promoters provided.

8.8 Concluding remarks

Antimicrobial use in poultry will need to continue, as the need to treat and control certain bacterial disease outbreaks for health and welfare concerns will always exist. Continued use can induce resistance in certain poultry bacterial pathogens or commensals, which in turn could impact therapeutic efficacies. However, there are far too many complex issues involved to simply associate food animal antimicrobial usage in poultry flocks with bacterial resistance development in human medicine. There needs to be continued development and use of properly designed and interpreted risk assessment models and other research results to help fill in the current multitude of data gaps.

References

1. Swann, M.M. (1969). *Report of the Joint Committee on the use of antibiotics in animal husbandry and veterinary medicine* (ed. University of Wales Aberystwyth Library). M Stationary Office, London, UK.
2. Animal Health Institute (AHI) (2002). Survey shows antibiotic use in animals decline. AHI News release, October 6, 2004. www.ahi.org. National Institute for Animal Agriculture.
3. DANMAP 2005. (2006). Consumption of antimicrobial agents and occurrence of antimicroibial resistance in bacteria from food animals, foods, and humans in Denmark (eds. Hever, O.E., Hammerum, A.M.) Danish Institute for Food and Veterinary Research Soeborg, ISSN pp. 1600–2052.
4. Casewell, M., Friis, C., Marco, E., *et al.* (2003). The European ban on growth-promoting antibiotics and emerging consequences for human and animal health. *J. Antimicrob. Chemother.* 52: 159–61.
5. Kunin, C.M. (1993). Resistance to antimicrobial drugs – a worldwide calamity. *Ann. Internal Med.* 118 (7): 557–61.
6. Wassenaar, T.M. (2005). Use of antimicrobial agents in veterinary medicine and implications for human health. *Crit. Rev. Microbiol.* 31: 155–69.
7. AVMA (2005). American Veterinary Medical Association's guidelines to judicious therapeutic use of antimicrobials in poultry. Available at www.avma.org/scienact/jtua/poultry/poultry00.asp
8. Ungemach, F.R., Müller-Barth, D. and Abraham, G. (2006). Guidelines for prudent use of antimicrobials and their implications on antibiotic usage in veterinary medicine. *Int. J. Med. Microbiol.* 296: 33–38.
9. BTK (Bundestierärztekammer), ArgeVET (Arbeitsgemeinschaft Leitender Veterinärbeamten) (2000). Leitlinien für den sorgfältigen Umgang mit antimikrobiell wirksamen Tierarzneimitteln. *Deutsches Tierärzteblatt*, 48 (Suppl 11): 1–12 (In German).
10. EFSA (2006). The Community summary report on trends and sources of zoonoses, Zoonotic agents, antimicrobial resistance and foodborne outbreaks in the European Union in 2005. *EFSA J.* 2006, p. 95.
11. EFSA (2004). The use of antimicrobials for the control of *Salmonella* in poultry. *EFSA J.* 115: 1–76.
12. DANMAP 2000 (2001). Consumption of antimicrobial agents and occurrence of antimicrobial resistance in bacteria from food animals, foods, and humans in Denmark. (eds. Bager, F., Emborg, H.D.) Danish Veterinary Laboratory Copenhagen, ISSN pp. 1600–2032.
13. Moore, J.E., Corcoran, D., Dooley, J.S.G., *et al.* (2005). Campylobacter. *Vet. Res.* 36: 351–82.
14. SCVPH (Scientific Committee on Veterinary Measures relating to Public Health) – EU SANCO (2003a). *Opinion on the human risk caused by the use of fluoroquinolones in animals.* Adopted on 26–27 March 2003. European Commission, Health and Consumer Protection, Directorate C, Scientific Opinons.
15. Unicomb, L., Ferguson, J., Riley, T.V. and Collignon, P. (2003). 'Fluoroquinolone resistance in *Campylobacter* absent from isolates', Australia. *Emerg. Infect. Dis.* 9 (11): 1482–3.
16. NARMS (2003). National Antimicrobial Resistance Monitoring System: Final Report. www.cdc.gov/narms.
17. Van Boven, M., Veldman, K.T., de Jong, M.C.M. and Mevius, D.J. (2003). Rapid selection of quinolone resistance in *Campylobacter jejuni* but not in *Escherichia coli* in individually housed broilers. *J. Antimicrob. Chemother.* 52: 719–23.
18. Blanco. J.E., Blanco, M., Mora, A. and Blanco, J. (1997). Prevalence of bacterial resistance to quinolones and other antimicrobials among avian *Escherichia coli* strains isolated from septicemic and healthy chickens in Spain. *J. Clin. Microbiol.* 35: 2184–5.

8 Poultry

19. Bass, L., Liebert, C.A., Lee, M.D., *et al.* (1999). Incidence and characterization of integrons, genetic elements mediating multiple-drug resistance, in avian *Escherichia coli. Antimicrob. Agents Chemother.* 43 (12): 2925–9.

20. Zhao, S., Maurer, J.J., Hubert, S., *et al.* (2005). Antimicrobial susceptibility and molecular characterization of avian pathogenic *Escherichia coli* isolates. *Vet. Microbiol.* 107: 215–24.

21. White, D.G., Piddock, L.J.V., Maurer, J.J., *et al.* (2000). Characterization of fluoroquinolone resistance among veterinary isolates of avian *Escherichia coli. Antimicrob. Agents Chemother.* 44: 2897–9.

22. Cormican, M., Buckely, V., Corbett-Feeney, G. and Sheridan, F. (2001). Antimicrobial resistance in *Escherichia coli* isolates from turkeys and hens in Ireland. *J. Antimicrob. Chemother.* 48: 587–8.

23. Aarestrup, F.M., Agersø, Y., Ahrens, P., *et al.* (2000). Antimicrobial susceptibility and presence of resistance genes in staphylococci from poultry. *Vet. Microbiol.* 74: 353–64.

24. Johansson, A., Greko, C., Engstrom, B.E. and Karlsson, M. (2004). Antimicrobial susceptibility of Swedish, Norwegian and Danish isolates of *Clostridium perfringens* from poultry, and distribution of tetracycline resistance genes. *Vet. Microbiol.* 99: 251–7.

25. Watkins, K.L., Shryock, T.R., Dearth, R.N. and Saif, Y.M. (1997). *In vitro* antimicrobial susceptibility of *Clostridium perfringens* from commercial turkey and broiler chicken origin. *Vet. Microbiol.* 54: 195–200.

26. Van den Bogaard, A.E., Willems, R., London, N., *et al.* (2002). Antibiotic resistance of faecal enterococci in poultry, poultry farmers and poultry slaughterers. *J. Antimicrob. Chemother.* 49: 497–505.

27. Hershberger, E., Oprea, S.F., Donabedian, S.M., *et al.* (2005). Epidemiology of antimicrobial resistance in enterococci of animal origin. *J. Antimicrob. Chemother.* 55: 127–30.

28. Jones, R. (1998). Antimicrobial activity of quinupristin/dalfopristin tested against over 28,000 recent clinical isolates from 200 medical centers in the United States and Canada. *Diag. Microbiol. Infect. Dis.* 30: 437–51.

29. Tejedor-Junco, M.T., Afonso-Rodriguez, O., Martin-Barrasa, J.L. and Gonzales-Martin, M. (2005). Antimicrobial susceptibility of *Enterococcus* strains isolated from poultry faeces. *Res. Vet. Sci.* 78: 33–8.

30. Popp, C. (2003). *Ornithobacterium rhinotracheale*: Typisierung, Pathogenität, Resistenzverhalten und Bekämpfung, Ph.D. Thesis, Veterinary Faculty, University of Berlin (in German).

31. Lister, S. (2005). Pathogenic agents involved in turkey respiratory diseases under field conditions, the UK perspective. *Proceedings 4th International Bayer Poultry Symposium, Istanbul 2005*, pp. 57–73.

32. Baywater, R. (2005). Results of a European survey of antimicrobial resistance in zoonotic and indicator bacteria from poultry. *Proceedings 4th International Bayer Poultry Symposium, Istanbul 2005*, pp. 10–16.

33. Saif, Y.M., Barnes, H.J., Glisson, J.R., Fadley, A.M., McDougald, L.M. and Swayne, D.E. (2003). In *Diseases of Poultry*, 11th edn, Section II, Bacterial disease (eds. Saif, Y.M., Barner, J.R., Glisson, A.M., Fadley, L.M., McDougald and Swayne, D.E.) Iowa State Press, pp. 567–863.

34. Hofacre, C. (2000). Present and future control methods for colibacillosis. *Proceedings of the XXI World`s Poultry Congress*, Montreal Canada, 20–24 August 2000, CD Rom.

35. Chaslus-Dancla, E., Baucheron, S., Biet, F., *et al.* (2002). Survey of resistance to antibiotics in avian pathogenic *Escherichia coli* (APEC) from three countries: a European collaboration. *Proceedings of the 11th European Poultry Congress*, Bremen.

Chapter 9

GUIDELINES FOR ANTIMICROBIAL USE IN CATTLE

Peter D. Constable, Satu Pyörälä and Geoffrey W. Smith

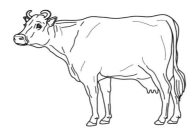

This chapter discusses the appropriate use of antimicrobials in seven common diseases of cattle; septicaemia, calf diarrhoea, septic arthritis, infectious diseases of the foot, pneumonia, metritis and mastitis. The seven disease conditions were selected because collectively they represent the majority of antimicrobial administration to cattle. Antimicrobials obviously play an important role as part of the treatment of many other diseases of cattle such as omphalophlebitis in calves, peritonitis, infectious bovine keratoconjunctivitis, listeriosis, pyelonephritis, cystitis, thrombophlebitis, abscesses, cellulitis and osteomyelitis.

9.1 Septicaemia

Antimicrobials are frequently used to treat septicaemia in ruminants. Septicaemia remains a common condition in neonates and is usually associated with Gram-negative bacteria such as *Escherichia coli*, *Klebsiella* spp, or *Salmonella enterica* subspp. *enterica serovars*. Aggressive treatment of septicaemia with bactericidal antimicrobials is indicated (1) because the case-fatality rate is high and the immune system in neonates is not as well developed as in adults. However, because neonatal septicaemia in calves is usually associated with insufficient colostrum ingestion or the presence of concurrent diseases such as diarrhoea or omphalophlebitis, improvement of hygienic and management conditions at the farm level represents an important tool to decrease the incidence of septicaemia and minimize the use of antimicrobials.

Potentiated sulfonamides (25 mg/kg, IV or IM every 24 h) are a first choice antimicrobial to treat neonatal septicaemia, with second choice antimicrobials being third- or fourth-generation cephalosporins (Table 9.1). Last choice antimicrobials are aminoglycosides and fluoroquinolones in countries where their use is permitted; aminoglycosides having a major disadvantage of prolonged slaughter withdrawal times because of sustained renal concentrations of up to 15 months. Doses higher than those approved have been suggested for some antimicrobials. For example, one study showed that ceftiofur at a dose of 5 mg/kg, IM every 24 h was associated with clinical improvement in an experimental model of salmonellosis in calves (2). This is more than double the approved dose of ceftiofur in the USA. However, the ceftiofur minimum inhibitory concentration (MIC) for 90% of the isolates (MIC_{90}) for *Salmonella* is 1 µg/ml as compared to 0.015–0.06 µg/ml for *Mannheimia haemolytica*, which is the primary target pathogen

Table 9.1 Guidelines to antimicrobial options for various septic arthritis pathogens in ruminants

Gram-positive bacteria

Arcanobacterium pyogenes	Penicillins
Chlamydia spp.	Oxytetracycline, fluoroquinolones
Erysipelothrix insidiosa	Penicillins, cephalosporins
Streptococcus spp.	Penicillins, cephalosporins
Staphylococcus aureus	Cephalosporins, tilmicosin, lincomycin, fluoroquinolones

Gram-negative bacteria

Coliform bacteria (*E. coli*)	Aminoglycosides, potentiated sulfonamides, third- or fourth-generation cephalosporins, fluoroquinolones
Salmonella spp.	Aminoglycosides, potentiated sulfonamides, third- or fourth-generation cephalosporins, fluoroquinolones
Histophilus somni	Oxytetracycline, third- or fourth-generation cephalosporins, tilmicosin, florfenicol
Prevotella melaninogenica	β-Lactams (primarily penicillin)

Mycoplasma spp.

Mycoplasma bovis	Oxytetracycline, florfenicol, spectinomycin, fluoroquinolones

of the label dose. As with other water-soluble drugs, ceftiofur also has a higher volume of distribution in neonatal calves as compared with adult cattle. Therefore, plasma concentrations are lower in neonates than adults following equivalent dose administration and a slightly higher dose is required for plasma concentrations to exceed the MIC of the target pathogen for the duration of therapy. Field studies comparing the efficacy of different antimicrobials in calves with septicaemia are lacking. Cefquinome (a fourth-generation cephalosporin) given at 2 mg/kg IM, every 24 h has been shown to be equally effective as gentamicin given at 3 mg/kg IM every 8 h (3). However, the use of third- and fourth-generation cephalosporins in cattle is questionable due to its high potential for selection of resistant bacteria of medical relevance, such as *Salmonella* resistant to ceftriaxone, because ceftriaxone is the drug of choice for treatment of severe forms of salmonellosis.

Septicaemia also occurs in adult cattle. For example, recent studies have demonstrated that a substantial proportion of cows with moderate-to-severe coliform mastitis are also bacteraemic (4) and some cattle with endocarditis, toxic metritis, peritonitis, pleuropneumonia or acute salmonellosis are also likely to be bacteraemic. In these animals, parenteral administration of antimicrobials is indicated. Ideally, the choice of antimicrobials in the 'toxic' cow should be based on culture and susceptibility results, which are almost never available when treatment is initiated. Therefore, the antimicrobial choice is generally based

on the initial clinical diagnosis and prediction as to the most likely pathogen. In many cases, the likely pathogen can be difficult or impossible to determine accurately based on physical examination findings alone (5) and therefore a broad-spectrum antimicrobial is often used in septic cattle. Resistance to many commonly used antimicrobials (such as amoxicillin, ampicillin, erythromycin, tylosin and sulfadimethoxine) has become common amongst Gram-negative bacteria, and these historically used antimicrobials rarely achieve plasma concentrations above the MIC of many major pathogens. First choice antimicrobials for the 'toxic' cow are oxytetracycline and potentiated sulfonamides, with last choice antimicrobials being third- (ceftiofur)- or fourth(cefquinome)-generation cephalosporins and fluoroquinolones, which should be regarded as reserve drugs in food animals (6).

9.2 Calf diarrhoea

9.2.1 Treatment

There are six major causes of diarrhoea in calves less than 21 days of age: enterotoxigenic *E. coli*, rotavirus, coronavirus, *Cryptosporidium parvum*, *Salmonella enterica* subspp. *enterica serovars* and nutritional. Clinical diarrhoea is more likely when calves are infected with more than one pathogen. Calves with diarrhoea have small intestinal overgrowth with *E. coli* bacteria, regardless of the inciting cause for the diarrhoea (7), and 20–30% of systemically ill calves with diarrhoea have bacteraemia, predominantly due to *E. coli* (3, 8, 9). The frequency of bacteraemia is considered sufficiently high that treatment of calves with diarrhoea that are sick (as indicated by decreased appetite and activity) should include routine treatment against bacteraemia, with emphasis on treating potential *E. coli* bacteraemia. A clinical sepsis score to predict bacteraemia (10) is not recommended to guide antimicrobial treatment decisions until further validation of the score in different calf-rearing scenarios. Bacteraemia should be suspected to be present in 100% of calves with clinical signs of *Salmonella* diarrhoea, although the prevalence of bacteraemia in affected calves does not appear to have been determined (2).

Antimicrobial treatment of diarrhoeic calves with systemic illness should be focused against *E. coli* in the blood (due to bacteraemia) and small intestine (due to bacterial overgrowth), as these constitute the two sites of infection. Faecal bacterial culture is not recommended in calves with diarrhoea, because faecal bacterial populations do not accurately reflect small intestinal or blood bacterial populations. Furthermore, the clinical breakpoints for definition of resistance have not been validated for calves with diarrhoea (7). Antimicrobial efficacy is therefore best evaluated by the clinical response to treatment. Epidemiological data on antimicrobial resistance can, and should, be used to guide antimicrobial choice at the herd or country level.

Antimicrobials should be administered to all calves with diarrhoea that exhibit systemic signs of illness (as indicated by inappetance, dehydration, lethargy or pyrexia) or have blood or mucosal shreds in their stool; the latter indicates breakdown of the blood–gut barrier and an increased risk of bacteraemia. Parenteral administration of antimicrobials is preferred to oral administration, with the ideal parenteral antimicrobial being bactericidal and predominantly Gram negative in spectrum, as well as being excreted in an active form in bile so that there is also an antimicrobial effect in the small intestine. Antimicrobials should not be administered to diarrhoeic calves that have a normal appetite, activity level, rectal temperature, hydration status and the absence of concurrent infections such as pneumonia or omphalophlebitis (11). Instead, these calves should be separated from other calves and their health status monitored frequently.

Success of antimicrobial therapy varies with the route of administration and whether the antimicrobial is dissolved in milk, oral electrolyte solutions or water. Oral antimicrobials administered as bolus, tablet or in a gelatin capsule may be swallowed into the rumen and exhibit a different serum concentration–time profile to antimicrobials dissolved in milk-replacer that are suckled by the calf. Antimicrobials that bypass the rumen are not thought to alterrumen microflora, potentially permitting bacterial recolonization of the small intestine from the rumen; however, it should be recognized that the normal intestinal flora is always exposed to varying amounts of antimicrobial drugs regardless of the type of administration (12). Individual antimicrobial treatment of sick calves increases the level of resistance in faecal *E. coli* isolates, but the persistence of this change in antimicrobial susceptibility is controversial (13, 14).

First choice antimicrobials for the treatment of diarrhoea in ill calves include parenteral amoxicillin or ampicillin (10 mg/kg, IM every 12 h) or potentiated sulfonamides (25 mg/kg, IV or IM every 24 h) or oral amoxicillin trihydrate (10 mg/kg every 12 h) alone or combined with the inhibitor clavulanate potassium (12.5 mg combined drug/kg every 12 h) (7, 15). Second choice antimicrobials are third-(ceftiofur)- and fourth (cefquinome)-generation cephalosporins; parenteral ceftiofur has evidence of efficacy in experimentally induced *Salmonella enterica* serovar Dublin infection (2). Last choice antimicrobials are fluoroquinolones in those countries where fluoroquinolone administration is permitted to treat calves with *E. coli* diarrhoea and salmonellosis. Parenteral fluoroquinolones should be administered only to critically ill calves, such as those calves requiring intravenous fluid administration. Oral and parenteral fluoroquinolones have documented efficacy in treating calves with diarrhoea and systemic illness (7). Aminoglycosides should not be administered orally because they are very poorly absorbed, and should not be administered parenterally because of prolonged withdrawal times for slaughter, potential for nephrotoxicity in dehydrated calves and minimal excretion in bile. Historic studies reported that some orally administered antimicrobials (e.g. penicillin, neomycin, tetracycline) may increase the incidence of diarrhoea, produce malabsorption and reduce growth rate (7).

9.2.2 Prevention

The use of oral antimicrobials to prevent diarrhoea should never be a substitute for better management.

9 Cattle

When confronted with a calf diarrhoea problem, veterinarians and agricultural producers should implement an effective vaccination programme, optimize colostral immunoglobulin administration and absorption, sanitize feeding utensils and decrease environmental contamination with enteric pathogens, in conjunction with the appropriate use of intravenous fluids and oral electrolyte solutions (16). In general terms, antimicrobials should not be used to prevent calf diarrhoea unless all other measures have been documented to be ineffective.

The main reasons for administering antimicrobials to prevent diarrhoea in calves are to decrease *E. coli* bacterial numbers in the small intestine, to prevent *E. coli* bacteraemia, which presumably occurs following translocation of bacteria from the small intestinal lumen (16), and to decrease faecal shedding of *Salmonella enterica* subsp. *enterica serovars* (17). It therefore follows that when antimicrobials are administered to calves to prevent diarrhoea, they should be effective against *E. coli* and *Salmonella enterica* in the intestine. The ideal antimicrobial should reach therapeutic concentrations in the small intestinal lumen for a long enough period, have some degree of drug penetration through the intestinal wall (18), and have a narrow Gram-negative spectrum of activity in order to minimize potential collateral damage to other enteric bacteria (19). In view of the increasing concern regarding transferable resistance amongst enteric bacteria and the small number of contemporary studies documenting antimicrobial efficacy in preventing diarrhoea (16), the administration of antimicrobials in milk-replacer and calf starter rations to increase weight gain should be reevaluated. Oral administration of antimicrobials to prevent diarrhoea is not permitted in many countries. However, four orally administered antimicrobials (chlortetracycline, oxytetracycline, tetracycline and neomycin) are approved to prevent calf diarrhoea in the USA (7). Feeding of antimicrobials in milk-replacer results in a four-fold reduction in the prevalence of faecal shedding of *Salmonella enterica* in preweaned calves (17). However, the possible benefits of this practice should be weighed against the risk for development of resistance. In some circumstances, antimicrobials are used prophylactically to hide the negative effects of poor management. This practice is no longer recommended in the EU, even though it is still used in some countries.

As a last resort, when all other control measures have been appropriately implemented and documented to be ineffective, the most appropriate antimicrobials for preventing diarrhoea in calves are orally administered chlortetracycline (7 mg/kg, every 12 h) and oxytetracycline; chlortetracycline decreases the mortality rate, and oxytetracycline and chlortetracycline decrease the duration of diarrhoea (20). A more recent study found that the onset and the overall morbidity of important diseases in calves during their first weeks of life (diarrhoea, respiratory disease, navel infection) was lower in calves receiving chlortetracycline HCl (22 mg/kg per day) and neomycin sulfate (22 mg/kg per day) in milk-replacer than in control calves without in-feed antibiotics (21). An important finding of this study was that antimicrobial treated calves had higher levels of multiple antimicrobial resistance in faecal *E. coli* isolates (13). Although this study did not exclusively consider diarrhoea as the primary outcome, these findings are valuable because they reflect the pattern of diseases in newborn calves in a specialized calf-rearing facility with high disease incidence. It should be noted that these dose rates are higher than the dose rates approved and used in the USA to prevent diarrhoea. Chlortetracycline and oxytetracycline have label requirements that treatment must be administered separately to feeding of milk or milk-replacer, which makes administration impractical. This requirement is because tetracyclines are irreversibly bound to calcium, leading to reduced oral bioavailability when fed with milk or milk-replacer (22,23). Fluoroquinolones, aminoglycosides and third- and fourth-generation cephalosporins should not be administered to calves in order to prevent diarrhoea because of the possibility of selecting unwanted types of resistance amongst enteric bacteria.

9.3 Septic arthritis

Septic or infectious arthritis is a common orthopaedic problem of calves and adult cattle. In calves, septic arthritis is most frequently caused by the haematogenous spread of bacteria and is often associated with the presence of omphalophlebitis. In adult animals, septic arthritis more commonly results from direct inoculation of bacteria into the joint cavity, or from the extension of infection from periarticular tissue. A wide variety of bacteria have been associated with septic arthritis in cattle including *E. coli*, *Arcanobacterium pyogenes*, *Erysipelothrix insidiosa*, *Histophilus somni* (formerly *Haemophilus somnus*), *Proteus mirabilis*, *Chlamydia* spp., *Salmonella enterica* subspp. *enterica serovars*, *Staphylococcus* species (including *S. aureus*), *Streptococcus* spp., *Prevotella* (formerly *Bacteroides*) *melaninogenica* and *Mycoplasma* spp.

Successful treatment of septic arthritis in cattle requires early and aggressive antimicrobial treatment coupled with lavage of the joint. In cases diagnosed early, parenteral antimicrobial therapy can be very effective, usually resulting in complete resolution of the joint damage and a return to normal function. During septic arthritis, the blood flow and hence the transport of antimicrobials to the joint is generally increased. Therefore, most antimicrobials will achieve therapeutic concentrations in the joint following parenteral administration. Local (articular) injection of antimicrobials is not indicated and can result in a local synovitis. More chronic cases of septic arthritis are accompanied by substantial accumulation of fibrin clots in the joint cavity and become further complicated by the advanced destruction of tissue adjacent to the joint. Therefore, the elimination of infection from the joint with parenteral antimicrobial alone can be difficult and additional treatments such as joint lavage, arthrotomies and long-term intra-articular antimicrobials can be indicated.

Selection of the appropriate antimicrobial for treating septic arthritis is ideally based on isolation of a specific pathogen from a large volume of joint fluid; however, cultures take several days to produce a result and are frequently unrewarding (no bacteria isolated). Therefore, therapy is almost always initiated without exact knowledge of the bacteria being targeted. For this reason, it is important that a broad-spectrum antimicrobial be selected since there is significant diversity in the types of bacteria that cause septic arthritis in cattle. The drug of choice must be able to target Gram-positive bacteria (such as *A. pyogenes*, *S. aureus* and haemolytic streptococci), Gram-negative bacteria (such as *E. coli*) and preferably *Mycoplasma* species. First choice antimicrobials for the initial treatment of septic arthritis in cattle include potentiated sulfonamides, oxytetracycline, ampicillin and amoxicillin (not if *M. bovis* is suspected) with second choice antimicrobials being third (ceftiofur)-or fourth (cefquinome)-generation cephalosporins (not if *M. bovis* is suspected). Other antimicrobials such

as, aminoglycosides, florfenicol, lincomycin and spectinomycin could be used (Table 9.1) but extensive withdrawal times for aminoglycosides precludes their use in food-producing animals. Another option would be to use a combination of antimicrobials to increase the spectrum of activity such as an aminoglycoside (i.e. gentamicin) together with a β-lactam (penicillin).

Fluoroquinolones would also seem be a good option in countries where their use is permitted in ruminants. A study of experimentally induced arthritis, using *Mycoplasma bovis* in calves, failed to show significant benefit following parenteral administration of enrofloxacin at a dose of 5 mg/kg every 24 h (24). However, another study involving 29 calves with naturally occurring septic arthritis caused by various bacterial pathogens demonstrated that parenteral treatment with marbofloxacin at a dose of 4 mg/kg every 24 h for 10 days resulted in a high rate of clinical and bacteriologic cures (25). In addition to the possible risks to human health, a potential concern of fluoroquinolones in treating septic arthritis is toxicity to cartilage, particularly in young rapidly growing animals. Parenteral administration at 5 times the recommended dose has induced cartilage lesions in several species including dogs and nonhuman primates (26). However this has not been demonstrated to be of any clinical relevance in ruminants and fluoroquinolone use is generally considered safe, although not in line with the principles of prudent antimicrobial use.

There appears to be some diversity between *M. bovis* isolates from cattle in Europe and North America. Isolates collected in the EU have been shown to be most susceptible to danofloxacin, with limited susceptibility to florfenicol, oxytetracycline and spectinomycin (27). In contrast, the majority of *M. bovis* isolates in the USA were highly susceptible to florfenicol, oxytetracycline and spectinomycin. Very few isolates were inhibited by tilmicosin, and none by erythromycin, ampicillin or ceftiofur (28).

Duration of antimicrobial therapy in cases of septic arthritis remains empirical. It is widely considered that long-term treatment (three to four weeks) is necessary for complete resolution of the infected joint. The duration of antimicrobial therapy in humans and horses has typically been four weeks. However, results of a study using an experimentally induced model of septic arthritis in calves suggest a shorter duration of treatment would be appropriate. In this study, the tarsus joint of calves was inoculated with *E. coli* and

9 Cattle

then they were subsequently treated with ceftiofur. Bacteriologic culture of joint fluid remained positive in all calves from days two to four after inoculation but was negative in all calves after one week of antimicrobial treatment (29).

9.4   Infections of the foot

Interdigital necrobacillosis (foot rot, necrotic pododermatitis, interdigital phlegmon) and digital dermatitis are common infections of the bovine foot that often require antimicrobial therapy. Interdigital necrobacillosis occurs worldwide in dairy and beef cattle and is primarily caused by the Gram-negative anaerobic bacteria *Fusobacterium necrophorum* and *Prevotella* (formerly *Bacteroides*) *melaninogenica*. Although some cases will resolve without treatment, early and aggressive therapy with parenteral antibiotics is generally indicated in cattle with interdigital necrobacillosis. Numerous antimicrobials have been used to successfully treat this condition. First choice antimicrobials include ampicillin, penicillin, oxytetracycline and sulfamethazine; these are first choice antimicrobials because of their cost and efficacy. Florfenicol is a second choice antimicrobial (treatment is considerably more expensive), whereas the third-generation cephalosporin ceftiofur is a last choice antimicrobial. Ceftiofur is commonly used to treat lactating dairy cattle with foot infections because ceftiofur has no or minimal milk discard time as compared to other drugs. In contrast, long-acting formulations of oxytetracycline or florfenicol are commonly used in beef cattle in order to minimize the number of injections needed. Treatment of interdigital necrobacillosis continues to be one of the primary reasons for therapeutic use of antimicrobial in cattle in Europe and the USA(11, 30).

Digital dermatitis (papillomatous digital dermatitis) is a common cause of lameness in dairy cattle and a significant animal welfare concern for the livestock industry. The bacteria most consistently isolated from active lesions are spirochetes of the genus *Treponema* that invade the epidermis and dermis. Numerous studies have demonstrated a clinical response to antimicrobials applied directly to the lesion as a topical spray treatment or under a bandage. The most commonly used topical treatments are oxytetracycline, lincomycin (with or without spectinomycin) and valnemulin, with oxytetracycline being the preferred first choice treatment. Topical application of these antimicrobials does not result in violative milk residues (31) and is strongly preferred to parenteral administration. Parenteral use of antimicrobials for treatment of digital dermatitis has not been shown to be consistently effective and would necessitate the discarding of milk. Ceftiofur, a third-generation cephalosporin (1.5–2.0 mg/kg IM daily for 3 days) is effective in treating digital dermatitis (32). A fourth-generation cephalosporin (cefquinome, 1 mg/kg IM daily) has been approved for treatment of digital dermatitis in the UK, and a small study suggested that a five-day treatment course was efficacious (33). Foot baths containing erythromycin are effective in preventing digital dermatitis and are commonly used in Europe (34).

9.5   Pneumonia

Pneumonia has three main clinical manifestations in cattle: shipping fever in feedlot cattle shortly after a period of transport and co-mingling, enzootic pneumonia in dairy calves up to six months of age associated with poor ventilation and overcrowding and chronic pneumonia in adult cattle. Two other clinical manifestations of pneumonia in cattle (bovine tuberculosis caused by *Mycobacterium bovis* and contagious bovine pleuropneumonia caused by *Mycoplasma mycoides*) have been successfully controlled or eradicated from many countries.

Shipping fever is caused primarily by *Mannheimia haemolytica* (formerly *Pasteurella haemolytica* biotype A serotype 1), although clinical disease can also be caused by *Histophilus somni* and *Pasteurella multocida*, with an uncertain contributory role of *Mycoplasma bovis* and other *Mycoplasma* species. Enzootic pneumonia is most frequently caused by *Pasteurella multocida* biotype A serotype 3 with *Mycoplasma bovis* playing an uncertain contributory role. Chronic pneumonia is usually associated with *Arcanobacterium pyogenes* (formerly *Actinomyces pyogenes*). The pathogenesis of pneumonia in shipping fever and enzootic pneumonia is similar in that impaired respiratory defense mechanisms result in explosive growth of pathogenic bacteria in the upper respiratory tract with subsequent colonization of the lower respiratory tract and clinical signs of pneumonia.

More antimicrobial agents are approved for the treatment of respiratory disease than any other disease of cattle. Factors that influence veterinarians in the selection of an antimicrobial to treat bovine pneumonia include susceptibility of the pathogenic strain causing pneumonia (geographic and herd-specific variation in *in vitro* susceptibility patterns exist), and the likelihood of exceeding the MIC of *M. haemolytica*, *Pasteurella multocida*, or *Histophilus somni* in lung parenchyma as well as the lower and upper respiratory passages. The likelihood is probably highest for florfenicol, ceftiofur, tilmicosin, tulathromycin and fluoroquinolones, and not expected for penicillin, ampicillin, amoxicillin, erythromycin and tylosin. Other factors include the benefit–cost ratio, the route of administration (intravenous injection requires more skill and restraint, whereas intramuscular injection may lead to carcass damage), frequency of administration (less frequent is strongly preferred), volume administered (lower injection volumes are preferred), safety (tilmicosin can be fatal when injected intravenously in cattle or administered parenterally to other species including humans) and slaughter or milk- withdrawal time. Other factors to be considered are persistence in the environment and risk for promoting transfer of antimicrobial resistance genes. For instance, a strong positive association was observed between ceftiofur usage and the occurrence of cephalosporin resistance in faecal *E. coli* isolates on a herd basis, but not on an individual cow basis (35). There are also reports suggesting transfer of antimicrobial resistant *Salmonella* from diseased cattle treated with ceftiofur to humans (36, 37).

Antimicrobials for pneumonia should be administered subcutaneously, intramuscularly or intravenously and not in feed or water because sick cattle have reduced feed and water intakes and are unlikely to consume an adequate mass of drug. Intratracheal injections have been performed in the belief that gravity will cause the antimicrobial to end up at the site of infection (anteroventral lung region); however, the antimicrobial has difficulty in gaining access to the diseased lung because of closure of bronchioles with inflammatory exudates.

Oxytetracyclines and spectinomycin are first choice antimicrobials for treating pneumonia. Second choice antimicrobials are florfenicol and the macrolides (particularly tilmicosin or tulathromycin, and to a lesser extent spiramycin and tylosin). Last choice antimicrobials include third (ceftiofur)- and fourth (cefquinome)-generation cephalosporins and fluoroquinolones (enrofloxacin, danofloxacin, marbofloxacin). Fluoroquinolones have the clinical advantage that they are effective for treating *Mycoplasma bovis* and other *Mycoplasma* spp., which are resistant to β-lactams because they lack a cell wall. Most cases of pneumonia in cattle are treated with long-acting oxytetracycline formulations, macrolides, florfenicol, third- or fourth-generation cephalosporins or fluoroquinolones. The antimicrobial agent should be changed no earlier than 48 h after starting treatment if there is an inadequate clinical response to treatment. Criteria used to gauge treatment efficacy include reduction in rectal temperature, increased rumen fill and a clean nose. Changing drugs too rapidly does not allow time for adequate concentrations to be achieved in the diseased lung, whereas failing to change drugs when needed can result in death or chronic pneumonia. Treatment should be given according to the label or as prescribed by a veterinarian and for at least 48 h after clinical signs abate, although the optimal time for treatment has not been determined. Discontinuing treatment too soon can result in relapses or incomplete cure. Mass medication of animals is done when there is a high incidence of shipping fever in a group of animals and the cost of medicating all animals in the group is less than the cost of treating sick animals individually (examining them, sorting them, etc.) or there is inadequate hospital pen space to house the sick animals.

The most important determinant of antimicrobial efficacy in treating pneumonia is attaining and maintaining an effective antimicrobial concentration at the site of infection, which is diseased parenchymal tissue in the lower respiratory tract, particularly the anteroventral region of the lung. This is a different requirement to that for metaphylaxis where the goal is to minimize, prevent or delay the explosive proliferation of *M. haemolytica* in the upper respiratory tract and associated horizontal transmission as well as lower respiratory tract infection. A delay in bacterial proliferation is suspected to allow additional time for vaccines administered on arrival at the feedlot to elicit an effective immune response. Metaphylaxis may also decrease the total amount of antimicrobials needed to treat large numbers of cattle with clinical signs of respiratory disease (38).

Antimicrobial susceptibility testing has frequently been recommended to guide the treatment of respiratory disease in cattle. The utility of periodic susceptibility testing to guide treatment decisions on feedlots has not been verified and is questionable, given that

9 Cattle

strains of *M. haemolytica* in a single outbreak of bovine respiratory disease vary between and within an animal (39). A major difficulty with susceptibility testing is obtaining a representative culture of bacteria from the lower respiratory tract of cattle with pneumonia (40). The gold standard method is culturing affected anteroventral lung parenchyma at necropsy; however, cattle dying of pneumonia have usually been treated with antimicrobials, which increases the percentage of resistant isolates (41–43). Necropsy sampling is therefore strongly biased towards treatment failures. A practical method for obtaining a representative culture of the lower respiratory tract bacteria in untreated cattle is therefore needed.

Antemortem culture of the bovine respiratory tract has used nasal swabs, guarded deep nasopharyngeal swabs, guarded tracheal swabs, bronchoalveolar lavage and transtracheal washes. Currently, endoscopic-assisted bronchoalveolar lavage and transtracheal wash provide gold standard methods for obtaining a lower respiratory tract culture in live cattle. Unfortunately, both techniques are rarely performed because they are time consuming and require specific training and appropriate restraint of the animal, or expensive and fragile equipment. Nasal swabs are commonly used to collect samples from cattle in the field because the technique is rapid and inexpensive; however, nasal swabs should not be used to identify the presence of lower respiratory pathogens in individual cattle. This is because bacterial populations in the upper respiratory tract differ from those in the lower respiratory tract (44, 45). Deep nasopharyngeal swabbing using sterile equine uterine culture swabs (76 cm long) shows promise as a practical method for obtaining isolates that reflect lower airway infection with *M. haemolytica*, but not *M. bovis* (46).

9.6 Metritis

Postpartum septic metritis occurs primarily in cows within two to ten days of parturition and is characterized clinically by severe toxaemia and a copious foul smelling uterine discharge, with or without retention of the placenta. The predominant bacteria in the uterus of cows with metritis vary with time since parturition; in general, *E. coli* predominates in the first five days after parturition, whereas *Arcanobacterium pyogenes*, *Bacteroides* spp. and *Fusobacterium necrophorum* predominate after this time (47, 48).

Staphylococcus spp., *Streptococcus* spp., *Pseudomonas aeruginosa*, *Proteus* spp. and occasionally *Clostridium* spp. are also present; the latter can occasionally result in tetanus if *Cl. tetani* proliferates.

Cows with retained fetal membranes but without systemic illness should be monitored but treatment with antimicrobial agents is not indicated. Antimicrobial treatment with oxytetracycline (10 mg/kg BW IM, daily) before placental shedding delays detachment of the placenta; this finding is consistent with the concept that intrauterine bacterial infection facilitates placenta detachment (48).

Cows with retained fetal membranes accompanied with systemic signs of illness (inappetance, decreased milk production, pyrexia) should be treated with antimicrobial agents daily for several days or until recovery occurs. Death can occur in untreated animals. Because of the mixed bacterial flora in the postpartum uterus with a retained placenta, broad-spectrum parenteral antimicrobials should be administered for several days until recovery is apparent (49). First choice antimicrobials include intramuscular ampicillin (10 mg/kg BW), intramuscular procaine penicillin (22 000 U/kg BW every 24 h) and intravenous oxytetracycline (11 mg/kg BW every 24 h). Oxytetracycline administration should be confined to the first five to seven days postpartum when *E. coli* predominates, as it is likely to be ineffective against *A. pyogenes* in the endometrium. Oxytetracycline at 30 mg/kg BW IV as a single dose in cows with retained fetal membranes resulted in concentrations of the antimicrobial in uterine secretions, placenta and cotyledon for 32–36 h (50). Two IM injections of oxytetracycline at 25 mg/kg BW resulted in lower peak concentrations, but these were maintained for 144 h. Parenteral oxytetracycline appears to decrease endotoxin production, as indicated by the severity of leukopenia in cattle with retained placenta (48).

A last choice antimicrobial is subcutaneous ceftiofur (2.2 mg/kg BW every 24 h); ceftiofur increases the cure rate and milk yield and decreases rectal temperature when administered to dairy cows with fever and vaginal discharge or dystocia (51). Parenteral ceftiofur decreased the pregnancy rate and increased the cure rate, compared to parenteral ampicillin, in cattle that were also treated with intrauterine ampicillin and cloxacillin (52). Subcutaneous administration of ceftiofur (1 mg/kg BW) achieves concentrations of ceftiofur derivatives in uterine tissue and lochial fluid that exceeds MICs for common metritis pathogens (53).

There is limited evidence that the intrauterine infusion of antimicrobial agents has a beneficial effect in the treatment of postpartum septic metritis. As a result, intrauterine infusion should only be performed in systemically ill cows with toxic metritis. Nevertheless, a wide variety of antimicrobial agents have been used for intrauterine medication for retained placenta and metritis in cows, although β-lactam-resistant antimicrobials should be administered because the uterine lumen can contain β-lactamase-producing bacteria (47, 48). Intrauterine infusion of tetracyclines (5–6 g) are commonly used in systemically ill cows with toxic metritis and this appears to be the most effective local treatment. However, tetracyclines should be administered as a powder dissolved in an appropriate volume of 0.9% NaCl because vehicles such as propylene glycol can irritate the endometrium. Intrauterine infusion of oxytetracycline decreases lochial odour and the incidence of fever in cattle with retained placenta (54). In cattle with retained placenta, intrauterine administration of 1 g of ampicillin and 1 g of cloxacillin for three consecutive days was also effective in decreasing the incidence of fever in the first 10 days postpartum (55). For comparison, intrauterine administration of a povidone-based oxytetracycline solution (5 g daily until expulsion) combined with fenprostalene (1 mg, SC) in cattle with retained placenta did not alter the time to detachment of the placenta but increased the frequency of pyometra (56); this finding was consistent with the concept that intrauterine bacterial infection facilitates placenta detachment (48). Intrauterine infusion of 0.5 g of the first-generation cephalosporin cefapirin improved the reproductive performance but only when administered after 26 days in milk (57). Intrauterine infusion of 1 g of the third-generation cephalosporin ceftiofur in 20 ml of sterile water once between 14 and 20 days of lactation had no effect on reproductive performance but decreased the risk of culling and increased the time to culling (58).

9.7 Mastitis

The bovine mammary gland is a difficult target for antimicrobial treatment. Penetration of a substance into milk when administered parenterally, or absorption and distribution throughout the udder when infused intramammarily (IMM), depends on its pharmacokinetic characteristics. These are lipid solubility, degree of ionization, extent of binding to serum and udder proteins and the type of vehicle. Antimicrobial treatment of dairy cows creates residues into milk, and residue avoidance is an important aspect of mastitis treatment.

Pharmacodynamics of the antimicrobial is another aspect that should be considered. Milk should not interfere with antimicrobial activity. The activity of macrolides, tetracyclines and trimethoprim–sulfonamides has been shown to be reduced in milk (59, 60). Selecting a substance with a low MIC value for the target pathogen is preferable, particularly when the antimicrobial is administered systemically. The antimicrobial should preferably have bactericidal action, as phagocytosis is impaired in the mammary gland (61).

Antimicrobial susceptibility determined *in vitro* has been considered as a prerequisite for treatment, but efficacy *in vitro* does not guarantee efficacy *in vivo* when treating bovine mastitis (62, 63). Antimicrobial resistance amongst mastitis pathogens has not yet emerged as a clinically relevant issue, but geographical regions may differ in this respect. The biggest problem is the widespread resistance of staphylococci, particularly *Staphylococcus aureus*, to penicillin G (64, 65). Coagulase-negative staphylococci tend to be more resistant than *S. aureus* and easily develop multi-resistance (65). Mastitis streptococci have remained susceptible for penicillin G, but emerging resistance to macrolides and lincosamides has been detected (65). Antimicrobial susceptibility of coliform bacteria varies (66, 67).

The most common route of the administration of antimicrobials in mastitis is the IMM route. The advantages of this route are high concentrations of the substance achieved in the milk and low consumption of the antimicrobial as the drug is directly infused into the diseased quarter. For example, the concentration of penicillin G in milk after systemic administration is 100–1000 fold lower than after IMM administration (68–70). Disadvantages of IMM administration are uneven distribution throughout the udder (71, 72) and risk for contamination when infusing the product via the teat canal. The efficacy of IMM treatment varies according to the causing pathogen, with the best therapeutic response being shown for mastitis caused by streptococci, coagulase-negative staphylococci and *Corynebacterium* spp.

9.7.1 Clinical mastitis

Mastitis is the most common reason for antimicrobial treatment of dairy cows, and such treatment may have an impact on public health. Treatment of clinical mastitis should take national and international prudent use guidelines into account (6, 73) and should be targeted towards the causative bacteria whenever possible. In acute situations, treatment must be initiated based on herd data and personal experience. Rapid on-farm bacteriological diagnosis would facilitate the selection of the most appropriate antimicrobial. Selective diagnostic media which allow rapid (overnight) diagnosis are available in many countries, which are important in decision making for the individual cow. Treatment protocols and drug selection for each farm should be made by veterinarians familiar with the farm. Use of on-farm written protocols for mastitis treatment can promote the judicious use of antimicrobials and reduce the use of antimicrobials (74). Procedures for residue avoidance should be routine in mastitis treatment. The therapeutic response of the cows can be monitored using individual somatic cell count data if available, or using the California Mastitis Test, and selective bacteriological culturing in herds with contagious mastitis.

The systemic (parenteral) route of administration has been suggested to be more efficient than IMM for treatment of clinical mastitis, as antimicrobials theoretically have better penetration of udder tissue (72, 75). However, it is difficult to attain and maintain therapeutic concentrations in milk or udder tissue following systemic administration, and very few substances have optimal pharmacokinetic and pharmacodynamic characteristics for systemic mastitis treatment (Figure 9.1). Commonly used broad-spectrum antimicrobials, such as oxytetracycline, trimethoprim–sulfonamide and ceftiofur combinations frequently do not produce therapeutic concentrations in milk and as a result have variable efficacy for the treatment of clinical mastitis (76–80); the exception being severe clinical mastitis due to coliform bacteria (67, 81, 82), presumably due to a marked increase in the permeability of the blood–milk barrier or therapeutic effects of combating bacteraemia. Macrolides have ideal pharmacokinetics (69, 83), but poor efficacy has been reported when used for the systemic treatment of clinical mastitis (80, 84). One substance used for systemic treatment is penicillin G, which as weak acid penetrates poorly into mammary gland. Due to the very low MIC values of susceptible organisms, therapeutic concentrations can be achieved in milk (68, 69). Efficacy of systemic penicillin G treatment has been shown in clinical trials (84–86). Penethamate is a more liphophilic penicillin G formulation and diffuses better than penicillin G procaine into milk (87). Combinations of penicillin and aminoglycosides should not be used, as there is no scientific evidence on a better efficacy of the combination and aminoglycosides are known to produce long-lasting residues (88).

The important clinical question regarding treatment is whether the antimicrobial should accumulate in milk or udder tissue (Tables 9.2 and 9.3; 89).

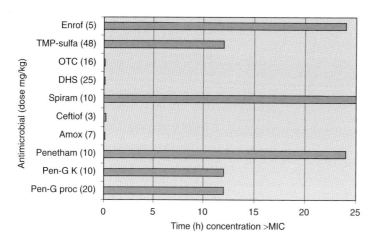

Figure 9.1 Duration of concentrations in milk with systemic administration of some commonly used antimicrobials (parenteral dose stated in parentheses in mg/kg). Concentrations refer to normal milk. Mastitis may affect the concentrations so that milk concentrations of bases (e.g. macrolides) decrease and acids (e.g. β-lactams) increase. The table must be interpreted with care as the concentrations shown are total concentrations. Only the unbound, free drug is active against microbes. Data has been compiled from different sources.

This site of accumulation may depend on the causative agent: streptococci are known to stay in the milk compartment, but *S. aureus* bacteria penetrate udder tissue and cause deep infection. The only type of mastitis where systemic treatment would be clearly advantageous may be mastitis caused by *S. aureus* (90). In severe mastitis due to coliform bacteria, parenteral administration of antimicrobials has been suggested in order to treat bacteraemia (4). Although the efficacy of the antimicrobial treatment in coliform mastitis has been questioned (91, 92), it is clear that systemic

Table 9.2 Where to target antimicrobial therapy in clinical mastitis due to different pathogens (89)

	Milk/ducts	Udder tissue	Cow
Streptococcus agalactiae	+++	–	–
Other streptococci	+++	+	–
Staphylococcus aureus	+	+++	–
Coagulase negative staphylococci	+++	–	–
Coliforms	+	–	+++

antimicrobial treatment can be beneficial in cases of severe *E. coli* mastitis with heavy bacterial growth in the udder. Enrofloxacin, ceftiofur and cefquinome have shown efficacy in experimental or clinical trials (82, 93–95). There is no evidence that administering bactericidal antimicrobials to cows with severe coliform mastitis causes the release of massive amounts of endotoxin (93).

Use of narrow-spectrum antimicrobials is preferable when treating clinical mastitis (Table 9.3). First choice antimicrobials for treating mastitis due to streptococci and penicillin-susceptible staphylococci are β-lactam antimicrobials, particularly penicillin G. Broad-spectrum antimicrobials such as third or fourth-generation cephalosporins should not be used as first alternatives for mastitis, as they may increase emergence of broad-spectrum β-lactam resistance. Systemic treatment is recommended in clinical mastitis due to *S. aureus* and in severe cases of coliform mastitis, preferably in combination with IMM treatment (96). Too short a duration of standard treatment is probably an important reason for poor cure rates in mastitis therapy. Extended treatment (an industry term that really means appropriate duration of treatment) improves cure rates, and duration of treatment should generally be extended in

9 Cattle

Table 9.3 Suggestions for antimicrobial treatment of clinical mastitis due to different pathogens. The availability of substances on the market mentioned in the table may differ between countries

Microorganism	Species	Drug of choice	Alternative	Comments
Streptococci	*S. agalactiae* *S. dysgalactiae* *Streptococcus uberis*	Penicillin G		Intramammary (IMM) treatment preferable.
	Enterococci	According to susceptibility testing		Prognosis for bacteriological cure poor.
Staphylococci	*Staphylococcus aureus* Coagulase-negative staphylococci β-Lactamase –	Penicillin G		Combination treatment in *S. aureus* mastitis
	Staphylococcus aureus Coagulase-negative staphylococci β-Lactamase +	No antimicrobials	Cloxacillin Macrolides Lincosamides	IMM and/or systemic treatment depending on the drug used. Cloxacillin selects for methicillin-resistant *S. aureus*
Coliforms	*Escherichia coli*	No antimicrobials	Fluoroquinolones Cephalosporins	Antimicrobials necessary in serious cases and during puerperal period

mastitis caused by *S. aureus* and *Streptococcus uberis* (90, 97). Clinical mastitis episodes should be treated for at least three days; this recommended treatment duration is longer than most label recommendations in the USA. All mastitis treatment should be evidence based, in other words, the efficacy of each product and treatment length should be demonstrated by scientific studies.

9.7.2   Subclinical mastitis

Treating subclinical mastitis with antimicrobials is generally not economical during lactation (98) because of high treatment costs and poor efficacy. In a US study with a large number of subclinical mastitis cases (99), the overall bacteriological cure rate for antimicrobial treatment was 75% and that for no treatment 68%. The marginal benefit applied for streptococcal mastitis only; in mastitis due to *S. aureus*, antimicrobials were equal to no treatment. Treatment of subclinical mastitis will not affect the incidence of mastitis in the herd unless other preventive measures are taken. Studies on treating cows based on high somatic cell counts have generally shown that no effect on milk production has been achieved. In herd problems caused by very contagious bacteria such as *S. aureus* or *Streptococcus agalactiae*, treatment of subclinical mastitis is advised. Models for economical analysis of treatment of subclinical mastitis have been proposed, but should be interpreted with caution as have been studied for one substance and country only (100, 101).

9.7.3   Dry cow therapy

Treatment of all dairy cows at drying-off has been practiced for decades; such treatment serves a two-fold purpose of eliminating a large number of sub-clinical infections and preventing new infections in the early dry period. Blanket dry cow therapy still provides one of the corner stones in mastitis control in many countries. The practice of blanket dry cow therapy has recently been questioned, since bulk milk tank somatic cell counts have markedly decreased and the principal causative agents of mastitis has changed from contagious to environmental. Selective dry cow therapy (i.e. identification and treatment of cows with intramammary infection) is an increasingly attractive method to decrease routine antimicrobial use in dairy cattle (102). Refinement of currently available screening tests for intramammary infection (such as somatic cell count, California Mastitis test results or electrical conductivity) that produces a test with adequate sensitivity and specificity will make selective dry cow therapy a routine recommendation for herds (103). It is not economical to treat cows infected by the so-called minor pathogens (104). Systemic administration of antimicrobials has been proposed for dry cow therapy, but no scientific evidence has been presented to support the better efficacy of this practice. An internal teat sealer for prevention of new infections shows promise as a non-antibiotic alternative for preventing new intramammary infections during the dry period. In some countries, prepartum intramammary antimicrobial therapy has been introduced as a means to control mastitis in heifers. This cannot be regarded as a prudent use of antimicrobials; furthermore, the advantages from this practice have been questioned (105).

9.8   General conclusions

Important considerations when administering antimicrobials as part of the treatment of diseased cattle are: (1) administering as directed on the label or by a veterinarian whenever possible; (2) selecting an antimicrobial agent with an appropriate spectrum of activity; (3) using a dosage protocol that *attains* and *maintains* an effective therapeutic concentration at the *site of infection*; (4) treating for an appropriate duration; (5) avoiding adverse local or systemic effects and violative residues; and (6) minimizing the potential for transfer of antimicrobial resistance genes. Recommended dosages of antimicrobial agents administered intravenously, intramuscularly, subcutaneously, or orally in cattle are stated in Table 9.4. The overarching philosophy is that veterinarians should use and prescribe antimicrobials conservatively in order to minimize potential adverse effects on animal or human health (12). Animal use of fluoroquinolones and third- or fourth-generation cephalosporins should be restricted whenever possible in cattle because these antimicrobial classes are very important in the treatment of severe and invasive infections in humans (6).

Table 9.4 Examples of dosages of antimicrobial agents administered intravenously, intramuscularly, subcutaneously or orally in cattle[a]

Drug	Dose(s)	Indication
Amoxicillin trihydrate	10–15 mg/kg IM/PO q 12 h	Oral only to suckling calves with diarrhoea, Postpartum metritis Septic arthritis
	12.5 mg/kg PO q 12 h	When combined with clavulanate potassium and administered to suckling calves with diarrhoea
Ampicillin trihydrate	10–15 mg/kg IM/PO q 12 h	Postpartum metritis Septic arthritis
	1 g ampicillin and 1 g cloxacillin intrauterine	Postpartum metritis
Cefquinome	1 mg/kg IM q 24 h	Treatment of respiratory disease (last choice) Digital dermatitis in cattle (last choice)
Ceftiofur crystalline free acid	3 mg/kg SC in ear once	Treatment of respiratory disease (last choice)
Ceftiofur HCl suspension	1.1–2.2 mg/kg IM/SC q 24 h for 3–5 days	Treatment of respiratory disease (last choice) Acute interdigital necrobacillosis (last choice)
Ceftiofur sodium	2.2 mg/kg SC q 24 h	Postpartum metritis (last choice) Acute coliform mastitis (last choice)
	1.1–2.2 mg/kg IM/SC q 24 h for 3–5 days	Treatment of respiratory disease (last choice) Acute interdigital necrobacillosis (last choice)
	1.5–2.0 mg/kg IM q 24 h	Digital dermatitis in cattle (last choice)
	5 mg/kg IM q 24 h	Salmonellosis in calves (last choice)
Chlortetracycline HCl	7–11 mg/kg PO q 12 h	In milk replacer to suckling calves
Danofloxacin	1.25 mg/kg IV/SC/IM q 24 h for 3–5 days (EU)	Treatment of respiratory disease (last choice)
Difloxacin	2.5 mg/kg q 24 h for 3-5 days	Treatment of respiratory disease (last choice)
Enrofloxacin	7.5–12.5 mg/kg IV/SC once	Septicaemia (last choice), Calf diarrhoea (last choice),
	2.5–5.0 mg/kg IV/SC q 24 h for 3–5 days	Treatment of respiratory disease (last choice)
	5 mg/kg IV q 24 h IV/SC	Acute coliform mastitis (last choice)
Erythromycin	8.8–10 mg/kg IM	Treatment of respiratory disease.
Florfenicol	20 mg/kg IM, repeat at 48 h	Treatment of respiratory disease.
	40 mg/kg IM once	
Gentamicin	2.2–6.6 mg/kg IM q 12–24 h	Septicaemia in calves. Last choice because of prolonged slaughter withdrawal. Voluntary ban on use in food-producing animals
Marbofloxacin	2 mg/kg IV/IM/SC q 24 h for 3–5 days	Treatment of respiratory disease (last choice)
Neomycin sulfate	22 mg/kg PO q 12 h	In milk replacer to suckling calves, rarely indicated alone, possibly indicated when combined with chlortetracycline in milk replacer
Oxytetracycline	10 mg/kg IV q 24 h	Post partum metritis, acute interdigital necrobacillosis, lacerations/abscesses, respiratory disease, infectious bovine keratoconjunctivitis (pinkeye), tick-borne fever, anaplasmosis
	20 mg/kg IM q 48 h	Long acting formulation for acute interdigital necrobacillosis, lacerations/abscesses, respiratory disease, infectious bovine keratoconjunctivitis (pinkeye), anaplasmosis

Continued

Table 9.4   (Continued)

Drug	Dose(s)	Indication
Penethamate	10–15 mg/kg IM q 24 h	Clinical mastitis due to streptococci and penicillin susceptible staphylococci
Penicillin G: procaine	20 000 U/kg IM q 24 h	Clinical mastitis due to streptococci and penicillin susceptible staphylococci Septic arthritis Postpartum metritis
Penicillin G: sodium/ potassium	9 500 U/kg IV q 12 h	Clinical mastitis due to streptococci and penicillin susceptible staphylococci
Spectinomycin	10–15 m/kg q 24 h SC for 3–5 days	Respiratory disease
Spiramycin	10 mg/kg IV q 24 h	Clinical mastitis due to streptococci and staphylococci
Tetracycline	5–6 g intrauterine	Postpartum metritis
Tilmicosin	10 mg/kg SC once	Respiratory disease in beef cattle >1 month of age or dairy cattle <20 months of age
Trimethoprim- sulfonamide	25 mg/kg IV/IM q 24 h	Septicaemia in cattle, diarrhoea in calves
Tulathromycin	2.5 mg/kg SC once	Treatment of respiratory disease
Tylosin	10–20 mg/kg IM	Treatment of respiratory disease in beef and non-lactating dairy cattle

[a] It should be noted that the dose rates may not be the same than those approved for these products in different countries. The withdrawal times should be adjusted accordingly if off-label doses are used. Clinical efficacy of this dosing has not been shown for all indications.

9 Cattle

References

1. Aldridge, B.M., Garry, F.B. and Adams, R. (1993). Neonatal septicemia in calves: 25 cases (1985–1990). *J. Am. Vet. Med. Assoc.* 203: 1324–9.
2. Fecteau, M.E., House, J.K., Kotarski, S.F. *et al.* (2003). Efficacy of ceftiofur for treatment of experimental salmonellosis in neonatal calves. *Am. J. Vet. Res.* 64: 918–25.
3. Thomas, E., Roy, O., Skowronski, V., *et al.* (2004). Comparative field efficacy study between cefquinome and gentamicin in neonatal calves with clinical signs of septicemia. *Revue Méd. Vét.* 155: 489–93.
4. Wenz, J.R., Barrington, G.M., Garry, F.B., *et al.* (2001). Bacteraemia associated with naturally occurring acute coliform mastitis in dairy cows. *J. Am. Vet. Med. Assoc.* 219: 976–81.
5. Smith, G.W., Constable, P.D. and Morin, D.E. (2001). Ability of hematologic and serum biochemical variables to differentiate Gram-negative and Gram-positive mastitis in dairy cows. *J. Vet. Intern. Med.* 15: 394–400.
6. OIE (2006). Guidelines on the responsible and prudent use of antimicrobial agents in veterinary medicine. Available at: http://www.oie.int/eng/normes/mcode/en_ chapitre_3.9.3.htm Accessed 20 February.
7. Constable, P.D. (2004). Antimicrobial use in the treatment of calf diarrhea. *J. Vet. Intern. Med.* 18: 8–17.
8. Fecteau, G., Van Metre, D.C., Pare, J., *et al.* (1997). Bacteriological culture of blood from critically ill neonatal calves. *Can. Vet. J.* 38: 95–100.
9. Lofstedt, J., Dohoo, I.R. and Duizer, G. (1999). Model to predict septicemia in diarrheic calves. *J. Vet. Intern. Med.* 13: 81–8.
10. Fecteau, G., Paré, J., Van Metre, D.C., *et al.* (1997). Use of a clinical sepsis score for predicting bacteremia in neonatal dairy calves on a calf rearing farm. *Can. Vet. J.* 38: 101–104.
11. Ortman, K. and Svensson, C. (2004). Use of antimicrobial drugs in Swedish dairy calves and replacement heifers. *Vet. Rec.* 154: 136–40.
12. Morley, P.S., Apley, M.D., Besser, T.E., *et al.* (2005). Antimicrobial drug use in veterinary medicine. *J. Vet. Intern. Med.* 19: 617.
13. Berge, A.C.B., Moore, D.A. and Sischo, W.M. (2006). Field trial evaluating the influence of prophylactic and therapeutic antimicrobial administration on antimicrobial resistance of fecal *Escherichia coli* in dairy calves. *Appl. Environ. Microbiol.* 72: 3872–8.
14. Sato, K., Bartlett, P.C. and Saeed, M.A. (2005). Antimicrobial susceptibility of *Escherichia coli* isolates from dairy farms using organic versus conventional production methods. *J. Am. Vet. Med. Assoc.* 226: 589–94.
15. White, G., Piercy, D.W.T. and Gibbs, H.A. (1981). Use of a calf salmonellosis model to evaluate the therapeutic properties of trimethoprim and sulphadiazine and their mutual potentiation *in vivo*. *Res. Vet. Sci.* 31: 27–31.

16. Constable, P.D. (2003). Use of antibiotics to prevent calf diarrhea and septicemia. *Bovine Practitioner* 37(2): 137–42.

17. Berge, A.C.B., Moore, D.A. and Sischo, W.M. (2006). Prevalence and antimicrobial resistance patterns of *Salmonella enterica* in preweaned calves from dairies and calf ranches. *Am. J. Vet. Res.* 67: 1580–8.

18. Ziv, G., Nouws, J.F.M., Groothuis, D.G., *et al.* (1977). Oral absorption and bioavailability of ampicillin derivatives in calves. *Am. J. Vet. Res.* 38: 1007–13.

19. Reisinger, R.C. (1965). Pathogenesis and prevention of infectious diarrhea (scours) of newborn calves. *J. Am. Vet. Med. Assoc.* 147: 1377–86.

20. Dalton, R.G., Fisher, E.W. and McIntyre, W.I.M. (1960). Antibiotics and calf diarrhea. *Vet. Rec.* 72: 1186–99.

21. Berge, A.C.B., Lindeque, P., Moore, D.A., *et al.* (2005). A clinical trial evaluating prophylactic and therapeutic antibiotic use on health and performance of preweaned calves. *J. Dairy Sci.* 88: 2166–77.

22. Schifferli, D., Galeazzi, R.L., Nicolet, J., *et al.* (1982). Pharmacokinetics of oxytetracycline and therapeutic implications in veal calves. *J. Vet. Pharmacol. Ther.* 5: 247–57.

23. Palmer, G.H., Bywater, R.J. and Stanton, A. (1983). Absorption in calves of amoxycillin, ampicillin, and oxytetracycline in milk replacer, water, or an oral rehydration formulation. *Am. J. Vet. Res.* 44: 68–71.

24. Belli, P., Poumarat, F., Perrin, M. and Martel, J.L. (1993). Evaluation of the *in vivo* activity of enrofloxacin in experimental *Mycoplasma bovis* infection of calves. *Med. Vet.* 10: 85–91.

25. Grandemange, E., Gunst, S., Woehrle, F. and Boisrame, B. (2002). Field evaluation of the efficacy of Marbocyl(R) 2% in the treatment of infectious arthritis of calves. *Irish Vet. J.* 55: 237–40.

26. Gough, A.W., Kasali, O.B., Siglar, R.E. and Baragi, V. (1992). Quinolone arthropathy – acute toxicity to immature articular cartilage. *Toxicol. Pathol.* 20: 436–9.

27. Ayling, R.D., Baker, S.E., Peek, M.L., Simon, A.J. and Nicholas, R.A. (2000). Comparison of *in vitro* activity of danofloxacin, florfenicol, spectinomycin and tilmicosin against recent field isolates of *Mycoplasma bovis*. *Vet. Rec.* 146: 745–7.

28. Rosenbusch, R.F., Kinyon, J.M., Apley, M., *et al.* (2005). *In vitro* antimicrobial inhibition profiles of *Mycoplasma bovis* isolates recovered from various regions of the United States from 2002 to 2003. *J. Vet. Diag. Invest.* 17: 436–41.

29. Francoz, D., Desrochers, A., Fecteau, G., Desautels, C., Latouche, J.S. and Fortin, M. (2005). Synovial fluid changes in induced infectious arthritis in calves. *J. Vet. Intern. Med.* 19: 336–43.

30. Sawant, A.A., Sordillo, L.M. and Jayarao, B.M. (2005). A survey on antibiotic usage in dairy herds in Pennsylvania. *J. Dairy Sci.* 88: 2991–9.

31. Britt, J.S., Carson, M.C., vanBredow, J.D. and Condon, R.J. (1999). Antibiotic residues in milk samples obtained from cows after treatment for papillomatous digital dermatitis. *J. Am. Vet. Med. Assoc.* 215: 833–6.

32. Guterbock, W.M., Borelli, C.L. and Read, D.H. (1996). Evaluation of four therapies of papillomatous digital dermatitis in dairy cattle. *Bovine Proc.* 28: 240–1.

33. Laven, R.A. (2006). Efficacy of systemic cefquinome and erythromycin against digital dermatitis in cattle. *Vet. Rec.* 159: 19–20.

34. Laven, R.A. and Proven, M.J. (2000). Use of an antibiotic footbath in the treatment of bovine digital dermatitis. *Vet. Rec.* 147: 503–6.

35. Tragesser, L.A., Wittum, T.E., Funk, J.A., Winokur, P.L. and Rajala-Schultz, P.J. (2006). Association between ceftiofur use and isolation of *Escherichia coli* with reduced susceptibility to ceftriaxone from fecal samples of dairy cows. *Am. J. Vet. Res.* 67: 1696–1700.

36. Zhao, S., Qaiyumi, S., Friedman, S., *et al.* (2003). Characterization of *Salmonella enterica* serotype Newport isolated from humans and food animals. *J. Clin. Microbiol.* 41: 5366–71.

37. Fey, P.D., Safranek, T.J., Rupp, M.E., *et al.* (2000). Ceftriaxone-resistant *Salmonella* infection acquired by a child from cattle. *N. Engl. J. Med.* 342: 1242–9.

38. Schwarz, S., Kehrenberg, C. and Walsh, T.R. (2001). Use of antimicrobial agents in veterinary medicine and food animal production. *Int. J. Antimicrob. Agents* 17: 431–7.

39. Murphy, G.L., Robinson, L.D. and Burrows, G.E. (1993). Restriction endonuclease analysis and ribotyping differentiate *Pasteurella haemolytica* serotype A1 isolates from cattle within a feedlot. *J. Clin. Microbiol.* 31: 2303–8.

40. Constable, P.D. (2004b). Use of susceptibility testing in veterinary medicine. *Proceedings 37th Annual Convention, American Association Bovine Practitioners* 37: 11–17.

41. Hjerpe, C.A. and Routen, T.A. (1976). Practical and theoretical considerations concerning treatment of bacterial pneumonia in feedlot cattle, with special reference to antimicrobic therapy. *Proc. Ann. Conv. AABP*, San Francisco 9: 142–7.

42. Martin, S.W., Meek, A.H. and Curtis, R.A. (1983). Antimicrobial use in feedlot calves: its association with culture rates and antimicrobial susceptibility. *Can. J. Comp. Med.* 47: 6–10.

43. Allen, J.W., Viel, L., Bateman, K.G., *et al.* (1992). Changes in the bacterial flora of the upper and lower respiratory tracts and bronchoalveolar lavage differential cell counts in feedlot calves treated for respiratory diseases. *Can. J. Vet. Res.* 56: 177–83.

44. Allen, J.W., Viel, L., Bateman, K.G., *et al.* (1991). The microbial flora of the respiratory tract in feedlot calves: associations between nasopharyngeal and bronchoalveolar lavage cultures. *Can. J. Vet. Res.* 55: 341–6.

45. Thomas, A., Dizier, I., Trolin, A., *et al.* (2002). Comparison of sampling procedures for isolating pulmonary mycoplasmas in cattle. *Vet. Res. Comm.* 26: 333–9.

46. Godinho, K.S., Sarasola, P., Renoult, E., *et al.* (2007). Use of deep nasopharyngeal swabs as a predictive diagnostic

9 Cattle

method for natural respiratory infections in calves. *Vet. Rec.* 160: 22–5.

47. Dohmen, M.J.W., Joop, K., Sturk, A., *et al.* (2000). Relationship between intra-uterine bacterial contamination, endotoxin levels, and the development of endometritis in postpartum cows with dystocia or retained placenta. *Theriogenology* 54: 1019–32.

48. Konigsson, K., Gustafsson, H., Gunnarsson, A., *et al.* (2001). Clinical and bacteriological aspects on the use of oxytetracycline and flunixin in primiparous cows with induced retained placenta and post-partal endometritis. *Reprod. Dom. Anim.* 36: 247–56.

49. Bretzlaff, K.N., Ott, R.S., Koritz, G.D., *et al.* (1983). Distribution of oxytetracycline in genital tract tissues of postpartum cows given the drug by intravenous and intra-uterine routes. *Am. J. Vet. Res.* 44: 764–9.

50. Cohen, R.O., Ziv, G., Soback, S., *et al.* (1993). The pharmacology of oxytetracycline in the uterus of postparturient dairy cows with retained foetal membranes. *Israel J. Vet. Med.* 48: 69–79.

51. Zhou, C., Boucher, J.E. and Dame, K.J. (2001). Multilocation trial of ceftiofur for treatment of postpartum cows with fever. *J. Am. Vet. Med. Assoc.* 219: 805–8.

52. Drillich, M., Beetz, O., Pfützner, A., *et al.* (2001). Evaluation of a systemic antibiotic treatment of toxic puerperal metritis in dairy cows. *J. Dairy Sci.* 84: 2101–17.

53. Okker, H., Schmitt, E.J., Vos, P.L.A.M., *et al.* (2002). Pharmacokinetics of ceftiofur in plasma and uterine secretions and tissues after subcutaneous postpartum administration in lactating dairy cows. *J. Vet. Pharmacol. Ther.* 25: 33–8.

54. Callahan, C.J., Horstman, L.A. and Frank, D.J. (1988). A comparison of fenprostalene and oxytetracycline as treatment for retained fetal membranes in dairy cows. *Bovine Pract.* 23: 21–3.

55. Drillich, M., Mahistedt, M., Reichert, U., *et al.* (2006). Strategies to improve the therapy of retained fetal membranes in dairy cows. *J. Dairy Sci.* 89: 627–35.

56. Stevens, R.D., Dinsmore, R.P. and Cattell, M.B. (1995). Evaluation of the use of intrauterine infusions of oxytetracycline, subcutaneous injections of fenprostalene, or a combination of both, for the treatment of retained fetal membranes in dairy cows. *J. Am. Vet. Med. Assoc.* 207: 1612–5.

57. Leblanc, S.J., Duffield, T.F., Leslie, K.E., *et al.* (2002). The effect of treatment of clinical endometritis on reproductive performance in dairy cows. *J. Dairy Sci.* 85: 2237–49.

58. Scott, H.M., Schouten, M.J., Gaiser, J.C., *et al.* (2005). Effect of intrauterine administration of ceftiofur on fertility and risk of culling in postparturient cows with retained fetal membranes, twins, or both. *J. Am. Vet. Med. Assoc.* 226: 2044–52.

59. Fang, W. and Pyörälä, S. (1996). Mastitis causing *Escherichia coli*: serum sensitivity and susceptibility to selected antibacterials in milk. *J. Dairy Sci.* 79: 76–82.

60. Louhi, M., Inkinen, K., Myllys, V. and Sandholm, M. (1992). Relevance of sensitivity testings (MIC) of *S. aureus*

to predict the antibacterial action in milk. *J. Vet. Med. B* 39: 253–62.

61. Sordillo, L. (2005). Factors affecting mammary gland immunity and mastitis susceptibility. *Livestock Prod. Sci.* 98: 89–99.

62. Constable, P.D. and Morin, D.E. (2002). Use of antimicrobial susceptibility testing of bacterial pathogens isolated from the milk of dairy cows with clinical mastitis to predict response to treatment with cephapirin and oxytetracycline. *J. Am. Vet. Med. Assoc.* 221: 103–8.

63. Constable, P.D. and Morin, D.E. (2003). Treatment of clinical mastitis. Using antimicrobial susceptibility profiles for treatment decisions. In: Sears P. Guest Editor, *Bovine Mastitis. Vet. Clin. North Am. Food Anim. Practice* 19: 139–55.

64. Olsen, J.E., Christensen, H. and Aarestrup, F.M. (2006). Diversity and evolution of blaZ from *Staphylococcus aureus* and coagulase-negative staphylococci. *J. Antimicr. Chemother.* 57: 450–60.

65. Pitkälä, A., Haveri, M., Pyörälä, S, Myllys, V. and Honkanen-Buzalski, T. (2004). Bovine mastitis in Finland 2001 – prevalence, distribution of bacteria and antimicrobial resistance. *J. Dairy Sci.* 87: 2433–41.

66. Lehtolainen, T., Shpigel, N., Pohjanvirta, T., Pelkonen, S. and Pyörälä, S. (2003). *In vitro* antimicrobial susceptibility of *Escherichia coli* isolates originating from clinical mastitis in Finland and Israel. *J. Dairy Sci.* 86: 3927–32.

67. Morin, D.E., Shanks, R.D. and McCoy, G.C. (1998). Comparison of antibiotic administration in conjunction with supportive measures versus supportive measures alone for treatment of dairy cows with clinical mastitis. *J. Am. Vet. Med. Assoc.* 213: 676–84.

68. Franklin, A., Holmberg, O., Horn af Rantzien, M. and Åström, G. (1984). Effect of procaine benzylpenicillin alone or in combination with dihydrostreptomycin on udder pathogens *in vitro* and in experimentally infected bovine udders. *Am. J. Vet. Res.* 45: 1398–1402.

69. Franklin, A., Horn af Rantzien, M., Obel, N., Östensson, K., Åström, G. and Rantzien, M.H. (1986). Concentrations of penicillin, streptomycin, and spiramycin in bovine udder tissue liquids. *Am. J. Vet. Res.* 47: 804–7.

70. Moretain, J.P. and Boisseau, J. (1989). Excretion of penicillins and cephalexin in bovine milk following intramammary administration. *Food Add. Contamin.* 6: 79–90.

71. Ehinger, A.M. and Kietzmann, M. (2000). Tissue distribution of oxacillin and ampicillin in the isolated perfused bovine udder. *J. Vet. Med. A* 47: 157–68.

72. Ullberg, S., Hansson, E. and Funke, H. (1958). Distribution of penicillin in mastitic udders following intramammary injection – an autoradiographic study. *Am. J. Vet. Res.* 19: 84–92.

73. Anonymous (2003). Use of antimicrobial agents in animals. Report of the working group on antimicrobial agents. Ministry of Agriculture and Forestry in Finland. MAFF Publications 9, 2003. Available at: http://www.mmm.fi/julkaisut/tyoryhmamuistiot/2003/tr2003_9a.pdf. Accessed 20 February.

9 Cattle

74. Raymond, M.J., Wohlre, R.D. and Call, D.R. (2006). Assessment and promotion of judicious antibiotic use on dairy farms in Washington State. *J. Dairy Sci.* 89: 3228–40.

75. Ziv, G. (1980). Drug selection and use in mastitis: systemic vs. local therapy. *J. Am. Vet. Med. Assoc.* 176: 1109–15.

76. Duenas, M.I., Paape, M.J., Wettemann, R.P. and Douglass, L.W. (2001). Incidence of mastitis in beef cows after intramuscular administration of oxytetracycline. *J. Anim. Sci.* 79: 1996–2005.

77. Erskine, R.J. and Barlett, P.C. (1996). Intramuscular administration of ceftiofur sodium versus intramammary infusion of penicillin/novobiocin for treatment of *Streptococcus agalactiae* mastitis in dairy cows. *J. Am. Vet. Med. Assoc.* 208: 258–60.

78. Kaartinen, L., Löhönen, K., Wiese, B., Franklin, A. and Pyörälä, S. (1999). Pharmacokinetics of sulphadiazine-trimethoprim in lactating dairy cows. *Acta Vet. Scand.* 40: 271–8.

79. Lents, C.A., Wettemann, R.P., Paape, M.J., *et al.* (2002). Efficacy of intramuscular treatment of beef cows with oxytetracycline to reduce mastitis and to increase calf growth. *J. Anim. Sci.* 80: 1405–12.

80. Owens, W.E., Nickerson, S.C. and Ray, C.H. (1999). Efficacy of parenterally or intramammarily administered tilmicosin or ceftiofur against *Staphylococcus aureus* mastitis during lactation. *J. Dairy Sci.* 82: 645–7.

81. Shpigel, N.Y., Winkler, M., Ziv, G., *et al.* (1998). Relationship between *in vitro* sensitivity of coliform pathogens in the udder and the outcome of treatment for clinical mastitis. *Vet. Rec.* 142: 135–7.

82. Erskine, R.J., Barlett, P.C., VanLente, J.L. and Phipps, C.R. (2002). Efficacy of systemic ceftiofur for severe clinical mastitis in dairy cattle. *J. Dairy Sci.* 85: 2571–5.

83. Sanders, P., Moulin, G., Guillot, P., *et al.* (1992). Pharmacokinetics of spiramycin after intravenous, intramuscular and subcutaneous administration in lactating cows. *J. Vet. Pharmacol. Ther.* 15: 53–61.

84. Pyörälä, S. and Pyörälä, E. (1998). Efficacy of parenteral administration of three antimicrobial agents in treatment of clinical mastitis in lactating cows: 487 cases (1989–1995). *J. Am. Vet. Med. Assoc.* 212: 407–12.

85. Waage, S. (1997). Comparison of two regimens for the treatment of clinical bovine mastitis caused by bacteria sensitive to penicillin. *Vet. Rec.* 141: 616–20.

86. Taponen, S., Jantunen, A., Pyörälä, E. and Pyörälä, S. (2003). Efficacy of targeted 5-day parenteral and intramammary treatment of clinical *Staphylococcus aureus* mastitis caused by penicillin-susceptible or penicillin-resistant bacterial isolate. *Acta Vet. Scand.* 44: 53–62.

87. Ziv, G. and Storper, M. (1985). Intramuscular treatment of subclinical staphylococcal mastitis in lactating cows with penicillin G, methicillin and their esters. *J. Vet. Pharmacol. Ther.* 8: 276–83.

88. Whittem, T. and Hanlon, D. (1997). Dihydrostreptomycin or streptomycin in combination with penicillin in dairy cattle therapeutics: a review and re-analysis of published data, Part 1: Clinical pharmacology. *New Zealand Vet. J.* 45: 178–84.

89. Erskine, R.J. (2003). Antibacterial therapy of clinical mastitis – part I. Drug selection. Part II Administration. *North Am. Vet. Conf. Proceedings* 17: 13–16.

90. Barkema, H., Schukken, Y.H. and Zadoks, R.N. (2006). Invited review: the role of cow, pathogen, and treatment regimen in the therapeutic success of bovine *Staphylococcus aureus* mastitis. *J. Dairy Sci.* 89: 1877–95.

91. Jones, G.F. and Ward, G.E. (1990). Evaluation of systemic administration of gentamicin for treatment of coliform mastitis in cows. *J. Am. Vet. Med. Assoc.* 197: 731–5.

92. Pyörälä, S., Kaartinen, L., Käck, H. and Rainio, V. (1994b). Efficacy of two therapy regimes for treatment of experimentally induced *Escherichia coli* mastitis in the bovine. *J. Dairy Sci.* 77: 453–61.

93. Dosogne, H., Meyer, E., Sturk, A., *et al.* (2002). Effect of enrofloxacin treatment on plasma endotoxin during bovine *Escherichia coli* mastitis. *Inflammation Res.* 51: 201–5.

94. Rantala, M., Kaartinen, L., Välimäki, E., *et al.* (2002). Efficacy and pharmacokinetics of enrofloxacin and flunixin meglumine for treatment of cows with experimentally induced *Escherichia coli* mastitis. *J. Vet. Pharm. Ther.* 25: 251–8.

95. Shpigel, N.Y., Levin, D., Winkler, M., *et al.* (1997). Efficacy of cefquinome for treatment of cows with mastitis experimentally induced using *Escherichia coli*. *J. Dairy Sci.* 80: 318–23.

96. Taponen, S., Dredge, K., Henriksson, B., *et al.* (2002). Efficacy of intramammary treatment with procaine penicillin G vs. procaine penicillin plus neomycin in bovine clinical mastitis caused by penicillin-susceptible, gram-positive bacteria – a double blind field study. *J. Vet. Pharm. Ther.* 26: 193–8.

97. Oliver, S.P., Almeida, R.A., Gillespie, B.E., *et al.* (2004). Extended ceftiofur therapy for treatment of experimentally-induced *Streptococcus uberis* mastitis in lactating dairy cattle. *J. Dairy Sci.* 87: 3322–9.

98. Shephard, R.W., Malmo, J. and Pfeiffer, D.U. (2000). A clinical trial to evaluate the effectiveness of antibiotic treatment of lactating cows with high somatic cell counts in their milk. *Aust. Vet. J.* 78: 763–8.

99. Wilson, D.J., Gonzalez, R.N., Case, K.L., Garrison, L.L. and Grohn, Y.T. (1999). Comparison of seven antibiotic treatments with no treatment for bacteriological efficacy against bovine mastitis pathogens. *J. Dairy Sci.* 82: 1664–70.

100. Swinkels, J.M., Hogeveen, H. and Zadoks, R.N. (2005a). A partial budget model to estimate economic benefits of lactational treatment of subclinical *Staphylococcus aureus* mastitis. *J. Dairy Sci.* 88: 4273–87.

101. Swinkels, J.M., Rooijendijk, J.G.A., Zadoks, R.N. and Hogeveen, H. (2005b). Use of partial budgeting to determine the estimate economic benefits of antibiotic treatment of chronic subclinical mastitis caused by *Streptococcus uberis* or *Streptococcus dysgalactiae*. *J. Dairy Res.* 72: 75–85.

9 Cattle

102. Østerås, Edge V.L. and Martin, S.W. (1999). Determinants of success or failure in the elimination of major mastitis pathogens in selective dry cow therapy. *J. Dairy Sci.* 82: 1221–31.

103. Huijps, K. and Hogeveen, H. (2007). Stochastic modeling to determine the economic effects of blanket, selective, and no dry cow therapy. *J. Dairy Sci.* 90: 1225–34.

104. Robert, A., Seegers, H. and Bareille, N. (2006). Incidence of intramammary infections during the dry period without or with antibiotic treatment in dairy cows – a quantitative analysis of published data. *Vet. Res.* 37: 25–48.

105. Borm, A.A., Fox, L.K., Leslie, K.E., *et al.* (2006). Effects of prepartum intramammary antibiotic therapy on udder health, milk production, and reproductive performance in dairy heifers. *J. Dairy Sci.* 89: 2090–8.

9 Cattle

Chapter 10

GUIDELINES FOR ANTIMICROBIAL USE IN HORSES

J. Scott Weese, Keith Edward Baptiste, Viveca Baverud and Pierre-Louis Toutain

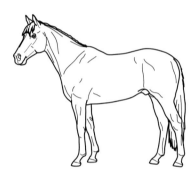

Prudent antimicrobial therapy is a critical component of equine medicine. Antimicrobials are widely used for treatment of known or suspected bacterial infections, and for prevention of post-operative and secondary infections. Most horses are companion or athletic animals with a close human–animal bond. Due to their affective and economic value, antimicrobial combinations and expensive drugs that are otherwise rarely used in veterinary medicine are frequently used. Empirical treatment is also very common. However, the emergence of multi-drug resistant bacteria in horses is of increasing concern and various veterinary organizations have recently developed general ethical guidelines to encourage prudent antimicrobial use (1, 2).

Although the basic principles of equine antimicrobial therapy are no different to those in other animal species, there are some special considerations. Some horses are food-producing animals, and inherent concerns about antimicrobial residues and antimicrobial resistance in food products need to be considered if equine meat is destined for human consumption. As hindgut fermenters, horses are particularly susceptible to adverse gastrointestinal consequences of antimicrobial administration. The fragility and the economic and emotional value of neonatal foals encourage antimicrobial treatment; however, the pharmacodynamics of antimicrobials in foals is poorly understood. The large size of most horses can result in economic constraints to optimal therapy if the most appropriate drugs are more expensive than other options. The size and temperament of a horse may influence selection of treatment options based on the ability of veterinarians or owners to safely administer drugs via different routes. In some countries, lay people have ready access to certain antimicrobials and veterinarians may encounter cases that have been treated with one or more drugs, often with inappropriate dosing regimens. All these factors need to be taken into consideration when prescribing or administering antimicrobials to a horse.

10.1 Adverse effects of antimicrobials

A variety of adverse effects can occur as a result of antimicrobial therapy, including colitis, allergic reaction, immune-mediated disease and arthropathy. Clinically, the main adverse effect is antimicrobial-associated colitis. This syndrome develops in temporal association with antimicrobial therapy and may be caused by changes in the composition of the intestinal microflora. While the relative risk of colitis with different antimicrobials has not been assessed objectively, it seems clear that there is great variation. Drugs that have low oral absorption or are excreted in bile or enterocytes, pose a higher risk because of the drug levels achieved in the intestinal tract. Drugs with activity against anaerobes are also considered more likely to cause colitis.

Absolute prevention of colitis is impossible. The realistic goal is to reduce the risk through appropriate use of antimicrobials. The oral route of administration should only be used for drugs with proven efficacy and safety in horses. Drugs such as lincomycin, clindamycin and oral penicillins are considered very high risk and should never be used in horses. Other antimicrobials, such as oxytetracycline and erythromycin, are also considered risky but can be usefully employed in certain conditions. For example, oxytetracycline is the drug of choice of Potomac Horse Fever (PHF). Erythromycin is highly effective for treatment of *Rhodococcus equi* infection in foals but can cause severe colitis in adults, even following minimal exposure (3). It is important to remember that there is some degree of risk with any antimicrobial administered by any route. The likelihood and consequences of antimicrobial-associated colitis should be carefully considered when deciding whether antimicrobials are necessary, as well as in the selection of the most appropriate drug for a certain disease or pathogen.

There are regional differences in the apparent incidence of adverse effects due to antimicrobials. This is perhaps best illustrated by the high incidence of *Clostridium difficile* associated diarrhoea in mares in Sweden exposed to low levels of erythromycin while their foals are being treated for *R. equi* pneumonia (4). This phenomenon is reported less commonly (or rarely) in other areas. Fatal colitis has also been reported anecdotally following the administration of doxycycline to horses in Europe, but is not considered a serious problem in North America. However, one out of

six horses died of acute colitis in a study on doxycycline pharmacokinetics carried out in the USA (5).

Enrofloxacin has been associated with arthropathy in foals and should be avoided in this age group. This is consistent with findings in other animals. However, complete scientific documentation on the adverse effect of enrofloxacin in foals has never been published and thus there is a lack of critical review on this topic.

10.2 Drug interactions

The likelihood of negative drug interactions in horses is less important than in humans. In contrast, drug–food interactions are frequent in horses and certain dietary conditions (e.g. fed versus fasted conditions, before or after meal, type of food, etc.) need to be controlled carefully when administering antimicrobial drugs orally. Drug–drug interactions may be of pharmacodynamic or pharmacokinetic origin. Interactions between antimicrobial drugs are more commonly of pharmacodynamic nature. For example, the synergistic effect derived from the combination of penicillins and aminoglycosides has been well documented in human medicine both *in vitro* and *in vivo*. However, synergy has not been validated *in vivo* for other antimicrobial combinations commonly used in equine medicine, in particular the combination of erythromycin with rifampicin used for treatment of *R. equi* infection in foals. It would be interesting to compare under controlled *in vivo* conditions the efficacy of this antimicrobial combination with that of erythromycin alone at different stages of the infection.

Although pharmacodynamic interaction between antimicrobial and non-antimicrobial drugs is theoretically possible, very little equine-specific information is available on this type of interaction. For aminoglycosides, a neuromuscular blockade may be expected, especially during anaesthesia, since aminoglycosides inhibit prejunctional release of acetylcholine. However, it has been shown that a single high dose of gentamicin (6 mg/kg BW) does not cause significant neuromuscular blockade when administered to healthy horses anaesthetized with halothane (6). Other drug combinations that should be avoided in equine medicine include

- β-lactams (penicillins/cephalosporins) with tetracyclines. The inhibition of cell wall synthesis exerted by β-lactams requires bacterial replication and is affected by the bacteriostatic effect of tetracyclines.

- Procaine penicillin and trimethoprim/sulfonamides. Trimethoprim/sulfonamides inhibit folic acid synthesis in the bacterial cell but many bacteria can break down the procaine portion of penicillin to *para*-aminobenzoic acid, a precursor of folic acid, thus counteracting the effect of these antimicrobials.
- Fluoroquinolones and rifampin. Rifampicin results in inhibition of bacterial autolysin synthesis, which is necessary for the antibacterial effect of fluoroquinolones (7).
- Trimethoprim/sulfonamides and rifampin. The latter drug seems to increase trimethoprim/sulfonamides elimination.
- Trimethoprim/sulfonamides and alpha-2 agonist drugs. This antimicrobial association appears to enforce the effect of alpha-2 agonist drugs, thereby enhancing cardiac arrhythmias.

10.3 Antimicrobial resistance in bacteria isolated from horses

For some equine pathogens, *in vitro* susceptibility or resistance to certain antimicrobial agents is highly predictable. For example, β-haemolytic streptococci are almost always susceptible to penicillins and *R. equi* is usually susceptible to erythromycin, at least based on *in vitro* measurement. Surveys on antimicrobial susceptibility of equine bacterial pathogens failed to detect erythromycin resistance in *R. equi* (Tables 10.1a and b) and the genetic basis of macrolide resistance has never been described in this species. Such microbiological information is clinically relevant since penicillins and erythromycin are the first choice drugs for treatment of infections caused by β-hemolytic streptococci and *R. equi*, respectively. Organisms such as *Pseudomonas aeruginosa*, *Klebsiella* and *Enterobacter* are intrinsically resistant to penicillins. In contrast, resistance in other species such as *Escherichia coli* and *Staphylococcus aureus* is highly unpredictable and *in vitro* susceptibility testing is extremely useful to generate local data that can be used to guide antimicrobial choices as well as to evaluate the effects of antimicrobial use. It is important to consider local patterns of antimicrobial resistance when developing a treatment regimen. Resistance patterns may differ greatly between geographic regions (Tables 10.1a and b), and even between farms in close proximity.

Resistance data that are not generated at the hospital/farm level must be interpreted with caution. Since culture and susceptibility testing are not usually

Table 10.1a Susceptibility patterns (% susceptible)[a] of selected bacteria from clinical specimens from horses admitted to the Ontario Veterinary College, Canada

Organism	N	Pen	Amp	Ceft	Enro	Ery	Rif	TMS	Gent	Ami	Tet	Chl
Streptococcus zooepidemicus	164	97	99	100	63	93	98	45	88	9	26	80
Streptococcus equi	26	97	97	100	67	92	89	72	100	0	80	100
Escherichia coli	102	2	40	84	91	2	0	42	71	90	48	70
Actinobacillus equuili	28	52	63	100	92	39	46	57	100	65	86	95
Staphylococcus aureus	70	29	26	77	97	79	88	66	49	96	66	88
Rhodococcus equi	11	9	18	36	64	100	83	27	100	100	36	50
Klebsiella spp.	52	0	0	73	90	0	6	21	37	80	38	65
Salmonella spp.	146	0	33	67	65	0	0	40	44	73	63	37
CoNS	34	56	59	74	86	73	80	65	76	93	77	86
Pseudomonas spp.	63	5	10	22	44	5	9	16	56	90	33	21
Enterococcus spp.	54	43	55	10	16	19	11	22	43	16	30	67
Acinetobacter spp.	28	4	18	7	81	0	7	18	21	74	25	43
Citrobacter spp.	18	0	0	61	94	6	0	56	24	60	33	50
Enterobacter spp.	72	0	3	38	65	0	18	19	20	70	31	42

[a]Antimicrobial susceptibility testing performed by the Kirby–Bauer Disk Diffusion method following CLSI guidelines by the Animal Health Laboratory, University of Guelph.
CoNS, coagulase-negative staphylococci; Pen, penicillin; Amp, ampicillin; Ceft, ceftiofur; Enro, enrofloxacin; Ery, erythromycin; Rif, rifampicin; TMS, trimethoprim/sulfamethoxazole, Gent, gentamicin; Tet, oxytetracycline; Ami, amikacin; Chl, chloramphenicol.

Table 10.1b Occurrence of susceptibility among bacterial isolates from horses. The isolates are from clinical samples submitted to the Department of Bacteriology at the National Veterinary Institute; Uppsala, Sweden

Organism	N	Origin of isolates	Percentage of susceptible isolates (highest MIC value for susceptibility mg/L)							
			Pen (≤1)	Amp (≤2)	Ceft (≤2)	Enro (≤0.25)	Ery (≤0.5)	TMS (≤0.5/9.5)	Gent (≤4)	Tet (≤4)
Streptococcus zooepidemicus	175	Respiratory tract	100	100	100	0	NT	41	NR	97
Streptococcus equi	50	Respiratory tract	100	100	100	0	NT	98	NR	100
Escherichia coli	161	Female genital tract	NR	31	100	96	NT	81	98	94
Actinobacillus spp.	149	Diverse	87	87	NT	98	0	95	42	97
Staphylococcus aureus	516	Diverse	56	56	100	92	NT	92	94	97
Rhodococcus equi	20	Respiratory tract	5	10	NT	10	100	0	100	
Pseudomonas aeruginosa	37	Diverse	0	0	5	8	NT	5	81	2

Antimicrobial susceptibility testing was determined by broth microdilution.

NR, not relevant; NT, not tested.

Data collected and modified from SVARM, Swedish Veterinary Antimicrobial Resistance Monitoring. The National Veterinary Institute, Uppsala, Sweden, 2001 and 2005 and further from the database of clinical specimens investigated at the Department of Bacteriology, SVA.

Pen, penicillin; Amp, ampicillin; Ceft, ceftiofur; Enro, enrofloxacin; Ery, erythromycin; Rif, rifampicin; TMS, trimethoprim/sulfamethoxazole, Gent, gentamicin; Tet, oxytetracycline.

performed prior to initial treatment, data published in the scientific literature are usually based on refractory infections that have previously been treated with one or more antimicrobials. Additionally, most studies are based on horses attending referral hospitals, which are more likely to have received antimicrobial treatment and therefore carry resistant bacteria. These selection biases tend to overestimate the actual levels of antimicrobial resistance and have to be considered for a correct interpretation of data on prevalence of resistance. Methodological differences (i.e. methods and criteria used for measurement and definition of resistance) should also be taken into account when comparing results reported from different laboratories, particularly from different countries, as such differences could account for some of the variation observed.

The emergence of multi-drug resistant bacteria is a global problem in horses, as in other animals. Specific pathogens of concern include multidrug-resistant *Salmonella*, methicillin-resistant *Staphylococcus aureus* (MRSA), multidrug-resistant *Pseudomonas* (particularly *P. aeruginosa*) and multidrug-resistant *Enterococcus* (e.g. vancomycin-resistant enterococci). Multidrug resistance in equine bacteria increases the risk of treatment failure and leads to higher costs to horse owners because of prolonged hospitalization and use of expensive antimicrobials, including drugs of critical importance in human medicine (see Chapter 4).

Much of the present concern about the emergence of multidrug-resistant bacteria in horses involves MRSA (8,9). MRSA infections are difficult to treat because limited treatment options exist. While most often associated with skin and soft-tissue infections, fatal MRSA infections can develop, including septicaemia. A difficult aspect in controlling the spread of MRSA is the fact that these bacteria can colonize the nasal passages or gastrointestinal tract without any outward signs. This complicates infection control because a silent reservoir of infected horses can be present in the population. Antimicrobial therapy has been identified as a risk factor for hospital-associated (10) and community-associated MRSA colonization, highlighting the need for prudent antimicrobial therapy in veterinary hospitals and on farms. Transmission between horses and humans, in both directions, has been reported and cases of zoonotic infections have occurred in equine personnel (11). It should be noted that detection of MRSA is difficult due to variable *in vitro* expression of the gene (*mecA*) encoding methicillin resistance. MRSA can be promptly detected only by using certain β-lactam drugs (i.e. oxacillin or cefoxitin) that are not always included in the equine panels for antimicrobial susceptibility testing. Thus, it is likely that the occurrence of this important multi-drug-resistant pathogen is presently overlooked in many equine practices.

10.4 Empirical antimicrobial therapy and diagnostic submissions

Empirical antimicrobial therapy is routinely employed for most infections in horses, although it is generally recognized that submission of culture specimens and use of proper laboratory techniques for bacterial isolation and antimicrobial susceptibility testing are critical for successful treatment of individual patients, identification of population (herd, region) problems and detection of changes in pathogen distribution or resistance patterns. Unless the nature of the disease is such that there is no contraindication to delaying therapy, empirical therapy at the first visit is a common practice in equine medicine. In some situations, it may not be required or even appropriate to collect a diagnostic specimen. For example, nasal swabs (except in suspected cases of strangles with presence of purulent exudate) and swabs from contaminated wounds have limited diagnostic value due to the presence of high numbers of bacterial contaminants. In other cases, representative diagnostic specimens cannot be collected because of the impossibility to access the infection site (i.e. abdominal abscesses) or economic constraints. At times, bacteriological analysis may lead to false-negative results because of intermittent shedding of the pathogen, presence of fastidious or unculturable organisms, failure to use specialized microbiological media, improper sample collection, improper sample storage or shipping or prior antimicrobial therapy. However, in many other circumstances, the importance of bacteriological culture and antimicrobial susceptibility testing cannot be disregarded.

Disease conditions that are not life-threatening but prone to relapse or treatment failure (e.g. cystitis) and caused by pathogens with unpredictable antimicrobial susceptibility (e.g. Gram-negative bacteria) should be treated empirically with narrow-spectrum

antimicrobials and culture specimens should be collected prior to initiation of therapy. A variety of potentially life-threatening infections can be encountered, such as severe pneumonia, pleuropneumonia, peritonitis, septic arthritis and neonatal septicaemia. Only in these situations is empirical use of broad-spectrum antimicrobials or antimicrobial combinations (i.e. penicillin and aminoglycoside) justified while awaiting culture results. There are also disease conditions in which empirical antimicrobial therapy is not recommended. Mild upper respiratory tract infection (i.e. likely viral in origin), diarrhoea in adult horses and mild superficial wounds (not involving a joint or tendon sheath) do not typically need anti-microbials. Supportive care, close monitoring and wound management should be adequate.

10.5 Antimicrobial prophylaxis

The general principles of perioperative prophylaxis that were addressed in Chapter 1 also apply to horses. There is no need to administer antimicrobials for uncomplicated procedures such as castration and many orthopaedic procedures, including those performed in field situations. The risk of infection and potential consequences of infection must be considered when deciding whether antimicrobial prophylaxis is indicated. It is important to emphasize that antimicrobials should not be used in place of good surgical technique, a proper surgical environment, good management and optimal infection control practices (12). No specific recommendations exist for horses, but in human medicine it is recommended to administer antimicrobials approximately 1 h before surgery so that therapeutic levels are present at the surgical site at the time of first incision. Often, a single perioperative dose is all that is required, and prolonged treatment after surgery is often not necessary. Commencing antimicrobial prophylaxis after surgery is generally regarded as inefficacious.

10.6 Disease- and pathogen-specific guidelines

A system-based approach to antimicrobial therapy is outlined in the following paragraphs. The guidelines provided in this section strike a balance between prudent antibiotic use and recommendations from the scientific literature. However, the equine literature is not always based on objective scientific studies. Clinical reports, antimicrobial susceptibility data and clinical experience are often used to formulate published recommendations because of the relative paucity of scientific data. As such, the scientific literature tends to be dominated by recommendations that promote the use of broad-spectrum drugs and antimicrobial combinations, especially penicillin with gentamicin. There is a need for more research to rationalize the use of antimicrobials in equine medicine.

The following tables provide recommendations for specific diseases/syndromes and pathogens. The tables have been drafted considering a combination of factors, including expected pathogens, expected susceptibility patterns and typical patient factors. The recommended doses for antimicrobial agents used in equine medicine are listed in Table 10.2. The scientific quality of the literature on which these tables are based is highly variable, as there is a general paucity of well-controlled studies on antimicrobial efficacy in horses. Many antimicrobial recommendations, particularly multiple drug combinations, have been passed down through the literature but are not based on any objective data. A common example of this is the combination of penicillin, gentamicin and metronidazole, which is sometimes used for the treatment of life-threatening conditions such as pleuropneumonia and peritonitis. This triple antimicrobial combination is considered the most broad-spectrum coverage possible for equine pathogens, with the exception of resistant organisms and *Mycoplasma* spp. However, this triple combination tends to be employed based on fears of missing a pathogen involved, economic value of the horse or lack of knowledge about the disease. The combination of a β-lactam with an aminogylcoside is a very broad-spectrum combination for sensitive organisms. However, some anaerobes, notably some strains of *Clostridium* and *Bacteroides* are not affected by β-lactams. Metronidazole treatment improves anaerobic coverage with better pharmacodynamic and pharmacokinetic characteristics for long-acting penetration into difficult to reach body sites. Nevertheless, most infections in horses are caused by aerobic Gram-positive and Gram-negative bacteria, and thus this triple antimicrobial combination does not represent improved coverage. In fact, it is possible that the more antimicrobial treatments that disrupt the intestinal anaerobic population, the more likely the horse could develop antimicrobial-associated colitis. Thus, it would be more prudent to put thought and effort into finding the cause(s) and choose antimicrobials with better pharmacodynamic and pharmacokinetic characteristics against Gram-positive and Gram-negative infections. Equine anaerobic infections in most cases are more likely associated with mixed chronic infections (e.g. >5 days) in body sites that can develop into low oxygen tension sites (e.g. pleura, peritoneum, deep wounds).

Our recommendations should be considered general guidelines that do not supersede information obtained through culture and susceptibility testing from the individual patient. Most of them are disease-specific recommendations that can be used in situations where the specific agent or its susceptibility pattern is unknown, when samples are not submitted to laboratory diagnosis or while culture results are pending. Only few pathogen-specific recommendations are provided to guide antimicrobial selection when the causative agent has been identified and *in vitro* susceptibility data are available, as this situation is rather infrequent in clinical practice. In some situations, multiple options are presented in each category (first, second and last choice). This is because recommended drugs within the same category are presumed to be similarly appropriate and other factors such as cost, route of administration and patient factors (e.g. age, concurrent disease) should be considered for selecting the best antimicrobial option. Furthermore, not all of the suggested antimicrobials are available in all jurisdictions and the use of certain compounds (i.e. chloramphenicol) is banned in some countries.

10.6.1 Respiratory infections

Respiratory tract diseases are common in horses, and one of the most frequent reasons for antimicrobial administration (Table 10.3). Causes for respiratory tract diseases are multi-factorial. Recommended treatments are variable and some references still endorse the use of broad-spectrum antimicrobials for equine respiratory tract diseases, even to cover the possibility of secondary bacterial pneumonia from a primary viral infection, despite the absence of data supporting these approaches. It is important for equine clinicians to remember that most respiratory diseases in horses are non-infectious or viral and do not require antimicrobial treatment. Furthermore, secondary bacterial pneumonia is rare. The use of broad-spectrum

Table 10.2 Recommended dosages of antimicrobial agents used in horses

Drug	Dose(s)	Comment
Amikacin	Foals: 21–25 mg/kg IV/IM q24 h Adults: 10 mg/kg IV/IM q24 h	Nephrotoxic. Monitoring of drug levels is ideal in compromised animals. Not recommended in combination with phenylbutazone.
	Intra-articular: 250–500 mg/d/joint q24 h Intrauterine: 2 g	Watch total systemic dose. Buffer with equal volume 7.5% sodium bicarbonate.
Ampicillin sodium	10–20 mg/kg IV q6–8 h Intra-uterine: 1–3 g	
Ampicillin trihydrate	20 mg/kg IM q12 h	
Azithromycin	10 mg/kg PO q24 h for 5 d then q48 h	
Cefazolin	20 mg/kg IV q6 h 20–25 mg/kg IM q8 h Intra-articular: 500 mg/d/joint	
Cefepime	Foals: 11 mg/kg IV q8 h Adults: 6 mg/kg IV q8 h	
Cefotaxime	25–40 mg/kg IV q6–8 h	
Cefoxitin	20 mg/kg IM/IV q8 h	
Cefquinome	Foals: 1 mg/kg IM/IV q12 h Adults: 1 mg/kg IM/IV q24 h	
Ceftiofur	2.2–4.4 mg/kg IV/IM q12 h	4.4 mg/kg has been recommended for foals and Gram-negative infections.
	Regional perfusion: 20 ml of 50 mg/ml q24 h Intra-uterine: 1 g	Synovial infection.
Ceftriaxone	25 mg/kg IV q12 h	
Cefalexin	30 mg/kg PO q8 h	Safety unclear.
Chloramphenicol	35–50 mg/kg PO q6–8 h	Human health concerns. Illegal in some jurisdictions.
Clarithromycin	7.5 mg/kg PO q12 h	
Dihydrostreptomycin	10 mg/kg IM q12 h	
Doxycycline	10 mg/kg PO q12 h; 20 mg/kg PO q24 h	High risk of colitis in some areas, particularly Europe.
Enrofloxacin	5 mg/kg IV q24 h 7.5–10 mg/kg PO q24 h; 7.5–10 mg/kg IV for *Pseudomonas* infections	Not for use in growing animals. Should always be reserved as second-line treatment based on culture and susceptibility. Not recommended in combination with rifampin.
Erythromycin	Estolate: 25 mg/kg PO q6 h Phosphate: 37.5 mg/kg PO q12 h	Hyperthermia may develop in hot weather. High risk of colitis in adult horses.
Gentamicin	6.6 mg/kg IV/IM	Nephrotoxic. Monitoring of drug levels is ideal in compromised animals. Not recommended in combination with phenylbutazone.
	Aerosol: 20 ml of 50 mg/ml q24 h	For treatment of bacterial pneumonia. Efficacy unknown.

10 Horses

Continued

Table 10.2 (Continued)

Drug	Dose(s)	Comment
	Intraosseus perfusion: 2.2 mg/kg in 0.1 ml/kg saline	Infections of synovial structure and bones in distal limb.
	Intra-articular: 150 mg/d/joint	
	Intra-uterine: 1–2 g	Buffer with equal volume 7.5% sodium bicarbonate.
Imipenem-cilastatin	10–20 mg/kg slow IV q6 h	Very rarely indicated.
Marbofloxacin	2 mg/kg PO/IM/IV	
Metronidazole	Colitis:15 mg/kg PO q8 h	Teratogenic.
	Other: 20–25 mg/kg PO q 6 h; 20 mg/kg per rectum	Stop if anorexia develops.
Oxytetracycline	6.6 mg/kg slow IV q12–24 h	High risk of colitis.
Penicillin: benzathine	Not recommended	Does not produce therapeutic levels and should not be used.
Penicillin: procaine	20 000 IU/kg IM q12 h	Once daily dosing may be required in some regions for regulatory purposes.
Penicillin: sodium/ potassium	20 000 IU/kg IV q6 h	
	Intra-uterine: 5–10 million IU	
Rifampin	10 mg/kg PO q12–24 h	Causes discolouration of urine and tears. Should never be used alone.
Ticarcillin	Intra-uterine: 6 g	
Trimethoprim- sulfonamide	24–30 mg/kg IV/PO q12 h	Slow IV infusion.
	30 mg/kg for donkeys	Not recommended with detomidine.

antimicrobials for respiratory tract diseases based on clinical signs alone (e.g. fever, cough, nasal discharge) can no longer be justified. There are a number of diagnostic techniques (e.g. trans-tracheal wash, tracheal aspirate, broncho-alveolar lavage, lung biopsy) that are simple and safe to perform whereby representative samples can be obtained for culture and sensitivity (13). Regardless of the causal agent of a lower respiratory tract infection, adequate stall rest in a well-ventilated stable and supportive care, including good-quality hay and water, are the most important components of recovery. Exercise during clinical disease and recovery may worsen the clinical disease. Stall rest for three weeks after clinical resolution has been used as guideline for bacterial lower airway diseases.

The direct delivery of antimicrobials to the lower airways through nebulization has been an enticing method to deliver maximal drug concentrations to the site of infection, gaining rapid onset of action, while minimizing systemic exposure. Aerosol particle sizes between 1 and 5 μm are thought to be ideal for therapy, using ultrasonic or jet nebulizers. Aminoglycosides

are the most commonly reported aerosolized antimicrobial agents because they remain bioactive when aerosolized, and are poorly absorbed across epithelial surfaces, thus remaining within the pulmonary tree where they exert concentration-dependent effects (14). However, inhalation antimicrobial therapy has remained controversial in human medicine because of the potential risk of pulmonary contamination with environmental bacteria, and poor drug delivery to consolidated regions of the lung. Irritation from the drug may induce bronchoconstriction, and aerosol administration on surfaces containing large numbers of diverse bacteria may select for antimicrobial resistant bacteria. For most nebulizer systems, it has been estimated that approximately 10% of the drug reaches the lungs during disease, due to the excessive mucus secretions, bronchospasm and higher, more turbulent air flow rates with tachypnoea.

R. equi pneumonia is a common reason for antimicrobial use in foals. Treatment of *R. equi* infections is no longer simple given the emergence of macrolide and rifampin resistance strains as well as the

Table 10.3 Antimicrobial recommendations for selected respiratory tract diseases

Disease/syndrome	Pathogen	First choice	Second choice	Last choice	Comments
Bacterial pneumonia	S. equi sub. zooepidemicus Staphylococcus Actinobacillus E. coli Klebsiella spp. Others	Penicillin[a]	Ceftiofur[a] TMS	Macrolides[a] TMS with aminoglycoside	Important to perform culture and sensitivity.
	Bordetella bronchiseptica	Gentamicin Amikacin	Tetracycline	Macrolide	Prolonged treatment may be required.
Guttural Pouch Empyema	Various, incl. Streptococcus	Penicillin	Ceftiofur		Guttural pouch flushing more important. Systemic antimicrobials are rarely indicated. Administration of both local and systemic benzylpenicillin appears to improve treatment success rate with S. equi.
Lung abscess	Streptococcus Actinobacillus E. coli	Penicillin[a]	TMS	Macrolides[a] with rifampicin	Consider surgical drainage in cases refractory to treatment.
Mycoplasma felis pneumonia		Tetracycline	Macrolides	Enrofloxacin	
Pleuropneumonia	S. equi sub. zooepidemicus Staphylococcus Actinobacillus E. coli Anaerobes	Penicillin[a,b]	Ceftiofur[a] Macrolides	Enrofloxacin[b]	Supportive care and pleural fluid drainage are important adjunctive therapies.
Pneumonia in foals	Rhodococcus equi.	Macrolides with rifampicin	Azithromycin with rifampicin	TMS	Risk of clostridial colitis to mares in certain geographic regions.
Sinusitis	Streptococcus Staphylococcus	None	None	None	Antimicrobials are not necessary with adequate removal and flushing of purulent debris.
Strangles	Streptococcus equi sub. equi.	Penicillin	Ceftiofur	TMS	Simple, first-time cases of strangles that are not systemically ill do not require antimicrobial treatment.
Streptococcus zooepidemicus		Penicillin	Ceftiofur	TMS	Conflicting reports of efficacy of trimethoprim sulfa for S. zooepidemicus.

TMS, trimethoprim/sulfonamides.
[a] Combination with an aminoglycoside is optional if Gram-negative pathogens are suspected.
[b] Combination with metronidazole is optional if anaerobic pathogens are suspected.

10 Horses

10.6.3 Musculoskeletal infections

The musculoskeletal system can present a variety of challenges for antimicrobial therapy (Table 10.5). It is difficult to reach therapeutic antimicrobial levels in many tissues, such as bone, tendon, tendon sheath and joints following oral or parenteral antimicrobial administration. Alternative approaches such as intra-articular therapy, intra-osseous infusion and regional perfusion may be useful in many situations to provide very high local antimicrobial levels. The tendency for abscess formation in soft tissues presents further challenges that inhibit antimicrobial penetration and activity.

Septic arthritis is a major problem in equine medicine. Direct culture is often unrewarding. The use of enrichment culture is important, and optimally synovial fluid samples should be inoculated into blood culture broth shortly after collection. Samples in blood culture broth are incubated for up to one week, thereby greatly increasing sensitivity. Sterile technique is critical because this enrichment process can detect very low numbers of bacteria, including contaminants. Empirical therapy is important because of the low sensitivity of direct culture, the time delay associated with enrichment culture and possible consequences of disease. Gram staining of synovial fluid should be performed to provide basic information about the likely pathogen. Prompt treatment is required, including antimicrobials and ancillary procedures such as joint lavage, to reduce the risk of performance- or life-threatening damage within the joint. A distinct advantage in the treatment of septic arthritis is the ease of local (intra-articular) therapy in most situations. Intra-articular injection of antimicrobials is a very common practice when treating septic arthritis because of the ability to provide very high drug levels at the infected site. This is an easy procedure for most joints, and is often combined with joint lavage. Concerns regarding the potential for development of chemical arthritis following injection of antimicrobials have been addressed; however, this has not been demonstrated to be a clinically relevant concern, particularly considering the severe potential sequelae associated with septic arthritis. Some antimicrobials are irritating and may produce chemical synovitis, so only drugs known to be safe and effective (e.g. amikacin, gentamicin, ceftiofur, cefazolin, sodium/potassium penicillin) should be injected into joints. Since antimicrobials injected into joints will be absorbed into the circulation, the total amount injected should be considered, particularly when multiple joints are being treated and when the same drug is being used parenterally. In situations where neonatal foals are being treated for multiple septic joints, aminoglycosides should not be used both parenterally and intra-articularly because excessive drug levels may result.

Osteomyelitis is more difficult to treat because of the difficulty in producing high enough antimicrobial levels and the presence of organic debris at the infection site. The deep site of many infections may complicate the collection of proper culture specimens. Bone biopsy is the best method to obtain a positive culture. Combination therapy may be required including parenteral therapy plus surgical intervention and local therapy. Antimicrobials can be impregnated into a variety of materials, including polymethylmethacrylate (PMMA) beads or plaster of Paris (17). These materials can then be surgically implanted in an infected area with the antimicrobial being eluted over time. This can result in prolonged high drug levels at the site of infection with minimal systemic exposure and lower drug cost compared to systemic therapy. However, elution rates are variable and depend on the antimicrobial, dose and characteristics of the implant site. This approach is most often used in cases of osteomyelitis, deep wound infections and fracture site infections.

Regional perfusion involves administration of antimicrobials into the occluded vasculature of the infected limb, resulting in high local tissue antimicrobial levels including synovial fluid, soft tissues and bone. Antimicrobials are injected either into a superficial vein or into the medullary bone cavity. Therapeutic antimicrobial levels may be achieved in poorly vascularized tissues where therapeutic levels cannot be reached with systemic treatment. β-Lactams and aminoglycosides are most commonly used. Irritating drugs should not be used. While uncommonly used, subcutaneous placement of an infusion pump delivers high antimicrobial levels at the site of infection for prolonged periods. Pumps can be filled weekly and produce therapeutic levels for weeks or months. This approach is probably most useful for osteomyelitis and fracture-site infections.

Biofilms can complicate certain infections, particularly those involving orthopaedic implants and other invasive devices (18). Biofilms are communities of bacteria that adhere to inert surfaces (i.e.

Table 10.5 Antimicrobial recommendations for selected musculoskeletal diseases

Disease/syndrome	Pathogen	First Choice	Second choice	Last choice	Comments
Clostridial myositis	*Clostridium perfringens*	Penicillin	Metronidazole Oxytetracycline	Chloramphenicol	Surgical debridement/aeration is important.
Pigeon fever	*Corynebacterium pseudotuberculosis*	Penicillin	TMS	Chloramphenicol Erythromycin	Surgical drainage alone is often the best option. The incidence of serious colitis following erythromycin therapy is high, particularly in some areas.
Fistulous withers	*Brucella abortus*, *Streptomyces* spp., others	Oxytetracycline Gentamicin	Doxycycline	TMS	
Osteomyelitis	*Staphylococcus Streptococcus, Salmonella, E. coli, Klebsiella, Acinetobacter, Enterobacter*	Penicillin with aminoglycoside	Ceftiofur with aminoglycoside	Enrofloxacin	Regional limb perfusion, intra-osseus perfusion or antimicrobial impregnated materials may be useful.
Septic arthritis	*Staphylococcus, S. zooepidemicus, E. coli, Actinobacillus, R. equi*	Penicillin with aminoglycoside Intraarticular amikacin	Ceftiofur Cefoxitin	Enrofloxacin Chloramphenicol TMS	Intra-articular therapy and lavage are important.
Septic tenosynovitis	Various, particularly *Staphylococcus* spp., *Streptococcus* spp. and Enterobacteriaceae	Penicillin with aminoglycoside Intrasynovial amikacin Regional limb perfusion	Ceftiofur	Cefoxitin[a]	Lavage is critical
Ulcerative lymphangitis	*C. pseudotuberculosis, P. aeruginosa, Streptococcus, Staphylococcus, Pasteurella*	Penicillin with aminoglycoside	TMS	Ceftiofur[a]	
Deep wounds	Various, including anaerobes	Penicillin with gentamicin	Ceftiofur TMS Metronidazole (anaerobes)		
Wounds: deep penetrating foot wounds	Various, including anaerobes	Penicillin with aminoglycoside	Ceftiofur with aminoglycoside Metronidazole (anaerobes)	Oxytetracycline[b]	

TMS, trimethoprim/sulfonamides.
[a] Combination with aminoglycoside is optional.
[b] Combination with metronidazole is optional if anaerobes are suspected.

10 Horses

Table 10.6 Antimicrobial recommendations for selected ophthalmologic diseases

Disease/syndrome	Pathogen	First choice	Second choice	Last choice	Comments
Bacterial conjunctivitis	Various	Topical antimicrobials[a]			Conjunctivitis is not usually caused by bacterial infection.
Corneal laceration/ perforation	Various	Penicillin with aminoglycoside	Ceftiofur with aminoglycoside	TMS	Concurrent aggressive medical and surgical treatment required.
Corneal ulceration	Various	Topical antimicrobials[a]	Topical antimicrobials and systemic penicillin and aminoglycoside; topical antimicrobials and systemic trimethoprim sulfonamide	Doxycycline if keratomalacia is present	May also use antimicrobial impregnated collagen shields or contact lenses.
Stromal abscess	Various	Topical ciprofloxacin with systemic penicillin. Topical ciprofloxacin with systemic TMS.	Topical chloramphenicol with penicillin and/or aminoglycoside. Topical chloramphenicol with TMS		Not always caused by bacterial infection. Concurrent medical and surgical procedures are important.

TMS, trimethoprim/sulfonamides.

[a]A wide range of topical antimicrobials may be used, including cefazolin, ciprofloxacin, triple antimicrobial (bacitracin/neomycin/ polymixin), chloramphenicol, gentamicin, fusidic acid, tobramycin and amikacin. The most appropriate formulation should be chosen depending on the results of bacteriological culture. It should be considered that certain ophthalmic antimicrobials target specific bacterial groups. For example, fusidic acid and polymixin are mainly active against *S. aureus* and Gram-negative, respectively.

implants) and dead tissue (i.e. bony sequestra). Sessile bacteria that are resident in biofilms are largely resistant to antimicrobials, phagocytes and antibodies. The potential role of biofilms in infections of these types should be considered, particularly if there is poor response to initial treatment.

10.6.4 Ophthalmologic infections

Ophthalmologic conditions present some unique challenges, based on the types of infection and ability of drugs to access certain areas. However, topical therapy facilitates treatment greatly in many cases (Table 10.6). The blood–ocular barriers (i.e. blood–retinal barrier that is equivalent to the blood–brain barrier (BBB) and blood–aqueous barrier) affect the ability of most systemic drugs to penetrate into the eye (posterior and anterior segments, respectively), thereby limiting the usefulness of this route. Certain antimicrobials (i.e. chloramphenicol, sulfonamides) penetrate this barrier better than others. Most drugs will penetrate better in the presence of inflammation, but many will also bind to proteins present in inflammatory exudates. Systemic, subconjunctival, intraocular and topical administration are potential routes of administration. Topical therapy alone may involve direct application to the eye, administration via a subpalpebral lavage system (19) or through the use of an antimicrobial-impregnated collagen shield or contact lenses. Topical therapy alone is often adequate for corneal ulcers, however a combination of different routes may be indicated for more serious conditions. Not all antimicrobials are safe for topical or intraocular use. Intravenous administration is preferred over intramuscular or oral administration because higher plasma levels attained by this route of administration may result in higher ocular levels.

A variety of bacteria and fungi can be part of the normal ocular microflora. These include *Staphylococcus aureus,* coagulase-negative staphylococci, *Moraxella equi, Streptococcus zooepidemicus, Corynebacterium* spp, *Bacillus* spp., *Aspergillus* spp., *Penicillium* spp.,

Table 10.7 Antimicrobial recommendations for selected urinary tract conditions

Disease/syndrome	Pathogen	First choice	Second choice	Last choice	Comments
Cystitis	*E. coli* *Proteus* *Pseudomonas, Klebsiella,* *Enterobacter,* *Streptococcus* *Staphylococcus*	Penicillin Ampicillin TMS	Ceftiofur	Penicillin with aminoglycoside Enrofloxacin	Sulfamethoxazole should not be used as it is largely excreted in an inactive form.
Pyelonephritis	Various, particularly Gram-negative	Ampicillin TMS	Ceftiofur	Penicillin with aminoglycoside; Enrofloxacin	

TMS, trimethoprim/sulfonamides.

Alternaria spp. and *Cladosporium* spp. (20). Various antimicrobial ointments or solutions are available on the market and should be selected on the basis of the target pathogen (Table 10.6).

10.6.5 Urinary tract infections

Urinary tract infections are less common in horses than other animals. Cystitis is the most common bacterial infection of the urinary tract, and is often associated with bladder dysfunction or other predisposing factors (Table 10.7). As such, recurrent infections can be encountered. Pyelonephritis is uncommon, however proper therapy is essential because of the potential consequences of disease. The advantage of treating urinary tract disease is the ability of many antimicrobials to reach high concentrations in urine, including penicillin, cephalosporins and trimethoprim–sulfonamides. As a result, pathogens that are reported as resistant *in vitro* may be susceptible *in vivo*. However, the underlying bladder wall (i.e. biophase for infection) is protected against xenobiotics, including drugs, by the uppermost cells of the urothelium at the inner surface of the bladder, known as umbrella cells. One important point to note is that while many sulfonamides concentrate in urine, this is not true for all. Sulfamethoxazole is largely metabolized before urinary excretion, and is therefore less likely to be effective in urinary tract disease. In addition, urine pH may influence local antibacterial activity.

Another important advantage with lower urinary tract disease is the relative ease of collecting culture specimens. Aseptically collected catheterized samples should be used for culture, and submitted in a sterile container. Urine swabs should be avoided because of the much smaller volume of material for culture and the fact they do not allow for quantitative culture. Semi-quantitative culture is useful to determine the clinical relevance of results, as contamination can occur even with catheterized samples. Growth from a catheterized sample of >1000 colony forming units (CFU/ml) is considered abnormal, while a suspicious growth is 500–1000 CFU/ml. For free-flow samples, >40 000 CFU/ml is considered abnormal with 20–40 000 CFU/ml suspicious (21).

Urinary tract disease often requires longer treatment than other body sites, possibly due to the location of bacteria within the bladder wall or biofilm. Cystitis is often treated for seven to ten days initially, and re-culture is indicated a few days following cessation of treatment. In refractory or severe cases, culturing a few days after the onset of antimicrobial therapy can be useful to detect early treatment failure, with the understanding that negative results do not necessarily indicate successful treatment. Pyelonephritis should be treated for a minimum of two weeks.

While less common in horses compared to household pets, recurrent urinary tract infections may be problematic. It is essential to determine the underlying cause for recurrent disease, and differentiate relapse from re-infection. If there is an underlying problem such as an anatomical defect, urolith or neurological dysfunction, antimicrobial therapy alone is unlikely to be successful.

10 Horses

10.6.6 Cardiovascular infections

Bacterial infections of the cardiovascular system are uncommon (Table 10.8). Injection- or intravenous catheter-associated thrombophlebitis is likely the most common problem; however, most cases of thrombophlebitis are probably inflammatory versus infection. Therefore, antimicrobials are not indicated in all cases and should be reserved for situations where there is a high likelihood of infectious thrombophlebitis or associated abscessation. Bacterial endocarditis and pericarditis are rare but potentially life-threatening conditions requiring appropriate therapy. Blood culture should be performed in cases of endocarditis to identify the cause, while culture of blood and pericardial fluid should be performed in cases of suspected bacterial pericarditis. Pericardial

fluid should be inoculated into blood culture broth immediately after collection. Pericardial drainage and lavage are important adjunctive treatments for pericarditis. Surgical incision and drainage is required if thrombophlebitis progresses to abscessation.

10.6.7 Neurological infections

Bacterial infections of the central nervous system are uncommon, but can have a devastating impact (Table 10.9). Accessibility to the site of infection for collection of diagnostic specimens, and administration of antimicrobials, is highly variable. The BBB and blood–cerebrospinal fluid barriers have a major impact on the penetration of most drugs. In general, drugs that are lipid soluble, non-ionized, not highly protein bound and small molecular size, penetrate

Table 10.8 Antimicrobial recommendations for selected cardiovascular infections

Disease/syndrome	Pathogen	First Choice	Second choice	Last choice
Endocarditis	*Streptococcus, Actinobacillus, Pasteurella*	Penicillin with gentamicin[a]	Ceftiofur	
Pericarditis	*Streptococcus* spp., *Actinobacillus* spp.	Penicillin with gentamicin	Ceftiofur	
Thrombophlebitis	Various opportunists	Penicillin with gentamicin	Ceftiofur	TMS

TMS, trimethoprim/sulfonamides.
[a] Combination with rifampicin is optional.

Table 10.9 Antimicrobial recommendations for selected neurological diseases

Disease/syndrome	Pathogen	First choice	Second choice	Last choice	Comments
Bacterial meningitis	*E. coli* Actinobacillus Streptococcus Others	Ampicillin with aminoglycoside	Cefotaxime Ceftriaxone	TMS Enrofloxacin	Ceftiofur does not cross intact blood–brain barrier.
Brain abscess	*Streptococcus* Other	TMS	Chloramphenicol Penicillin with chloramphenicol	Ceftiofur Erythromycin	
Spinal abscess	*Streptococcus* Other	TMS	Chloramphenicol Penicillin[a]	Ceftiofur Erythromycin	
Temporohyoid osteoarthritis/otitis interna-media	*Streptococcus* Actinobacillus Other	TMS	Ceftiofur	Enrofloxacin	
Tetanus	*Clostridium tetani*	Metronidazole	Penicillin		

TMS, trimethoprim/sulfonamides.
[a] Combination with aminoglycoside is optional.

10 Horses

better. Nevertheless, even drugs with these properties often poorly penetrate the CNS because the main determinant of the BBB passage is the presence of efflux pumps (i.e. P glycoprotein, MRP, etc.). Inflammation can result in increased drug penetration, however this cannot necessarily be relied on, so treatment choices should be based on knowledge of the aetiologic agent and drug penetration. Aminoglycosides penetrate poorly even in the presence of inflammation, however they are often used in combination therapy. Unlike other third-generation cephalosporins, central nervous system (CNS) penetration of ceftiofur is poor (22).

Bactericidal drugs are preferable because of the poor immune response within the CNS. As a result, intravenous administration is required because of the ability to provide high peak blood levels. Intrathecal administration of antimicrobials has been described, however there is little evidence of efficacy. Bacteriostatic drugs may be useful in some cases of brain abscess and spinal abscess, particularly drugs such as chloramphenicol that have other desirable properties.

10.6.8 Hepatobiliary infections

Bacterial infections of the hepatobiliary system are uncommon in horses (Table 10.10). Ascending infection via the bile duct and haematogenous infection can both occur. Accordingly, enteric bacteria are most commonly involved (23). Liver abscesses are similarly uncommon and develop by haematogenous spread or ascending infection of umbilical remnants.

10.6.9 Reproductive infections

Bacterial infections of the reproductive tract are relatively common, particularly in broodmares (Table 10.11). Many infections are associated with breeding, parturition, uterine motility defects and conformational defects. Underlying risk factors for infection must be considered and addressed.

Systemic and local (intrauterine) approaches may be practical in some cases. Infections confined to the uterine lumen and superficial endometrium are best treated by intrauterine therapy. A variety of antimicrobials may be infused into the uterus, including sodium/potassium penicillin, gentamicin, amikacin, ceftiofur, ticarcillin and ampicillin (24–26). Typically, a volume of 50–250 ml is infused. Irritating drugs should be avoided in order to reduce the risk of causing chemical endometritis. Buffering of acidic drugs such as aminoglycosides with sodium bicarbonate has been recommended. Systemic therapy, with or without local therapy, is indicated if deeper tissues are involved.

Uterine lavage is often an important component of treatment because excessive uterine fluid can result in a marked dilutional effect, as well as containing organic debris that decreases the activity of most antimicrobials. Another benefit of lavage is to remove bacteria and bacterial by-products. Other adjunctive medical therapies, such as oxytocin administration, may also be important in many cases.

The external reproductive tract is not a sterile site and care must be taken to prevent contamination during sampling of the uterus, which should be

10 Horses

Table 10.10 Antimicrobial recommendations for selected hepatic disorders

Disease/syndrome	Pathogen	First choice	Second choice	Last choice	Comments
Cholangiohepatitis Cholangitis	Enteric bacteria, especially *E. coli*	Ampicillin with gentamicin	TMS Ceftiofur	Enrofloxacin	
Liver abscess	β-Haemolytic streptococci, *Rhodococcus equi*, *E. coli*	TMS	Penicillin with gentamicin Erythromycin[a]	Chloramphenicol	Poor prognosis.
Listeriosis	*Listeria monocytogenes*	Penicillin or ampicillin	Ceftiofur	Penicillin or ampicillin with rifampin Ceftiofur with rifampin	

TMS, trimethoprim/sulfonamides.
[a] Combination with rifampicin is optional.

10 Horses

Table 10.11 Antimicrobial recommendations for selected reproductive diseases

Disease/syndrome	Pathogen	First choice	Second choice	Last choice	Comments
Contagious equine metritis	*Taylorella equigenitalis*	Mares: General: Local treatment with gentamicin and washing with 4% chlorhexidine for 5 d. Metritis or positive uterine culture: Intrauterine sodium/potassium penicillin. Stallions: Topical gentamicin and 4% chlorhexidine for 5 d	Systemic gentamicin or penicillin		Best if mares are treated during oestrus. Concurrent uterine lavage may be required. External washing of the genitalia of importance for successful treatment.
Endometritis	Various	Intrauterine penicillin with aminoglycoside. Intrauterine ticarcillin	Systemic ceftiofur or TMS (intrauterine antimicrobials optional)	Systemic enrofloxacin	Address underlying causes.
Mastitis	*Streptococcus Staphylococcus E. coli*	Intramammary or systemic penicillin	Intramammary cephalosporin Systemic TMS	Ceftiofur	Concurrent stripping of the udder is important.
Nocardioform placentitis	Gram-positive filamentous branching bacteria	TMS	Ceftiofur		Effectiveness of any treatment uncertain. Most mares do not require treatment and do not have subsequent problems.
Placentitis	*S. zooepidemicus E. coli, P. aeruginosa, Klebsiella*	TMS	Penicillin with gentamicin	Ceftiofur	Gentamicin may not readily cross placenta.
Retained placenta	*E. coli Klebsiella S. zooepidemicus*	Penicillin with gentamicin	Ceftiofur	TMS	Uterine lavage and other concurrent medical therapies are required.
Seminal vesiculitis	*Staphylococcus Streptococcus Pseudomonas*	Infusion of buffered amikacin into seminal vesicular openings	Systemic penicillin with gentamicin[a]	Systemic enrofloxacin[a]	
Vaginitis	*E. coli S. zooepidemicus* Other	TMS	Penicillin and gentamicin	Ceftiofur	Eliminate underlying causes. Treatment not required in mild cases.

TMS, trimethoprim/sulfonamides.
[a] Amikacin infusion is optional.

performed during oestrus. In order to minimize contamination, the perineum should be carefully washed, and sampling should be performed with a gloved hand in the vagina and double-guarded, occluded swabs. The culture swabs are transported in transport media to the lab.

10.6.10 Skin infections

Normal skin has a complex endogenous microflora, whereby disease is prevented usually by a combination of factors, not the least of which is the physical barrier of the skin. Disruption of this normal barrier by a variety of means creates the potential for secondary bacterial infection (Table 10.12). Primary bacterial infections are much less common but may also occur. Cytological examination is often used for a presumptive diagnosis of bacterial skin disease. For example, identification of intracellular cocci is typically interpreted as a clinically relevant tentative diagnosis of coagulase-positive staphylococcal or streptococci. Culture is often used for severe or refractory cases. The skin is a readily accessible site for collection of samples, however interpretation of results can be difficult because of the complex normal microflora, including many potential opportunistic pathogens. Culture of moist lesions and crusts is not typically recommended because of the likelihood of growing contaminants. Cultures of superficial lesions can be taken directly from the skin but it should be remembered that false-positive results are common. More reliable results can be obtained from intact pustules or furuncles if samples are collected by sterile aspiration. As opposed to direct sampling of superficial lesions, samples should be collected from the surface of plaques, nodules and fistulous tracts by skin biopsy after aseptic preparation of the site.

An advantage of dermatological disease is the ability to treat the affected area topically with antiseptics or antimicrobials. This route allows for delivery of high antimicrobial levels at the affected site while reducing systemic exposure. Drugs such as mupirocin, fusidic acid, bacitracin/neomycin/polymixin B and silver sulfadiazine can be effective in many cases. Recently, questions have been raised over the use of mupirocin in animals because of the importance of this drug in MRSA decolonization therapy in humans, and the emergence of resistance in MRSA. It is unclear whether the use of topical antimicrobials such as mupirocin for short-term therapy of local infections contributes

to resistance in human isolates. However, due to the increasing importance of MRSA in both humans and horses, this aspect should be considered when choosing a topical antimicrobial. Topical therapy has some drawbacks, as it can be difficult, time-consuming and not properly or effectively applied by some owners. Local irritation is also a potential problem in some cases. Factors including the type of disease, pathogen involved, severity and ability of the owner to treat must be considered when deciding whether to use system, topical or combination therapy. Removal of debris by appropriate bathing is an important aspect of topical therapy as it facilitates contact of the antimicrobial or antiseptic with the infected skin surface. Clipping of the haircoat may also be indicated to facilitate drug contact.

Many skin infections are self-limiting, or respond to topical antiseptic (povidone iodine, chlorhexidine) therapy. The severity and chronicity of disease are often used to determine whether antimicrobials are indicated. If systemic antimicrobials are chosen, then an adequate duration of therapy is important. Skin infections tend to require longer treatment than many other types of infection, and three to eight weeks of therapy is often necessary. It is often stated that treatment should extend 7–10 days beyond apparent resolution of superficial infections, and 14–21 days beyond resolution of deep infections.

10.6.11 Other conditions

Antimicrobial therapy may be indicated for treatment of a variety of other conditions (Table 10.13). Among the most important of these is neonatal septicaemia. This is an important problem because of the incidence of disease, mortality rate, the potential for performance-limiting complications such as septic arthritis, and the likelihood of death if initial antimicrobial treatment is not effective. For these reasons, broad-spectrum antimicrobial therapy is indicated. Optimal drugs or drug combinations may vary greatly with geographic region. In some areas, a combination of penicillin and trimethoprim-sulfa can be quite effective, while in other areas the incidence of trimethoprim-sulfa resistance amongst Gram-negative pathogens is relatively high and penicillin-aminoglycoside combinations are more widely used. Knowledge of local suscep-tibility patterns and clinical experience can guide optimal use, both in terms of clinical effect and prudent use.

10 Horses

Table 10.12 Antimicrobial recommendations for selected dermatologic diseases

Disease/syndrome	Pathogen	First choice	Second choice	Third choice	Comments
Cellulitis	S. aureus E. coli	Ceftiofur	Penicillin with aminoglycoside TMS	Enrofloxacin	Surgical drainage may be required.
Dermatophilosis	Dermatophilus congolensis	Bath with povidone-iodine or chlorhexidine shampoo	Penicillin	TMS	Often self-limiting. It is important to keep the horse dry.
Folliculitis and furunculosis	Staphylococcus, mainly S. aureus	Bath with povidone-iodine or chlorhexidine shampoo	Topical mupirocin	TMS Ceftiofur Enrofloxacin	Often self-limiting. Remove underlying risk factors.
Pastern dermatitis (scratches, mud fever, grease heal)	May involve: S. aureus Staphylococci D. congolensis β-haemolytic streptococci	Topical treatment with povidone-iodine or chlorhexidine shampoo	Topical mupirocin	TMS Penicillin	Multifactorial disease, not always involving bacterial infection. Bacteria not often the primary cause. Need to address other factors.
Staphylococcal pyoderma	Staphylococcus spp., mainly S. aureus	Topical antimicrobials; antibacterial shampoos	TMS	Ceftiofur Enrofloxacin	

TMS, trimethoprim/sulfonamides.

Table 10.13 Antimicrobial recommendations for selected miscellaneous conditions

Disease/syndrome	Pathogen	First choice	Second choice	Last choice	Comments
Ehrlichiosis	*Anaplasma phagocytophylum*	Oxytetracycline	Doxycycline		
Lyme disease	*Borrelia burgdorferi*	Oxytetracycline	Doxycycline	Ampicillin	
Neonatal septicaemia	*E. coli, Klebsiella Actinobacillus equuili Streptococcus Staphylococcus*	Penicillin with aminoglycoside Ampicillin with aminoglycoside Penicillin with TMS	Ceftiofur Cefotaxime Ceftriaxone	Cefoxitin with aminoglycoside Ceftiofur with aminoglycoside	Blood culture, using enrichment media, should be performed.
Omphalophlebitis	Various, especially those listed under neonatal septicaemia	Penicillin with amikacin	Cefoxitin with amikacin	Cefotaxime	Antimicrobials alone are unlikely to be effective. Surgical resection or drainage is critical.

10.7 Concluding remarks

As multidrug-resistant pathogens continue to emerge and disseminate, concerns regarding prudent use of antimicrobials in horses will undoubtedly increase. Identification of highly resistant pathogens will stimulate an increased pressure to use certain antimicrobials that are of critical importance in human medicine. Since extra-label use of antimicrobials is largely uncontrolled in many areas, increased use of certain antimicrobials, particularly 'high-profile' drugs such as vancomycin, may occur in the future, leading to increased public and regulatory scrutiny of antimicrobial practices in equine medicine. Accordingly, prudent and rational antimicrobial use has to be considered as an important ethical aspect in equine practice and is likely to be become even more important in the future.

References

1. Morley, P.S., Apley, M.D., Besser, T.E., *et al.* (2005). Antimicrobial drug use in veterinary medicine. *J. Vet. Intern. Med.* 19: 617–29.
2. American Association of Equine Practitioners (2006). Ethical guidelines and position statements. Available at: http://www.aaep.org/ethics_prof_guide.htm. Acccessed March 8.
3. Gustafsson, A., Baverud, V., Gunnarsson, A., Horn af Rantzien, M.H., Lindholm, A. and Franklin, A. (1997). The association of erythromycin ethylsuccinate with acute colitis in horses in Sweden. *Equine Vet. J.* 29: 314–8.
4. Baverud, V., Franklin, A., Gunnarsson, A., Gustafsson, A. and Hellander-Edman, A. (1998). *Clostridium difficile* associated with acute colitis in mares when their foals are treated with erythromycin and rifampicin for *Rhodococcus equi* pneumonia. *Equine Vet. J.* 30: 482–8.
5. Davis, J.L., Salmon, J.H. and Papich, M.G. (2006). Pharmacokinetics and tissue distribution of doxycycline after oral administration of single and multiple doses in horses. *Am. J. Vet. Res.* 67: 310–6.
6. Hague, B.A., Martinez, E.A. and Hartsfield, S.M. (1997). Effects of high-dose gentamicin sulfate on neuromuscular blockade in halothane-anesthetized horses. *Am. J. Vet. Res.* 58: 1324–6.
7. Michelet, C., Avril, J.L., Arvieux, C., Jacquelinet, C., Vu, N. and Cartier, F. (1997). Comparative activities of new fluoroquinolones, alone or in combination with amoxicillin, trimethoprim-sulfamethoxazole, or rifampin, against intracellular *Listeria monocytogenes*. *Antimicrob. Agents Chemother.* 41: 60–5.
8. Baptiste, K.E., Williams, K., Williams, N.J., *et al.* (2005). Methicillin-resistant staphylococci in companion animals. *Emerg. Infect. Dis.* 11: 1942–4.
9. Weese, J.S., Archambault, M., Willey, B.M., *et al.* (2005). Methicillin-resistant *Staphylococcus aureus* in horses and horse personnel, 2000–2002. *Emerg. Infect. Dis.* 11: 430–5.
10. Weese, J.S., Rousseau, J., Willey, B.M., Archambault, M., McGeer, A. and Low, D.E. (2006). Methicillin-resistant *Staphylococcus aureus* in horses at a veterinary teaching hospital: frequency, characterization, and association with clinical disease. *J. Vet. Intern. Med.* 20: 182–6.
11. Weese, J.S., Caldwell, F., Willey, B.M., *et al.* (2005). An outbreak of methicillin-resistant *Staphylococcus aureus* skin infections resulting from horse to human transmission in a veterinary hospital. *Vet. Microbiol.* 114: 160–164.

10 Horses

12. ASHP Therapeutic Guidelines on Antimicrobial Prophylaxis in Surgery. (1999). American Society of Health-System Pharmacists. *Am. J. Health Syst. Pharm.* 56: 1839–88.

13. Hoffman, A.M. and Viel, L. (1997). Techniques for sampling the respiratory tract of horses. *Vet. Clin. North Am. Equine Pract.* 13: 463–75.

14. McKenzie, H.C., 3rd and Murray, M.J. (2004). Concentrations of gentamicin in serum and bronchial lavage fluid after once-daily aerosol administration to horses for seven days. *Am. J. Vet. Res.* 65: 173–8.

15. Giguere, S. and Prescott, J.F. (1997). Clinical manifestations, diagnosis, treatment, and prevention of *Rhodococcus equi* infections in foals. *Vet. Microbiol.* 56: 313–34.

16. McGorum, B.C., Dixon, P.M. and Smith, D.G.E. (1998). Use of metronidazole in equine acute idiopathic toxaemic colitis. *Vet. Rec.* 142: 635–8.

17. Cruz, A.M., Rubio-Martinez, L. and Dowling, T. (2006). New antimicrobials, systemic distribution, and local methods of antimicrobial delivery in horses. *Vet. Clin. North Am. Equine Pract.* 22: 297–322, vii–viii.

18. Trampuz, A. and Widmer, A.F. (2006). Infections associated with orthopedic implants. *Curr. Opin. Infect. Dis.* 19: 349–56.

19. Giuliano, E.A., Maggs, D.J., Moore, C.P., Boland, L.A., Champagne, E.S. and Galle, L.E. (2003). Inferomedial placement of a single-entry subpalpebral lavage tube for treatment of equine eye disease. *Vet. Ophthal.* 3: 153–6.

20. Andrew, S.E., Nguyen, A., Jones, G.L. and Brooks, D.E. (2003). Seasonal effects on the aerobic bacterial and fungal conjunctival flora of normal thoroughbred brood mares in Florida. *Vet. Ophthal.* 6: 45–50.

21. MacLeay, J.M. and Kohn, C.W. (1998). Results of quantitative cultures of urine by free catch and catheterization from healthy adult horses. *J. Vet. Intern. Med.* 12: 76–8.

22. Cervantes, C.C., Brown, M.P., Gronwall, R. and erritt, K. (1993). Pharmacokinetics and concentrations of ceftiofur sodium in body fluids and endometrium after repeated intramuscular injections in mares. *Am. J. Vet. Res.* 54: 573–5.

23. Davis, J.L. and Jones, S.L. (2003). Suppurative cholangiohepatitis and enteritis in adult horses. *J. Vet. Intern. Med.* 17: 583–7.

24. Pedersoli, W.M., Fazeli, M.H., Haddad, N.S., Ravis, W.R. and Carson, R.L., Jr. (1985). Endometrial and serum gentamicin concentrations in pony mares given repeated intrauterine infusions. *Am. J. Vet. Res.* 46: 1025–8.

25. Spensley, M.S., Baggot, J.D., Wilson, W.D., Hietala, S.K. and Mihalyi, J.E. (1986). Pharmacokinetics and endometrial tissue concentrations of ticarcillin given to the horse by intravenous and intrauterine routes. *Am. J. Vet. Res.* 47: 2587–90.

26. Love, C.C., Strzemienski, P.J. and Kenney, R.M. (1990). Endometrial concentrations of ampicillin in mares after intrauterine infusion of the drug. *Am. J. Vet. Res.* 51: 197–9.

10 Horses

Chapter 11

GUIDELINES FOR ANTIMICROBIAL USE IN DOGS AND CATS

Luca Guardabassi, Geoffrey A. Houser, Linda A. Frank and Mark G. Papich

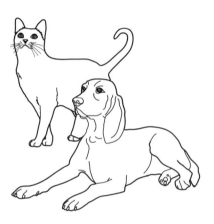

Guidance on prudent antimicrobial use is lacking in small animal practice. National guidelines on small animals are only available in a few countries and are generally limited to generic recommendations on antimicrobial choice. The present chapter is intended to fill this gap by providing small animal practitioners with a worldwide, comprehensive reference on rational and prudent antimicrobial usage. Disease- and pathogen-specific guidelines are given on all relevant aspects in everyday practice, including decisions on drug choice, route of administration and dosage, laboratory analysis, alternative medical or surgical treatment, customer communication and compliance. The guidelines (Section 11.3) are preceded by information on current trends in antimicrobial prescription (Section 11.1) and emergence of multi-resistant bacteria in pets (Section 11.2).

11.1 Current trends in antimicrobial prescription

According to a study conducted at a Finnish veterinary teaching hospital (1), most antimicrobials are prescribed for dogs (78%) and relatively lower amounts are given to cats (12%) and other pet animals (4%). Amoxicillin-clavulanate, first-generation cephalosporins, trimethoprim-sulfonamides (TMS), macrolides, lincosamides and fluoroquinolones are the antimicrobials most commonly prescribed to small animals. Patterns of usage vary extensively between geographical areas as well as between veterinary hospitals within the same region. National figures on antimicrobial prescriptions for companion animals are only available in Sweden (2) and in Denmark (3). Such figures indicate that the use of fluoroquinolones

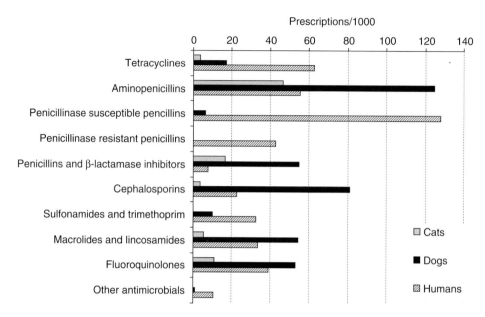

Figure 11.1 Sales of antimicrobials for systemic use for dogs, cats and humans in 2006 in Sweden, expressed as prescriptions/1000 individuals (based on data from Apoteket AB and Statistics Sweden).

or cephalosporins in dogs is comparatively higher than in cats and, surprisingly, even higher than in humans (Figure 11.1). These broad-spectrum antimicrobial drugs are often prescribed empirically in situations where their use may be not required (e.g. first-time superficial pyoderma or cystitis).

There is concern among small animal practitioners about the consequences of treatment failure, but too little awareness of the possible risks associated with overuse of antimicrobials. Indeed, various types of evidence indicate that antimicrobial therapy enhances colonization with multi-resistant bacteria in small animals, especially when broad-spectrum drugs are used. Multi-resistant *Staphylococcus intermedius* are isolated at significantly higher frequencies from dogs affected by recurrent pyoderma than from first-time cases without a history of antimicrobial treatment (4). Antimicrobial administration and hospitalization have been shown to be significant risk factors for carriage of multi-resistant *Escherichia coli*, with the association between usage and resistance being particularly significant in dogs treated with fluoroquinolones and cephalosporins (5). Even more conclusive evidence is provided by longitudinal experimental studies investigating the effects of antimicrobial therapy in dogs. Dogs treated with enrofloxacin have been shown to be

colonized and shed multi-resistant *E. coli* for longer periods compared with untreated dogs (6).

Antimicrobial usage is monitored and controlled more closely in food-producing animals than in companion animals. Whereas in the USA current regulations require that a food-animal drug must be shown *not* to produce a public health risk before it can be registered (see Chapter 5), there are no such requirements for antimicrobial drugs licensed for small animals. Regulatory authorities in Europe and the USA have registered fluoroquinolones and cephalosporins for treatment of relatively 'simple' infections – urinary tract infections (UTIs), skin infections and superficial wound infections in small animals. Some of the more recently approved drugs are third-generation cephalosporins. The status of being registered for simple infections and the focus of promotion and advertising of new drugs has driven the popularity for prescribing these agents for pets.

11.2 Emergence of multi-resistant bacteria in pet animals

Both animal and human health risks associated with the possible emergence of resistant bacteria in companion animals have been so far regarded as negligible. However, there is increasing evidence that clinically relevant resistance traits have emerged in bacteria isolated from small animals, especially dogs (7). The most important reasons for concern are, in order of importance, methicillin-resistant *S. aureus* (MRSA), methicillin-resistant *S. intermedius* (MRSI), and multi-resistant *E. coli*.

11.2.1 MRSA

Increasing numbers of reports have documented the occurrence of MRSA in dogs and cats. MRSA is a major concern in human medicine due to high mortality and morbidity worldwide. As in humans, pets can be asymptomatic carriers of MRSA on the skin and mucosal surfaces, but cases of canine and feline infections (mainly wound and post-surgical infections) are increasingly reported worldwide (8–15). In addition to resistance towards all pencillins and cephalosporins, these bacteria are frequently resistant to alternative systemic antimicrobials such as fluoroquinolones, aminoglycosides, tetracyclines, macrolides and lincosamides. Treatment of MRSA infections in animals is even more difficult than in humans since certain antimicrobial compounds employed in human medicine (e.g. vancomycin, linezolid, streptogramins, tigecycline) are expensive and all except for linezolid must be administered intravenously.

In addition to the veterinary problem, the emergence of MRSA in pets and other animals also has occupational health implications. Recent studies (11, 16–18) have reported MRSA carriage rates in veterinary staff (4–18%) that are significantly higher compared with those normally observed among healthy individuals in the community (≤0.1%). MRSA isolated from pets in Northern Europe usually belong to the epidemic clone EMRSA-15 (multi-locus sequence type 22), the most common cause of MRSA bacteraemia in humans. MRSA isolated from small animal practitioners usually belongs to this clone and transmission between epidemiologically related pets and veterinary staff or pet owners has been documented by molecular typing (11–13, 19). Distinct clones are reported in pets from other continents (20–23), probably reflecting geographical differences in the distribution of MRSA in the human community. MRSA carriage in pets has been associated with cases of MRSA infection in pet owners and veterinarians (20, 24, 25). Human-to-animal infection has also been documented (26, 27). Altogether, these data indicate that although MRSA in pets are likely to have originated from humans, these animals can act as reservoirs for the spread of MRSA in the community.

11.2.2 MRSI

Although resistance to fluoroquinolones or cephalosporins is still infrequent in *S. intermedius* (Table 11.1), both phenotypes have recently emerged. According to recent reports, the frequency of fluoroquinolone-resistant isolates from canine pyoderma ranges between 1% and 12% depending on the specific country/study (3, 28–31). Strains with high-level resistance

Table 11.1 Prevalences (%) of antimicrobial resistance in clinical *S. intermedius* isolates from dogs in different countries

Antimicrobial agent	Denmark (72) 2000–2005 *n*=201	England (83) 1980–1996 *n*=2296	France (30) 2002 *n*=50	Finland (84) 2002–2003 *n*=95	Sweden (3) 2005 *n*=121	Switzerland (85) 1999–2000 *n*=227	Canada (31) 2002–2003 *n*=255	USA (86) 1996–2001 *n*=97
Cefalothin/ cefalexin	1	1	0	N.D.	1	2	1	0
Chloramphenicol	13	N.D.	15	6	N.D.	30	N.D.	3
Erythromycin	28	9	14	25	22	37	10	23
Fluoroquinolones	1	N.D.	1	N.D.	2	4	5	0
Gentamicin	N.D.	N.D.	1	0	1	3	2	0
Lincosamides	27	14	11	20	18	N.D.	9	22
Penicillin	60	79	N.D.	55	84	76	75	55
Tetracycline	24	40	23	40	31	41	23	38
TMS[a]	3	9	N.D.	7	6	10	15	28

[a] Trimethoprim/sulfonamides.

11 Dogs & Cats

to cephalosporins may be regarded as MRSI, since resistance is mediated by the same gene (*mecA*) found in MRSA (32, 33). MRSI have been detected in dogs and cats in the USA, Canada, Slovenia, Germany and Sweden (31–38). These bacteria represent a serious therapeutic challenge in veterinary medicine. Clinical strains recently emerged in Europe that are commonly resistant to all oral antimicrobial formulations available for treatment of pyoderma and otitis (36–38). Similarly to MRSA, MRSI tend to be clonally distributed within countries, meaning that certain clones can be isolated from epidemiologically unrelated dogs and even from veterinary hospitals located at distant geographical areas within the same country (39).

Methicillin resistance has also been reported in the new emerging canine pathogen *S. schleiferi*, which has been associated with cases of recurrent pyoderma and otitis externa in dogs in the USA (40). A retrospective survey conducted at the University of Pennsylvania (41) has shown that the frequency of methicillin resistance in *S. schleiferi* is higher (49%) than in *S. aureus* (32%) and *S. intermedius* (17%). However, methicillin-resistant *S. schleiferi* are generally less resistant to other antimicrobial classes compared with *S. intermedius* and *S. aureus*. Methicillin resistance has been also described in *S. pseudintermedius*, a novel species associated with pets (42). A recent phylogenetic study has shown that *S. pseudintermedius*, not *S. intermedius*, is the common cause of canine pyoderma, whereas *S. intermedius* is the species associated with pigeons (39). Accordingly, the canine pathogen is likely to be reclassified as *S. pseudintermedius*.

11.2.3　Multi-resistant *E. coli*

Multi-resistant *E. coli* with extended-spectrum β-lactamase (ESBL) activity and/or fluoroquinolone resistance have been isolated from clinical infections in dogs in Italy, Portugal, Spain, USA, Canada and Australia (29, 43–50). Some strains may be resistant to all antimicrobial agents except amikacin and/or imipenem. The ESBL types reported in canine isolates are the same as those occurring in human clinical isolates (CTX-M, SHV and CMY). Although clinical isolates producing ESBL are still rare and not considered clinically significant at this time, their occurrence in dogs needs to be monitored carefully in the next years. ESBL-producing *E. coli* are resistant to all cephalosporins, which, together with fluoroquinolones, are critical drugs for treating recurrent UTIs in both pets and humans. Zoonotic

implications cannot be excluded since canine *E. coli* have been shown to be closely related to virulent strains causing UTIs in humans (51, 52).

11.3　Disease- and pathogen-specific guidelines

11.3.1　Skin infections

Canine pyoderma

Canine pyoderma is the number one reason for antimicrobial use in small animal practice. Three types of pyoderma are traditionally defined based on depth of pathological lesions: surface, superficial and deep pyoderma. All forms of canine pyoderma are typically associated with *S. intermedius*, although *S. aureus* and *S. schleiferi* may be rarely implicated in cases of recurrent infection. *S. intermedius* is a normal commensal of the dog and infection is secondary to underlying causes of different nature, mainly cornification defects and allergy. Due to the complex aetiology, therapy is a challenge and prevention of recurrent infection requires identification and elimination of the primary underlying cause. Amoxicillin/clavulanate, first-generation cephalosporins (cefalexin and cefadroxil) and fluoroquinolones (enrofloxacin, marbofloxacin, difloxacin and orbifloxacin) have favourable safety profiles and ensure clinical efficacy due to excellent activity against *S. intermedius* and distribution into the skin. These antimicrobial agents are very effective in treating canine pyoderma and are frequently used for empirical treatment. However, in view of the increasing risk of resistance, the majority of the authors think that these agents should only be used when resistance to other agents is likely. Since first-time infections are rarely associated with multi-resistant staphylococci, other antimicrobials can be chosen empirically in such cases. Common use of an antimicrobial is not a justification for recommending continuing use. Indiscriminate use could make these very valuable antimicrobials useless. In particular, efficacy of fluoroquinolones should be preserved for cases of recurrent or deep pyoderma and for severe, life-threatening infections associated with Gram-negative organisms.

Surface pyoderma

Surface pyoderma is not a true skin infection, but rather an inflammatory process associated with bacterial overgrowth on intertriginous areas where moisture and sebum have accumulated. Surface pyoderma generally does not require systemic antimicrobials; treatment should be directed at cleansing and removing the bacteria and sebum with mild topical antiseptics and/or antiseborrhoeics. Specially formulated shampoos containing chlorhexidine, benzoyl peroxide and other active ingredients are available to the clinician. Benzoyl peroxide can be irritating and drying and may bleach fabrics that come in contact with the product. If focal superficial lesions such as macules and papules are present, topical antimicrobials such as fusidic acid, mupirocin, chlorhexidine or benzoyl peroxide gel may be used. Fusidic acid should be preferred to mupirocin since the latter is used for MRSA decolonization in humans.

Superficial pyoderma

Superficial pyodermas are typically *S. intermedius* infections of the interfollicular epidermis (impetigo) or follicular epithelium (folliculitis). The most commonly administered first-line drugs are cephalosporins and amoxicillin/clavulanate. Both are associated with a high degree of success. However, lincomycin or clindamycin can be successfully employed empirically to treat first-time cases (Table 11.2). Lincomycin and clindamycin are almost identical with respect to mechanism of action and spectrum, but clindamycin is much more commonly used. Erythromycin is equally effective *in vitro* but requires three times daily administration and is frequently associated with anorexia and vomiting, which preclude the use of this antibiotic as first empiric choice. Trimethoprim-sulfonamides (TMS) can also be considered as first-line empirical drugs but their use should be avoided when long-term administration is required because dogs are susceptible to adverse effects (53, 54). When TMS are prescribed, the animal health status should be monitored and the pet owner should be informed about the possible risks, which include hypothyroidism, keratoconjunctivitis sicca, neutropenia, hepatopathy and polyarthritis.

Because of high levels of resistance in *S. intermedius* (Table 11.1), tetracyclines cannot be regarded as a good empiric choice. Doxycycline is more active than other tetracyclines against *S. intermedius* and can be administered once daily. However, the high plasma protein binding of doxycycline (>95%) (55) limits its diffusion into the skin. Remission rates of 53–73% have been reported in patients treated for six weeks with doxycycline (56), indicating that this

tetracycline can be used to treat infections caused by susceptible strains. Chloramphenicol resistance is less frequent than tetracycline resistance but the antibiotic is administered three times daily. In addition to the inconvenient frequency of administration, chloramphenicol is associated with drug interactions and bone marrow suppression. In people, it has been shown to cause aplastic anaemia. As a consequence, human formulations are no longer available commercially in some countries. An analogue compound, florfenicol, has excellent *in vitro* activity against *S. intermedius* but is not approved for use in dogs, has no pharmacokinetic advantages over chloramphenicol (requires three-times daily dosing) and only an injectable cattle formulation is available.

Topical therapy with antiseptics can be used as an adjunct to systemic antimicrobial therapy or can even be tried as a sole means of treatment. In one study, 50% of dogs with superficial pyoderma had lesions resolved when bathed three times weekly with either ethyl lactate or benzoyl peroxide shampoos (57). Identification of the underlying cause is essential to prevent recurrent infection. *S. intermedius* isolates from recurrent superficial pyoderma are significantly more resistant than those from first-time cases (4). In cases of recurrent infection, culture and susceptibility testing should be performed to guide drug selection. In addition to rational drug selection, the correct dose and length of treatment should be prescribed (Table 11.3). Therapy should be continued until at least one week past clinical resolution. This usually requires a minimum of three weeks of therapy and it can take up to six or eight weeks to achieve this endpoint. Discontinuation of therapy has potential consequences on selection of resistant bacteria, re-colonization and re-infection (Chapter 6). If infection persists and lesions recur within seven days after discontinuing therapy, it is likely that treatment was not long enough. Resampling and bacteriological culture are indicated in case of treatment failure.

A long-acting injectable (subcutaneous) third-generation cephalosporin, cefovecin, was recently registered in Europe for small animals (not available in the USA at the time of writing). It is intended as a single injection, which may be repeated at 14 days. Cefpodoxime proxetil is another oral third-generation cephalosporin recently registered in the USA and Europe. The duration of effective plasma and tissue concentrations is longer for cefpodoxime than other cephalosporins such as cefalexin. Consequently, it can be administered once daily instead of twice daily,

11 Dogs & Cats

11 Dogs & Cats

Table 11.2 Recommendations on antibacterial therapy of integumentary infections. Antimicrobial options are listed in order of preference within each category

Infection/ disease	Commonly isolated pathogen	First choice (empirical)	Second choice (based on culture)	Last resort	Comments
Surface pyoderma	S. intermedius	Generally does not require systemic antimicrobial therapy. Topical antimicrobials should be used if focal superficial lesions are observed.			Treatment with shampoos containing antiseptics such as chlorhexidine or astringent antimicrobial spray.
Localized pyoderma[a]	S. intermedius	Chlorhexidine gel / Benzol peroxide gel / Fusidic acid / Mupirocin	Amoxicillin, Doxycycline / Lincosamide[b] / TMS / Amox/clav / First-generation cephalosporin[c]	Fluoroquinolone[d]	To be combined with shampoos containing antiseptics. Identify and cure the primary cause
First-time superficial pyoderma (diffuse)[a]	S. intermedius	Lincosamide[b] and/or antiseptic shampoos	Amoxicillin / Doxycycline / TMS / Amox/clav / First-generation Cephalosporin[c]	Fluoroquinolone[d]	As above
Recurrent superficial or deep pyoderma[a]	S. intermedius	Amox/clav / First-generation Cephalosporin[c]	Amoxicillin / Doxycycline / Lincosamide / TMS	Fluoroquinolone[d] / Cefovecin[e] / Cefpodoxime[e]	As above
Otitis[f]	Gram+ cocci	Fusidic acid	Topical aminoglycoside[g]	Fluoroquinolone[d] (topical)	Flush with antiseptics (e.g. povidone-iodine, chlorhexidine or 2% acetic acid).
Otitis[f]	Gram– rods	Polymixin/Oxytetracycline	Topical aminoglycoside[g]	Fluoroquinolone[d] (topical)	As above.
Otitis[f]	P. aeruginosa	Polymixin / Silver sulfadiazine / Enrofloxacin (topical)[h]	Topical aminoglycoside[g]	Ticarcillin (topical)	To be combined with application of EDTA.
Bite wounds	Pasteurella Staphylococci Other	Amoxicillin	Doxycycline / TMS / Lincosamide[b] / Amox/clav	BAST	

Amox/clav, amoxicillin/clavulanate; TMS, trimethoprim/sulfonamide.
BAST, based on antimicrobial susceptibility testing.

[a] Cytology should always be done. Culture and antimicrobial susceptibility testing are recommended in all cases of deep and/or recurrent pyoderma, when infection fails to respond to empirical treatment, if mixed infection is shown by cytology and in immunosuppressed animals.
[b] Available lincosamides: clindamycin or lincomycin.
[c] Available first-generation cephalosporins: cefalexin and cefadroxil.
[d] Available fluoroquinolones: enrofloxacin, marbofloxacin, difloxacin and orbifloxacin.
[e] Third-generation cephalosporins should only be used for treated deep lesions contaminated with Enterobacteriaceae or in cases at high risk of non-compliance.
[f] Cytology is recommended to guide drug choice. Culture and antimicrobial susceptibility testing should be performed if rods are present.
[g] Topical aminoglycosides: gentamycin, neomycin, framycetin/gramicidin or amikacin.
[h] Choice based on clinical experience and drug availability.

Table 11.3 Recommended dosages of systemic antimicrobial agents used in small animals

Drug	Administration route	Dose(s)[a]	Dose interval	Comments
Amikacin	IV, IM, SC IV, IM, SC	Dog: 15–30 mg/kg Cat: 10–14 mg/kg	q24 h q24 h	Dog (avoid use in renal disease). Cat (avoid use in renal disease).
Amoxicillin/ clavulanate	PO	Dog: 12.5–25 mg/kg Cat: 62.5 mg per cat	q12 h	Dose listed is based on combined ingredients (amoxicillin + clavulanate).
Amoxicillin	PO	22 mg/kg	q8–12 h	For β-lactamase-producing strains, consider amoxicillin-clavulanate as an alternative.
Ampicillin	IM, SC, IV PO	10–20 mg/kg 20–40 mg/kg	q8 h q8 h	Dose is higher for oral dose because of low systemic absorption.
Ampicillin/ sulbactam	IV, IM	10–20 mg/kg	q8 h	Dose is listed for the ampicillin component. Note: sulbactam is not as effective for β-lactamase inhibition as clavulanate.
Azithromycin	PO	Dog: 3–5 mg/kg Cat: 5–10 mg/kg	q24 h to q48 h	Often, once daily administration is used for the first 3–5 days, then every 48 h thereafter.
Cefadroxil	PO	Dog: 22–20 mg/kg Cat: 22 mg/kg	Dog: q12 h Cat: q24 h	First-generation cephalosporin.
Cefazolin	IV, IM IV	20–35 mg/kg 22 mg/kg	q8 h q2 h (during surgery)	First-generation cephalosporin. Therapy. Prophylaxis.
Cefepime	IV, IM	40 mg/kg	q6 h	Fourth-generation cephalosporin.
Cefovecin	SC	Dog, cat: 8 mg/kg	q14d	Third-generation cephalosporin.
Cefpodoxime	PO	Dog: 5–10 mg/kg Cat: dose not established	q24 h	Third-generation cephalosporin.
Cefotaxime	IV, IM	50 mg/kg	q12 h	Third-generation cephalosporin.
Cefoxitin	IV, IM	30 mg/kg	q6–8 h	Second-generation cephalosporin.
Ceftiofur	SC	4.4 mg/kg	q24 h	Urinary tract infections only. Third-generation cephalosporin.
Cefalexin	PO	10–30 mg/kg	q12 h	Most common dose is 25 mg/kg q12 h PO. First-generation cephalosporin.
Chloramphenicol	PO	Dog: 40–50 mg/kg Cat: 12.5–20 mg/kg	Dog: q8 h Cat: q12 h	Prolonged use can lead to bone marrow depression, especially in cats.

Continued

11 Dogs & Cats

11 Dogs & Cats

Table 11.3 (Continued)

Drug	Administration route	Dose(s)[a]	Dose interval	Comments
Ciprofloxacin	PO	20 mg/kg	q24 h	Fluoroquinolone. Use of veterinary-labelled quinolones should be considered first.
Clarithromycin	PO	7.5 mg/kg	q12 h	Derivative of erythromycin. May cause GI problems in some animals.
Clindamycin	PO	Dog: 11–22 mg/kg Cat: 11 mg/kg up to 33 mg/kg	Dog: 11 mg/kg q12 h or 22 mg/kg q24 h Cat: q24 h	May cause GI problems in some animals.
Difloxacin	PO	Dog: 5–10 mg/kg	q24 h	Fluoroquinolone. Refer to precautions in text about using this class of drug. Do not use in cats (safety not established).
Dihydrostreptomycin	No dose established			
Doxycycline	PO	Dog, Cat: 3–5 mg/kg	q12 h	Treatment of Rickettsia or Ehrlichia may use 5 mg/kg q12 h.
Enrofloxacin	PO, IM	Dog: 5–20 mg/kg Cat: 5 mg/kg	q24 h	Fluoroquinolone. Refer to precautions in text about using this class of drug. In cats, do not exceed 5 mg/kg. Although not licensed for IV use in dogs, it has been given this route (cautiously) if necessary.
Erythromycin	PO	10–20 mg/kg	q8–12 h	Gastrointestinal problems, especially vomiting, are common.
Gentamicin	IV, IM, SC	Dog: 9–14 mg/kg Cat: 5–8 mg/kg	q24 h	Can be nephrotoxic; ensure adequate hydration and renal function before use.
Imipenem–cilastatin	IM, IV	5 mg/kg	q6–8 h	Penems are critically important drugs in human medicine. Do not use unless it is a life-threatening infection and susceptibility tests have shown resistance to any antimicrobials except penems.
Lincomycin	PO	15–25 mg/kg; for pyoderma 10 mg/kg has been used	q12 h	Use of lincomycin has been replaced in many hospitals by clindamycin, which is similar in activity, but has better pharmacokinetic characteristics.
Linezolid	Oral	Dog, cat: 10 mg/kg	q12 h	Critically important drugs in human medicine. Do not use unless it is a life-threatening infection and susceptibility tests have shown resistance to any antimicrobials except linezolid.

Drug	Route	Dose	Interval	Comments
Marbofloxacin	Oral	2.2–5.75 mg/kg	q24 h	Fluoroquinolone. Refer to precautions in text about using this class of drug.
Meropenem	SC, IV	8.5 mg/kg	q12 h SC or q8 h IV	Penems are critically important drugs in human medicine. Do not use unless it is a life-threatening infection and susceptibility tests have shown resistance to any antimicrobials except penems.
Metronidazole	Oral	Dog: 12–15 mg/kg Cat: 10–25 mg/kg	Dog: 15 mg/kg q12 h or 12 mg/kg q8 h Cat: q24 h	Do not exceed recommended doses per day or neurotoxicity is likely. Metronidazole is unpalatable in cats and metronidazole benzoate (ester) can be considered as an alternative.
Neomicin	Oral	10–20 mg/kg	q12 h	Not recommended as oral treatment for diarrhoea.
Nitrofuraontoin	Oral	10 mg/kg	Daily dose which can be divided into 4 times daily treatments	This drug is a urinary antiseptic and should not be used for systemic infections.
Orbifloxacin	Oral	2.5–7.5 mg/kg	q24 h	Fluoroquinolone. Refer to precautions in text about using this class of drug.
Ormethoprim-sulfadimethoxine	Oral	13.5 mg/kg	q24 h	Similar in activity as trimethoprim-sulfonamides.
Penicillin G	IM, IV	20000–40000 U/kg	q6–8 h	If IM route is used, less frequent intervals (q24 h) can be used.
Penicillin V	Oral	5 mg/kg	q12 h	Not recommended (not active orally due to poor absorption).
Rifampin	Oral	5 mg/kg	q12 h	Caution: may turn urine, saliva and tears orange colour.
Ticarcillin	IV, IM	50 mg/kg	q6h IV	Last resort drug against multi-resistant *Pseudomonas*. Do not use unless susceptibility tests have shown resistance to any antimicrobials except ticarcillin.
Trimethoprim-sulfadiazine	Oral	15 mg/kg	Once or twice daily, or 30 mg/kg once daily	Caution with use of sulfonamides in dogs (see Section *Canine pyoderma*).
Vancomycin	IV	15 mg/kg	q8 h, IV infusion for 30 min	Glycopeptide antibiotic of critical importance in human medicine. Do not use unless it is a life-threatening infection and susceptibility tests have shown resistance to any antimicrobials except glycopeptide. Give IV only, by slow infusion.

11 Dogs & Cats

aDoses listed in this table are taken from Papich 2007(89)

resulting in less antibiotic use in treated animals. These drugs have good activity against staphylococci, and are also registered for skin infections. Despite their convenient administration and pharmacokinetic properties, third-generation cephalosporins are active against a wide range of Gram-negative bacteria that are normally not associated with pyoderma, and their activity against *S. intermedius* is not superior to first-generation compounds. Furthermore, these drugs have potential for selection of both methicillin resistance in staphylococci and ESBL-producing organisms. Cefovecin and cefpodoxime proxetil are only recommended as first-line agents if there is a substantial problem with compliance. According to the label instructions of cefovecin in Europe, it is prudent to reserve third-generation cephalosporins for the treatment of clinical conditions, which have responded poorly, or are expected to respond poorly, to other classes of antimicrobials or first-generation cephalosporins. Use of the product should be based on susceptibility testing and take into account official and local antimicrobial policies.

Deep pyoderma

Deep skin infections occur when the follicular infection ruptures into the dermis, producing furunculosis and cellulitis. In addition to staphylococci, deep lesions can also be contaminated with *Pseudomonas* and *E. coli* organisms. Therefore, culture and susceptibility testing should be performed on all cases. Cephalosporins and amoxicillin/clavulanate are the drugs of choice for empirical treatment, which may be necessary whilst waiting for susceptibility test results. As a rule, treatment of deep pyoderma requires a longer course of treatment than superficial pyodermas. A minimum of four weeks should be considered with the endpoint being two weeks past clinical resolution of the lesions. This additional length of treatment is indicated because of the fibrosis or the granulomatous nature of the lesions. Dogs with deep pyoderma usually benefit from concurrent topical therapy such as whirlpool baths using dilute chlorhexidine and antibacterial shampoos. When lesions are localized, topical antimicrobials should be used instead of systemic drugs. For example, topical therapy with fusidic acid, mupirocin or benzoyl peroxide gel may be sufficient to treat focal deep infections over pressure points. In these situations, topical antimicrobials should be preferred as they exert a lower antimicrobial selective pressure on commensal bacteria.

Furthermore, moderately resistant organisms can be treated by achieving high antimicrobial concentrations locally.

11.3.2   Ear infections

Otitis externa is very common in the dog but rare in the cat. Inflammation of the external ear canal may be due to many causes and is frequently complicated by infection with bacteria, yeasts or both. Therefore, when managing otitis externa, it is important to identify the infectious agent as well as the underlying cause (e.g. allergy, foreign body, or chronic moisture from swimming or conformation). The keys to successful management of otitis externa are: (i) identification of the infectious agent via cytology; (ii) topical treatment with otic cleansers, to remove the excess wax, and medication; (iii) use of topical steroids when indicated to open the ear canal and decrease inflammation; (iv) frequent monitoring of the treatment progress; and (v) a maintenance plan consisting of regular ear cleaning once the infection has resolved to keep it from recurring.

The most common organisms associated with acute otitis externa are the yeast *Malassezia pachydermatis* and various bacterial species, most commonly *S. intermedius* and *Pseudomonas aeruginosa*, *Proteus*, *E. coli*, β-haemolytic streptococci, *Corynebacterium* and *S. schleiferi*. Acute otitis responds readily to most combination treatments that include a topical antifungal, antibacterial and corticosteroid agent. Topical products that are used for treatment of otitis are listed in Table 11.4. Both solutions, suspensions and ointments, may be effective. Because topical antimicrobials are administered in concentrated formulations (mg/ml), susceptibility tests that are based on achieved plasma concentrations (μg/ml) are misleading because they will greatly underestimate the drug's activity. As a general rule, solutions or suspensions are recommended for more stenotic canals, and a sufficient volume needs to be applied to ensure treatment of the infection in the horizontal ear canal (and bulla if the tympanic membrane is ruptured). Many cases of otitis externa are complicated by otitis media, which is confirmed by presence of a ruptured tympanic membrane. However, examination of the tympanic membrane is not always possible and the tympanic membrane may heal, leaving residual otitis media. Regardless of whether or not the tympanic membrane is ruptured, all infections of the ear canal

Table 11.4 Topical antibacterial options for treatment of otitis[a]

Antimicrobial drug	Topical concentration	Potential ototoxicity
Amikacin	50 mg/ml[b]	Yes
Gentamicin	3 mg/ml[c]	(Yes)[h]
Neomycin	3.2 mg/ml[c]	Yes
Enrofloxacin	10–20 mg/ml[d]	No
Fusidic acid	0.2 mg/ml[c]	No
Polymixin B	10 000 U/ml[e]	Yes
Tetracycline	2.2 mg/ml[c]	No
Ticarcillin	25 mg/ml[f]	No
Tobramycin	0.3%[c]	No
Silver sulfadiazine	0.5–1%[g]	No

[a] In case of *P. aeruginosa* infection, all products should be preceded by application of Tris EDTA and should be used twice daily.

[b] 3 ml amikacin (250 mg/ml) are mixed with 12 ml glycerine. Apply 0.5 ml twice daily into affected ear.

[c] Commercial products available.

[d] Dilute 1:6 in Tris EDTA or sterile water. Apply 0.5 ml twice daily into affected ear.

[e] Mix 50 ml saline into a vial containing 500 000 U polymixin B. This gives a final concentration of 10 000 U/ml and is stable for 60 days when refrigerated. Apply ½ ml twice daily into affected ear.

[f] Reconstitute the 3 g vial with 6 ml saline and freeze in 2 ml aliquots. These are stable for 3 months. Thaw one 2 ml aliquot and dilute with 40 ml saline (25 mg/ml), divide into 10 ml-aliquots and freeze. Remove one 10 ml aliquot at a time and apply ½ ml twice daily into affected ear.

[g] This product is supplied as a 1% cream or a micronized powder. This can be mixed as a suspension in sterile water at 0.5–1.0%.

[h] Gentamicin sulfate in the ear of dogs with intact or ruptured tympanic membranes was shown not to induce detectable alteration of cochlear or vestibular function (87).

are managed topically. Systemic antimicrobial therapy is more expensive and usually offers no benefit for otitis externa or media since it is difficult to achieve adequate concentrations in the ear tissue and middle ear, even if maximum doses are administered (58).

P. aeruginosa is the most common organism associated with chronic otitis externa and media in the dog and the most frustrating to deal with (59). *P. aeruginosa* is typically multi-resistant due to intrinsic resistance properties. The only oral drugs with activity against *P. aeruginosa* are fluoroquinolones. All other active drugs must be given by injection or topically. Based on various studies on *in vitro* susceptibility of canine *P. aeruginosa* isolates (60–62), the most effective antimicrobials include aminoglycosides (gentamicin, neomycin, tobramycin and amikacin), polymixin B, fluoroquinolones, ticarcillin, ceftazidime and imipenem.

Although *P. aeruginosa* isolates are often sensitive to gentamicin *in vitro*, treatment with topical products containing gentamicin or neomycin is rarely successful because aminoglycosides are inactivated by purulent material present in the ear canal. Furthermore, many gentamicin topical preparations are in an ointment base, which may be too viscous to penetrate through the stenotic ear canal, and the recommended dosage may be too small to achieve an adequate concentration in the horizontal ear canal.

Although resistance to fluoroquinolones can develop during therapy (63), topical treatment with enrofloxacin can be even successful with strains defined as resistant *in vitro* according to standard-setting committees such as the Clinical and Laboratory Standards Institute (CLSI, formerly NCCLS). In fact, such breakpoints are based on plasma concentrations obtained by oral dosing (μg/ml) and much higher concentrations can be achieved when enrofloxacin is administered topically (mg/ml). Fluoroquinolone resistance in *P. aeruginosa* is conferred by chromosomal mutations and overexpression of efflux pumps (64). Topical use of a calcium-chelating agent such as Tris-ethylene diamine tetra acetic acid (EDTA) may help to override the resistance attributed to the efflux pump by opening up pores in the bacteria and facilitating drug penetration (65–67). Because the ear canals are often stenotic, it is essential to open the canals to allow penetration of the topical treatments. This can be accomplished through systemic and/or topical corticosteroids. Often the systemic steroids are used initially followed by topical steroids once the canal is less stenotic and ulcerated.

11.3.3 Urinary tract infections (UTI)

Cystitis

Cystitis and lower UTIs are generally more common in the dog than in the cat, with a higher frequency in castrated bitches and males. The most common bacterium causing cystitis in the dog is *E. coli*, which has been estimated to account for 70–75% of cases, followed by staphylococci, *Proteus* and enterococci. Urine analysis including physico-chemical analysis and cytology is important to guide in the diagnosis as well as in the choice of the antimicrobial agent. The number of bacteria and the presence of granulocytes provide diagnostic evidence of infection. Urine should be collected by cystocentesis as this method avoids contamination with commensal bacteria from the urethra; concentrations above 1,000 CFU/ml should be regarded as infection. Measurement of urine pH combined with Gram staining and morphology of the bacteria present in the urine can enable prediction of the bacterial species involved. As a consequence of their metabolism, staphylococci and *Proteus* generally cause urine alkalinization, whereas *E. coli* and enterococci cause urine acidification. This information, combined with knowledge of the antimicrobial susceptibility patterns in the species, can lead to rational selection of the antimicrobial agents to be used.

Antimicrobial drugs should be selected based on the resistance profiles of urinary pathogens (Table 11.5) as well as on the drug concentrations that can be achieved in urine (Table 11.6). Avoid the use of drugs that are highly metabolized prior to excretion because the urine concentrations may not be active. Aminopenicillins (ampicillin and amoxicillin), trimethoprim and fluoroquinolones are eliminated by renal excretion and accumulate in urine at concentrations higher than in serum. The drugs can be efficacious *in vivo* even if the bacterial strain involved is regarded as intermediate based on antimicrobial

Table 11.5   Prevalences (%) of antimicrobial resistance in clinical *E. coli* isolates from dogs in different countries

Antimicrobial agent	Denmark (71) 2000–2005 n=201	Sweden (70) 2002–2003 n=121	Canada (31) 2002–2003 n=205	USA (45) 1990–1998 n=444
Ampicillin	22	15	33	42
Amoxicillin/clavulanate	4	ND	16	20
Cefalothin[a]	6	ND	39	42
Fluoroquinolones	7	8	3	18
Gentamicin	4	1	1	6
Tetracycline	26	10	14	31
Trimethoprim/sulfonamide	11/20[b]	14	8	23

ND, not determined.

[a] Cefalothin is the antibiotic used for testing susceptibility to first-generation cephalosporins.

[b] Sulfamethoxazole and trimethoprim were tested separately.

Table 11.6   Mean urine concentrations and *E. coli* minimum inhibitory concentrations (MICs) of antimicrobial agents used for treatment of urinary tract infections. Modified from Barsanti 2006 (88)

Antimicrobial agent	Dosage (mg/kg)	Route	Interval (h)	Concentration (mg/l)[a]	MIC (mg/l) *E. coli*[b]
Ampicillin	22	PO	8	309	NA
Cefalexin	8	PO	8	225	NA
Chloramphenicol	33	PO	8	124	2–16
Amikacin	5	SC	8	342	0.5–8
Gentamicin	2	SC	8	107	0.125–2
Enrofloxacin	2.5	PO	12	40	0.032–0.125
Nitrofurantoin	4.4	PO	8	100	4–32
Tetracycline	18	PO	8	138	NA
Trimethoprim	13	PO	12	26	0.125–2
Sulfonamides	13	PO	12	79	8–128

NA Not available.

[a] Concentrations were measured in healthy dogs. Patients with lower urinary tract infections may have bacteria in tissue layers of the urinary system, for which high urine concentrations may not be sufficient. Moreover, many patients with lower urinary tract infections have concurrent glucocorticoid therapy, diuretics, chronic renal failure, fluid therapy, or diabetes mellitus, all of which may dilute the urine.

[b] Antimicrobial wild-type MIC distributions of *E. coli* according to the European Committee on Antimicrobial Susceptibility Testing (EUCAST) (www.srga.org/eucastwt/WT_EUCAST.htm).

susceptibility testing. However, these interpretations should be made cautiously. With the exception of ampicillin (68), specific resistance breakpoints for urinary tract pathogens have never been standardized by CLSI. Thus, MICs should be interpreted using the same criteria as for systemic infections. One should not assume that concentrations in urine are sufficient to eradicate UTI with intermediate or resistant strains. In fact, uropathogenic bacteria may involve the deeper layers of the mucosa, the renal tissue or the prostate tissue. In these instances, it is the tissue concentration – which is correlated to the plasma concentration – that will be predictive of a bacteriologic cure (69).

Species-specific guidelines for treatment of UTIs in dogs and cats are presented in Table 11.7. Aminopenicillins and amoxicillin-clavulanate are the antimicrobial drugs of choice for empirical treatment of cystitis associated with enterococci and staphylococci respectively. Limited to the dog, TMS can be used empirically if bacilli are detected by microscopic examination. In *E. coli*, resistance to ampicillin and TMS ranges between 15–42% and 8–23% respectively (31, 45, 70, 71) (Table 11.5). When available, local patterns of antimicrobial resistance in *E. coli* should be considered in order to select the most appropriate drug for empirical treatment of UTI associated with this species.

Within sulfonamides, sulfamethoxazole is metabolized more extensively than sulfadiazine and the latter drug attains higher active concentrations in urine.

Treatment of acute bacterial cystitis requires a one to three week course of antimicrobials. Different approaches should be used for treating first case, uncomplicated and recurrent infections. Accurate clinical examination aimed at identification of underlying factors (e.g. cystic calculi, anatomical anomalies, metabolic diseases, nervous system abnormalities, bladder neoplasia, etc.) should be undertaken in cases of relapsing or persistent UTIs. Urine culture and susceptibility testing are recommended because previous exposure to antimicrobial drugs may predispose the patient to infection or re-infection with resistant bacteria. Antimicrobial therapy should be continued for six weeks and urine cultures should be performed five to seven days after therapy to confirm resolution of infection.

Pyelonephritis

Diagnosis of pyelonephritis is important because the prognosis of antimicrobial therapy is worse than for lower UTIs. Drug selection should be based on the antimicrobial susceptibility pattern of the pathogen

Table 11.7 Recommendations on antibacterial therapy of genito-urinary tract infections. Antimicrobial options are listed in order of preference within each category

Infection/ disease	Commonly isolated pathogen	First choice (empirical)	Second choice (based on culture)	Last resort	Comments
Cystitis	*S. intermedius* Enterococci Streptococci	Amoxicillin	Amox/clav Cephalosporin	Fluoroquinolone	Cytology should guide drug selection. 2–3 weeks treatment.
	E. coli *Proteus*	TMS (dog) Amoxicillin (cat)	Chloramphenicol Cephalosporin	Fluoroquinolone	
Pyelonephritis	As above, mainly *E. coli*	TMS or amox/clav	Cephalosporin	Fluoroquinolone	6 weeks treatment.
Acute prostatitis	As above	TMS Fluoroquinolone[a]	Erythromycin	Fluoroquinolone	4 weeks treatment.
Chronic prostatitis	As above	TMS Fluoroquinolone[a]	Erythromycin	Fluoroquinolone	6–8 weeks treatment.
Pyometra	As above	TMS (dog) Amoxicillin (cat)	BAST		5 days treatment. Surgical treatment required.

Amox/clav, amoxicillin/clavulanate; TMS, trimethoprim/sulfonamide.
BAST, based on antimicrobial susceptibility testing.
[a]Because many dogs are sensitive to the adverse effects of sulfonamides, especially when long treatment periods are required (e.g. prostatitis), fluoroquinolones should be considered as an alternative in these dogs.

11 Dogs & Cats

Table 11.8 Estimation of dose and dosage interval for antimicrobial therapy of pyelonephritis in patients with renal failure

New dose	Recommended dose × normal creatinine conc./patient's creatinine conc.
New interval I (hr)	Dosage interval × patient's creatinine conc./normal creatinine conc.

involved, generally *E. coli*. When possible, TMS or amoxicillin/clavulanic acid should be preferred to cephalosporins and fluoroquinolones. However, the use of either a third-generation cephalosporin or a fluoroquinolone may be considered in Gram-negative infections, as long-term therapy with sulfonamides has been associated with a risk of adverse effects (see Section 11.3.1). A six-week antimicrobial course is necessary for successful treatment. Aminoglycosides and nitrofurantoin should not be used because of nephrotoxicity and low serum levels (bacteraemia is common), respectively. If the animal presents signs of systemic illness, empirical treatment is justified and intravenous antimicrobial administration should be started in combination with supportive therapy. For cephalosporins and penicillin derivatives, dose and interval should be tuned proportionately to the loss of renal function (Table 11.8). There is no evidence that doses should be adjusted for fluoroquinolones.

Prostatitis

Urethral haemorrhagic discharge is frequent, but this clinical finding is also associated with non-infectious pathologies of the urogenital tract (e.g. cystic degeneration or prostatic hypertrophy). Thus, antimicrobials should only be prescribed if the diagnosis is confirmed on the basis of complete blood counts, urinalysis and urine culture. The organisms involved are the same as for cystitis but therapy is more difficult because the blood–prostatic barrier limits drug penetration. This is only true in chronic prostatitis since the blood–prostatic barrier is not intact during acute inflammation of the organ. To cross an intact blood–prostate barrier, a drug must be: (a) unionized or lipophilic, (b) have low protein binding, and (c) administered in high enough doses to provide a concentration gradient that drives the drug from the plasma to the prostate compartment. Drugs that are weak bases, although ionizable, are able to diffuse into the

prostate because they will be unionized at plasma pH. Antimicrobial drugs with good prostatic penetration are those with high lipid solubility such as TMS, macrolides and fluoroquinolones. However, macrolides are usually not appropriate because of poor activity against Gram-negative bacteria, which are commonly involved. Chloramphenicol and tetracyclines are ordinarily considered drugs with good tissue penetration but, according to research performed in dogs (72), penetrate the canine prostate poorly. Acute prostatitis requires four weeks of antimicrobial therapy whereas chronic prostatitis necessitates six to eight weeks.

11.3.4 Gastrointestinal and intra-abdominal infections

Bacterial infections in the oral cavity

Periodontal disease is typically a mixed infection associated with proliferation of spirochetes and Gram-negative anaerobic rods such as *Porphyromonas* and *Prevotella* species. Treatment requires tooth cleaning and extraction, tartar removal by ultrasonic scaling and root planning under general anaesthesia, and antiseptic treatment with chlorhexidine-based gels or solutions. Tetracycline-based preparations are available for topical antimicrobial application into single periodontal pockets (perioceutics). Systemic antimicrobial treatment should be limited to severe cases and immunosuppressed patients, and mainly directed against anaerobes (Table 11.9). Home dental care (tooth brushing) and client education play a major role in control and prevention of periodontal disease. Ulcerative stomatitis is a disease condition characterized by the presence of ulcers and secondary bacterial infection of the oral mucosa. Local irrigation with 1% hydrogen peroxide or 0.2% chlorhexidine is recommended. Serious anaerobic infections can be treated systemically as suggested for severe periodontitis.

Helicobacteriosis

Helicobacter pylori and *Helicobacter*-like organisms have been identified in biopsy specimens from dogs and cats, but their role in gastritis and ulcers has yet to be established. Some studies have found no association between *Helicobacter* infection and gastritis (73, 74) and antimicrobial combinations used in human medicine seem not to result in long-term eradication in dogs (75).

Table 11.9 Recommendations on antibacterial therapy of gastrointestinal and intra-abdominal infections. Antimicrobial options are listed in order of preference within each category

Infection/disease	Commonly isolated pathogen	First choice (empirical)	Second choice (based on culture)	Last resort	Comments
Gingivitis Periodontitis	Spirochetes Porphyromonas Prevotella	Chlorhexidine (topical)	Tetracycline (topical) Ampicillin Clindamycin	Metronidazole	Dental therapy and prophylaxis are essential. Systemic antimicrobial treatment should be limited to severe cases and immunosuppressed patients.
Ulcerative stomatitis	As above, mainly E. coli	Hydrogen peroxide with chlorhexidine (topical)	Amoxicillin Clindamycin	Metronidazole	Systemic antimicrobial treatment should be limited to severe cases and immunosuppressed patients.
Gastroenteritis	Salmonella	None	BAST		Bacterial gastroenteritis is usually self-limited and antimicrobials should only be used in case of clinical signs of systemic infection.
	Campylobacter	None	Erythromycin	Fluoroquinolones	
	C. difficile	None	Metronidazole		Bacterial gastroenteritis is usually self-limited and antimicrobials should only be used in case of clinical signs of systemic infection.
Acute peritonitis	Various	Cefoxitin or cefotetan	Aminoglycoside with penicillin, clindamycin or metronidazole	Fluoroquinolone with penicillin, clindamycin or metronidazole	Aggressive therapy, IV administration. Control source of infection and drainage are essential.
Cholangio-hepatitis	Various	Amoxicillin or doxycycline	BAST		May need surgery to restore bile flow.
Anal sacculitis	None	TMS or amoxicillin	BAST		Require topical treatment with chlorhexidine.

Amox/clav, amoxicillin/clavulanate; TMS, trimethoprim/sulfonamide.
BAST, based on antimicrobial susceptibility testing.

11 Dogs & Cats

Gastroenteritis

According to an Australian survey (76), 59% of small animal practitioners prescribe antimicrobial drugs for acute unspecified gastroenteritis. However, most cases of diarrhoea and vomiting in pets are not caused by bacteria but rather by viruses or non-infectious causes. Furthermore, even in bacterial gastroenteritis, infection is usually self-limiting and antimicrobial treatment has not been proven to have positive effects on patient recovery. Following a protocol generally employed in human medicine, empirical antimicrobial use should be limited to cases associated with signs of severe systemic infection (fever, depression and leucopenia or leucocytosis with a marked left shift). Where available, injectable formulations of TMS may be used in combination with supportive care (rehydration and fasting). When signs of acute sepsis are evident, administration of injectable, broad-spectrum antimicrobial combinations is recommended (see Section 11.3.10). Rectal swabs should be routinely submitted to laboratory analysis for identification of *Salmonella*, *Campylobacter* and toxigenic clostridia. When one of these organisms is detected, antimicrobial therapy can be used to eradicate pathogen carriage and avoid risks of zoonotic transmission. The choice of the antimicrobial agent should be based on antibiograms (Table 11.9) and therapeutic efficacy should be monitored after discontinuation of treatment.

Some forms of *chronic diarrhoea* in animals appear to be responsive to the macrolide tylosin and have been regarded as 'Tylosin-Responsive Chronic Diarrhoea in Dogs' (77). This syndrome is most likely caused by bacteria but the specific aetiology has not been identified. *Campylobacter jejuni* and *Clostridium perfringens* have been identified in some animals. Tylosin has been effective at improving clinical signs, whereas other antimicrobials (metronidazole, TMS, doxycycline) appear not to be effective (78). Metronidazole has been found to alter the indigenous bacterial population (78) and may have an immunosuppressive effect on the GI mucosa (decreased cell-mediated response) as well as adverse effects on the CNS (tremors, seizures and other). CNS problems may be prevented by avoiding high doses.

Peritonitis

Septic peritonitis is a life-threatening infection generally due to contamination from the gastrointestinal tract. Consequently, the bacteria involved are often a combination of Gram-negative bacilli, obligate anaerobes, and ocassionally *Enterococcus*. Samples of abdominal effusions should be obtained for culture and sensitivity testing. Cephamycins (cefoxitin and cefotetan) are an excellent empirical choice because of their activity against both anaerobic (including *Bacteroides*) and Gram-negative bacteria. Alternatively, aminoglycosides (gentamicin or amikacin) can be combined with drugs active against anaerobes (penicillin, metronidazole or clindamycin). In addition to medical therapy, the successful treatment of septic peritonitis requires surgical control of the source of infection and drainage. Although often recommended in veterinary literature and commonly practiced, there is a lack of evidence that peritoneal lavage with saline or mixtures of saline with antimicrobials are of any benefit to the patient.

11.3.5   Respiratory infections

Upper respiratory infections

Bacterial infections of the upper respiratory tract such as rhinitis, sinusitis, tonsillitis and pharyngitis are either self-limiting or secondary to underlying causes. Bacterial rhinitis requires flushing with physiological saline solution or antiseptic solutions to remove exudates and to keep the nasal cavity clean. Antimicrobial therapy is not required unless clinical signs are severe or persistent (Table 11.10). Similarly, studies on human cases have led to the conclusion that antimicrobials do not show any benefit on the resolution of acute bacterial sinusitis. Chronic bacterial sinusitis occurs in cats, mainly as a consequence of feline viral respiratory infections and leukaemia. In this disease also, the efficacy of antimicrobial therapy is limited because of the secondary nature of the bacterial infection, presence of biofilms in sinus cavities and poor drug penetration into the sinus. *Primary bilateral tonsillitis* in young, small-breed dogs has unclear aetiology. For all upper respiratory infections, systemic antimicrobials should only be used following bacterial culture and antibiogram (Table 11.10).

Bronchitis

Canine acute tracheobronchitis or *kennel cough* generally does not endanger the dog's life, is self-limiting, and there is no evidence that antimicrobial therapy speeds recovery. The causative pathogen, *Bordetella bronchiseptica*, resides on the surface of

Table 11.10 Recommendations on antibacterial therapy of respiratory infections. Antimicrobial options are listed in order of preference within each category

Infection	Commonly isolated pathogen	First choice (empirical)	Second choice (based on culture)	Last resort
Rhinitis Sinusitis Tonsillitis	Various	None	Doxycycline Amoxicillin Amox/clav	BAST
Acute bronchitis (kennel cough)	B. bronchiseptica	Self-limiting infection Antimicrobial therapy is not needed		
Chronic bronchitis	Various	None	BAST	
Pneumonia	Various	Amox/clav Cephalosporin[a] Fluoroquinolone[a]	BAST	Cephalosporin or fluoroquinolone with metronidazole
Pyotorax Pleuritis	Various	Penicillin with aminoglycoside	BAST	As above

Amox/clav, amoxicillin/clavulanate; TMS, trimethoprim/sulfonamide.
BAST, based on antimicrobial susceptibility testing.
[a]Third-generation cephalosporins or a fluoroquinolones are indicated in case of severe pneumonia. See Table 11.1 for available compounds.

the respiratory epithelium and many antimicrobials do not penetrate the blood–bronchus barrier sufficiently to be effective against this pathogen. Antimicrobials are only required if secondary bronchopneumonia or interstitial pneumonia is demonstrated by radiographic signs. *B. bronchiseptica* is often resistant to penicillins and cephalosporins (79). The recommended antimicrobial drugs are doxycycline, TMS and amoxicillin/clavulanate.

Bacteria usually play a secondary role in chronic bronchitis in dogs and cats. Collection of bronchoalveolar lavage (BAL) fluid is recommended to guide drug selection for therapy of chronic bronchitis, that is, a chronic cough for two months or longer without signs of respiratory distress or pneumonia. Bacterial counts higher than 10^3 CFU/ml BAL indicate bacterial infection. Antimicrobial agents should be prescribed on the basis of antimicrobial susceptibility testing.

Pneumonia

Bacterial pneumonia is more common in the dog than in the cat. *B. bronchiseptica* and *Streptococcus zooepidemicus* are the most common bacteria implicated in primary bacterial pneumonia in dogs. However, pneumonia is more frequently associated with opportunistic pathogens, which may include staphylococci, β-haemolytic streptococci (mainly groups C and G), *E. coli*, *Pasteurella multocida*, *P. aeruginosa*, *Klebsiella pneumoniae*, *Mycoplasma* and a variety of anaerobic organisms. Due to the large variety of organisms that can be implicated in bacterial pneumonia, it is important to select antimicrobial agents on the basis of bacterial identification and antimicrobial susceptibility testing. Furthermore, it is important to select drugs that are able to reach active concentrations in bronchial secretions such as erythromycin, clindamycin, chloramphenicol, TMS and fluoroquinolones. Although penicillins, cephalosporins and aminoglycosides will not achieve high drug concentrations in bronchial secretions, they will achieve adequate concentrations in the interstitial fluid of the lungs and airway mucosa. Therefore, these drugs may be effective for treating bronchopneumonia, but no well controlled studies of efficacy have been reported in veterinary medicine to determine which drug has the highest efficacy. If the infection is life-threatening, empirical antimicrobial treatment starting with IV administration may be needed.

Pyothorax and pleuritis

Periodical drainage of pleural exudates and saline lavage of the pleural cavity are essential to successful treatment of pyothorax. Without drainage and lavage, systemic antimicrobial therapy is ineffective. The efficacy of local antimicrobial therapy is controversial since most antimicrobial agents are rapidly adsorbed by the pleural mucosa. No single antimicrobial preparation can ensure success of therapy since pleural infections are usually associated with multiple organisms,

11 Dogs & Cats

often including distinct aerobic and anaerobic species. Cytology of pleural aspirates facilitates rational antimicrobial selection by providing information on bacterial Gram staining, morphology and intracellular location. Parental administration of penicillin G or ampicillin ensures activity against most anaerobic (except *Bacteroides*) and Gram-positive bacteria (except staphylococci). Other antimicrobials such as gentamicin or amikacin are necessary when infection is associated with Gram-negative bacilli. Antimicrobial therapy should be continued for four to six weeks and radiological monitoring can be usefully employed to monitor efficacy.

11.3.6   Eye infections

Conjunctivitis is a common disease in cats and a frustrating clinical problem to the veterinarian due to the frequent occurrence of recurrent episodes associated with carrier state of the pathogens most frequently involved, herpesvirus-1 (FHV-1) and *Chlamydophila felis*. The veterinarian should educate clients about the chronic nature of feline conjunctivitis and prepare them for the possibility of treatment failures, particularly in herpes-infected animals. The identification of cytoplasmic elementary bodies in conjunctival epithelial cells, a positive fluorescent antibody test on a conjunctival scraping, or a positive chlamydial culture, can all be used to confirm the diagnosis of *C. felis*. Infection control measures should be taken to avoid dissemination to other cats. Tetracyclines are first choice agents, as this obligate intracellular bacterium can be resistant to many common topical ophthalmic antimicrobials including bacitracin, neomycin and gentamicin. In case of recurrent episodes, systemic antimicrobial therapy should be considered to eliminate carriage. In the dog, infectious conjunctivitis is usually a secondary complication of entropion, keratoconjunctivitis sicca, penetration with foreign bodies and canine distemper. Macrolides and derivatives can be used for empirical treatment, taking the precaution to submit ocular swabs for bacteriological analysis. Cytology should be used to guide antimicrobial choice (Table 11.11). In case of deep corneal ulcerations, systemic antimicrobial treatment should be used.

11.3.7   Osteomyelitis

Osteomyelitis may be associated with a large variety of bacterial species, including Gram-positive, Gram-negative and anaerobic bacteria. Aspirates

of osteomyelitic lesions or material from sequestra, necrotic tissue or implants should be submitted to both aerobic and anaerobic culture, and sensitivity testing. If the ischaemic necrotic environment is not improved by drainage and surgical treatment, eradication of infection will not occur despite the administration of effective antimicrobials. Drug selection should be guided by bacteriological culture and susceptibility testing. Clindamycin, amoxicillin-clavulanate or cephalosporins may be appropriate first choices depending on the bacteria being involved. Long-term oral therapy (three to eight weeks or more) is usually necessary to control chronic cases of traumatic osteomyelitis. Local delivery of antimicrobials, such as placement of gentamicin-impregnated poly-methyl methacrylate (PMMA) at the site of infection, has also been used (80).

11.3.8   Arthritis

Infectious arthritis is relatively uncommon in small animals. Definitive diagnosis requires arthrocentesis and subsequent synovial fluid analysis. Macroscopic and cytological examination reveals signs consistent with suppurative inflammation with or without the presence of bacteria. *Staphylococcus* and *Streptococcus* are the most common isolates in septic arthritis due to surgery or penetrating wounds. Differential diagnosis is essential in case of polyarthritis, which may be consequent to bacteraemia, immune complex-mediated damage of articular tissues, or infections with *Anaplasma phagocytophilum,* various *Ehrlichia* spp. (e.g. Rocky Mountain spotted fever), *Borrelia burgdorferi, Leishmania*, and *Mycoplasma*. Synovial fluid or, when possible, joint capsule biopsies should always be submitted to laboratory analysis and susceptibility testing prior to the administration of antimicrobials (Table 11.11). Immediate inoculation onto culture or transport media may enhance bacterial detection.

11.3.9   Central nervous system (CNS) infections

Definitive diagnosis of bacterial CNS infection requires analysis and culturing of cerebrospinal fluid (CSF), but in practice antimicrobial therapy is often empirical. Antimicrobials capable of penetrating the blood–brain barrier in bactericidal concentrations are TMS, metronidazole and some fluoroquinolones. Other antimicrobials such as ampicillin and third-generation cephalosporins are capable of crossing the blood–brain barrier when inflammation of the

Table 11.11 Recommendations on antibacterial therapy of selected miscellaneous infections. Antimicrobial options are listed in order of preference within each category

Infection	Commonly isolated pathogen	First choice	Second choice	Comments
Conjunctivitis	Chlamydophila felis (cat); Gram-rods; Staphylococci; Streptococci	Doxycycline Tetracycline; Polymixin/oxytetracycline Fusidic acid Erythromycin	Chloramphenicol; Chloramphenicol Aminoglycoside Tetracycline	Differential diagnosis with herpes virus infections. Cytology should be used to guide drug selection. Erythromycin or derivatives can be used empirically if cocci are seen in the microscope.
Osteomyelitis	Various	Clindamycin Amox/clav Cephalosporin Gentamicin (local)	BAST	No antibiotic can cover all the possible types of bacteria. The choice depends on the likelihood of Gram-negative and anerobic bacteria being involved.
CNS infections	Various	TMS Amoxicillin or amox/clav	Metronidazole and/or fluoroquinolone	Metronidazole with fluoroquinolone is recommended only in case of life-threatening infections.
Arthritis	Various	BAST	BAST	Therapy should be continued for 3–8 weeks and monitored by cytology and culture.
Bacteraemia	Various	Ampicillin with aminoglycoside	BAST	
Anaplasmosis	Anaplasma phagocytophila	Doxycycline	Chloramphenicol	Resistance has never been described in this species.
Rocky Mountain fever	Ehrlichia rusticii	Doxycycline	Chloramphenicol	Resistance has never been described in this species.
Lyme disease	Borrelia burgdorferi	Doxycycline	Amoxicillin	
Leptospirosis	Leptospira interrogans	Penicillin G, amoxicillin	Doxycycline	Doxycycline is recommended to remove carriage after the acute phase.
Brucellosis		None	Dihydrostreptomycin with a tetracycline	Euthanasia is recommended since treatment is expensive and infection is difficult to be cured. Isolation and monitoring is required for at least 3 months.
Plague	Yersinia pestis	Streptomycin Gentamicin	Doxycycline Chloramphenicol	Suspected samples must be handled by a class 3 laboratory.
Tularaemia	Francisella tularensis	Gentamicin	Doxycycline Chloramphenicol	Suspected samples must be handled by a class 3 laboratory.

Amox/clav, amoxicillin/clavulanate; TMS, trimethoprim/sulfonamide.
BAST, based on antimicrobial susceptibility testing.

11 Dogs & Cats

meninges is present. TMS are a logical first choice if available in parenteral formulations. Alternatively, ampicillin administered intravenously may also be effective if meningeal inflammation is present. Although chloramphenicol can achieve bactericidal concentrations, this may not be the case with recommended dosages in dogs and cats (81). The use of fluoroquinolones or third generation cephalosporins combined with metronidazole should be reserved to life-threatening CNS infections or limited to failure of empirical treatment with TMS or ampicillin.

11.3.10   Bacteraemia and sepsis

Common causes of bacteraemia and sepsis include gastrointestinal, genitourinary tract, skin, wound, respiratory tract, abdomen, biliary tract and IV catheter-related infections. Bacteraemia may occur with routine dental prophylaxis, but current recommendations from dentists do not suggest that treatment with antibiotics is necessary, because this is only transient and resolves without systemic infection. Definitive diagnosis requires positive blood cultures (preferably two or three over a 24 h period) along with clinical signs and laboratory findings that are compatible with bacteraemia/sepsis. Samples should be obtained prior to antimicrobial administration. Clinical signs of bacteraemia warrant immediate parenteral (preferably IV) antimicrobial therapy against both Gram-positive and Gram-negative organisms. An aminoglycoside such as gentamicin or amikacin combined with ampicillin or cephalosporin can be selected for patients in which renal compromise and/or hypovolemia is not an issue. If the conditions are severe (e.g. temperature above 41°C), it is also acceptable to administer a fluoroquinolone alone or in combination with penicillin, ampicillin, potentiated ampicillin (e.g. ampicillin-sulbactam) or clindamycin, especially if anaerobic bacteria are suspected. Parenteral administration of antimicrobials should continue for five to seven days, followed by four to six weeks of oral administration. If the condition is refractory, there should be time for culture and susceptibility testing to indicate and justify appropriate drugs.

11.3.11   Antimicrobial prophylaxis

Antimicrobial prophylaxis can in no way function as a substitute for the maintenance of a proper surgical environment, the use of proper aseptic technique or the practice of effective non-traumatic surgical procedures. When evaluating the need for surgical wound prophylaxis, the USA National Research Council (NRC) wound classification system and the American Society of Anaesthesiologists preoperative assessment scores (82) should be taken into consideration together with other risk factors. These might include: the surgeons experience; whether or not veterinary students are involved; the need for IV and urinary catheters; contamination of the surgical site; drains; expected hospitalization time and and underlying disease. Perioperative prophylaxis is generally more effective than postoperative prophylaxis, although the latter is still frequently used in veterinary medicine.

We have identified at least five types of surgery where antimicrobial prophylaxis may be recommended as a routine practice: any surgery requiring more than 90 min, elective orthopaedic surgery, bowel surgery at risk of anastomotic leakage, severe skin or muscle lacerations, and dentistry associated with severe periodontal disease or immunocompromised patients. In long or elective orthopaedic surgery, IV administration of penicillin G, ampicillin or cefazolin prior to surgery and repeated after 90 min may be indicated. Wounds that fall into either the contaminated or dirty category according to the NRC classification can be treated by post-operative oral administration of amoxicillin/clavulanate or by perioperative injections of ampicillin-sulbactam or cefazolin. If anaerobic bacteria are suspected (e.g. deep puncture wounds), metronidazole can be added. Antimicrobial prophylaxis for bowel surgery should only be used when leakage is observed or expected. In this case, preoperative administration of intravenous ampicillin or metronidazole combined with an aminoglycoside or fluoroquinolone is indicated. In patients at risk, dental scaling or tooth extraction can be accompanied by prophylaxis mainly targeting anaerobes (penicillin G, ampicillin or clindamycin).

11.4   Final remarks

The recommendations presented in this chapter aim at minimizing and rationalizing the use of antimicrobials without affecting clinical efficacy. Although this is not an easy task, it is possible to use antimicrobials in a prudent and rational manner without consequences on clinical outcome. Achievement of this ambitious goal necessitates that (i) antimicrobials are only used when required; (ii) empirical treatment with broad-spectrum antimicrobials is limited to infections threatening the patient's life and otherwise untreatable by drugs with narrower spectrum; (iii) anamnesis, clinical signs, cytology and local data on antimicrobial susceptibility are used to predict the resistance profile of the pathogen involved and to select the most appropriate drug for empirical treatment; (iv) selected samples are submitted for laboratory analysis to confirm diagnosis, to monitor the efficacy of antimicrobial therapy, to evaluate the effects of antimicrobial policies and to generate local data on antimicrobial resistance; (v) disease-specific dosage regimens are prescribed taking into consideration drug pharmacokinetics and infection site; and (vi) pet owners are informed about the risk of treatment failure and the importance of prudent antimicrobial use and treatment compliance. The authors are aware that prudent antimicrobial use is more difficult to practice in countries where liability can be associated with treatment failure and adverse reactions. Furthermore, financial constraints may limit the availability of bacterial culture and susceptibility testing as aids to drug selection. However, the use of a 'best-guess' approach based on microscopy would facilitate choice of appropriate drugs targeting the relevant pathogen, thereby reducing the ecological impact on the commensal flora and the risk of selecting for resistance to last resort antibacterial drugs.

Acknowledgements

The authors thank Lina Petterson (Uppsala University, Sweden) and Christina Greko (National Veterinary Institute, Uppsala, Sweden) for kindly providing Figure 11.1.

References

1. Holso, K., Rantala, M., Lillas, A., et al. (2005). Prescribing antimicrobial agents for dogs and cats via university pharmacies in Finland – patterns and quality of information. Acta Vet. Scand. 46: 87–93.
2. SVARM (2005). Swedish veterinary antimicrobial resistance monitoring. The National Veterinary Institute (SVA), Uppsala, Sweden, 2006. Available at: www.sva.se.
3. DANMAP (2005). Use of antimicrobial agents and occurrence of antimicrobial resistance in bacteria from food animals, foods and humans in Denmark. ISSN 1600–2032 (www.danmap.org).
4. Holm, B.R., Petersson, U., Morner, A., et al. (2002). Antimicrobial resistance in staphylococci from canine

5. pyoderma: a prospective study of first-time and recurrent cases in Sweden. Vet. Rec. 151: 600–5.
5. Ogeer-Gyles, J., Mathews, K.A., Sears, W., et al. (2006). Development of antimicrobial drug resistance in rectal Escherichia coli isolates from dogs hospitalized in an intensive care unit. J. Am. Vet. Med. Assoc. 229: 694–9.
6. Trott, D.J., Filippich, L.J., Bensink, J.C. et al. (2004). Canine model for investigating the impact of oral enrofloxacin on commensal coliforms and colonization with multidrug-resistant Escherichia coli. J. Med. Microbiol. 53: 439–3.
7. Guardabassi, L., Schwarz, S. and Lloyd, D.H. (2004). Pet animals as reservoirs of antimicrobial-resistant bacteria. J. Antimicrob. Chemother. 54: 321–32.
8. Pak, S.I., Han, H.R. and Shimizu, A. (1999). Characterization of methicillin-resistant Staphylococcus aureus isolated from dogs in Korea. J. Vet. Med. Sci. 61: 1013–8.
9. Owen, M.R., Moores, A.P. and Coe, R.J. (2004). Management of MRSA septic arthritis in a dog using a gentamicin-impregnated collagen sponge. J. Small Anim. Pract. 45: 609–12.
10. van Duijkeren, E., Box, A.T., Heck, M.E., et al. (2004). Methicillin-resistant staphylococci isolated from animals. Vet. Microbiol. 103: 91–97.
11. Morris, D.O., Mauldin, E.A., O'Shea, K., et al. (2006). Clinical, microbiological, and molecular characterization of methicillin-resistant Staphylococcus aureus infections of cats. Am. J. Vet. Res. 67: 1421–5.
12. Loeffler, A., Boag, A.K., Sung, J., et al. (2005). Prevalence of methicillin-resistant Staphylococcus aureus among staff and pets in a small animal referral hospital in the UK. J. Antimicrob. Chemother. 56: 692–7.
13. O'Mahony, R., Abbott, Y., Leonard, F.C., et al. (2005). Methicillin-resistant Staphylococcus aureus (MRSA) isolated from animals and veterinary personnel in Ireland. Vet. Microbiol. 109: 285–96.
14. Baptiste, K.E., Williams, K., Willams, N.J., et al. (2005). Methicillin-resistant staphylococci in companion animals. Emerg. Infect. Dis. 11: 1942–4.
15. Boag, A., Loeffler, A. and Lloyd, D.H. (2004). Methicillin-resistant Staphylococcus aureus in small animal practice. Vet. Rec. 154: 366.
16. Strommenger, B., Kehrenberg, C., Kettlitz, C., et al. (2006). Molecular characterization of methicillin-resistant Staphylococcus aureus strains from pet animals and their relationship to human isolates. J. Antimicrob. Chemother. 57: 461–5.
17. Hanselman, B.A., Kruth, S.A., Rousseau, J., et al. (2006). Methicillin-resistant Staphylococcus aureus colonization in veterinary personnel. Emerg. Infect. Dis. 12: 1933–8.
18. Moodley, A., Nightingale, E.C., Stegger, M., et al. (2008). High risk for nasal carriage of methicillin resistant Staphylococcus aureus among Danish veterinary practioners. Scand. J. Work Environ. Health 34: (in Press).
19. Moodley, A., Stegger, M., Bagcigil, F., et al. (2006). PFGE and spa typing of methicillin-resistant Staphylococcus

11 Dogs & Cats

aureus isolated from domestic animals and veterinary staff in the UK and Ireland. *J. Antimicrob. Chemother.* 56: 692–7.

20. Weese, J.S., Dick, H., Willey, B.M., *et al.* (2006). Suspected transmission of methicillin-resistant *Staphylococcus aureus* between domestic pets and humans in veterinary clinics and in the household. *Vet. Microbiol.* 115: 148–55.

21. Rankin, S., Roberts, S., O'Shea, K., *et al.* (2005). Panton-Valentine leukocidin (PVL) toxin positive MRSA strains isolated from companion animals. *Vet. Microbiol.* 108: 145–8.

22. Malik, L., Coombs, G.W., O'Brien, F.G., *et al.* (2006). Molecular typing of methicillin-resistant staphylococci isolated from cats and dogs. *J. Antimicrob. Chemother.* 58: 428–31.

23. Boost, M.V., O'donoghue, M.M., Siu, K.H., *et al.* (2007). Characterisation of methicillin-resistant *Staphylococcus aureus* isolates from dogs and their owners. *Clin. Microbiol. Infect.* 13: 731–733.

24. Manian, F.A. (2003). Asymptomatic nasal carriage of mupirocin-resistant, methicillin-resistant *Staphylococcus aureus* (MRSA) in a pet dog associated with MRSA infection in household contacts. *Clin. Infect. Dis.* 36: 26–8.

25. van Duijkeren, E., Wolfhagen, M.J., Heck, M.E. and Wannet, W.J. (2005). Transmission of a Panton-Valentine leucocidin-positive, methicillin-resistant *Staphylococcus aureus* strain between humans and a dog. *J. Clin. Microbiol.* 43: 6209–11.

26. van Duijkeren, E., Box, A.T.A., Mulder, J., *et al.* (2003). Methicillin resistant *Staphylococcus aureus* (MRSA) infection in a dog in the Netherlands. *Tijdschrift voor Diergeneeskunde* 128: 314–5.

27. Vitale, C.B., Gross, T.L. and Weese, J.S. (2006). Methicillin-resistant *Staphylococcus aureus* in cat and owner. *Emerg. Infect. Dis.* 12: 1998–2000.

28. Lloyd, D.H., Lamport, A.I., Noble, W.C., *et al.* (1999). Fluoroquinolone resistance in *Staphylococcus intermedius*. *Vet. Dermatol.* 10: 249–51.

29. Cohn, L.A., Gary, A.T., Fales, W.H., *et al.* (2003). Trends in fluoroquinolone resistance of bacteria isolated from canine urinary tracts. *J. Vet. Diag. Invest.* 15: 338–43.

30. Ganiere, J.P., Medaille, C., Limet, A., *et al.* (2001). Antimicrobial activity of enrofloxacin against *Staphylococcus intermedius* strains isolated from canine pyodermas. *Vet. Dermatol.* 12: 171–5.

31. Authier, S., Paquette, D., Labrecque, O. and Messier, S. (2006). Comparison of susceptibility to antimicrobials of bacterial isolates from companion animals in a veterinary diagnostic laboratory in Canada between 2 time points 10 years apart. *Can. Vet. J.* 47: 774–8.

32. Jones, R.D., Kania, S.A., Rohrbach, B.W., *et al.* (2007). Prevalence of oxacillin- and multidrug-resistant staphylococci in clinical samples from dogs: 1,772 samples (2001–2005). *J. Am. Vet. Med. Assoc.* 230: 221–7.

33. Gortel, K., Campbell, K.L., Kakoma, I., *et al.* (1999). Methicillin resistance among staphylococci isolated from dogs. *Am. J. Vet. Res.* 60: 1526–30.

34. Zubeir, I.E., Kanbar, T., Alber, J., *et al.* (2007). Phenotypic and genotypic characteristics of methicillin/oxacillin-resistant *Staphylococcus intermedius* isolated from clinical specimens during routine veterinary microbiological examinations. *Vet. Microbiol.* 121: 170–6.

35. Vengust, M., Anderson, M.E., Rousseau, J., *et al.* (2006). Methicillin-resistant staphylococcal colonization in clinically normal dogs and horses in the community. *Lett. Appl. Microbiol.* 43: 602–6.

36. Kania, S.A., Williamson, N.L., Frank, L.A., *et al.* (2004). Methicillin resistance of staphylococci isolated from the skin of dogs with pyoderma. *Am. J. Vet. Res.* 65: 1265–8.

37. SVARM (2006). *Swedish veterinary antimicrobial resistance monitoring.* The National Veterinary Institute (SVA), Uppsala, Sweden, 2006. Available at: www.sva.se.

38. Loeffler, A., Linek, M., Moodley, A., *et al.* (2007). First report of multi-resistant, mecA-Positive *Staphylococcus intermedius* in Europe: 12 cases from a veterinary dermatology referral clinic in Germany. *Vet. Dermatol.* 18: 412–421.

39. Bannoehr, J., Ben Zakour, N.L., Waller, A.S., *et al.* (2007). Population genetic structure of the *Staphylococcus intermedius* group: insights into *agr* diversification and the emegency of methicillin-resistant strains. *J. Bacteriol.* 189: 8685–92.

40. Frank, L.A., Kania, S.A., Hnilica, K.A., *et al.* (2003). Isolation of *Staphylococcus schleiferi* from dogs with pyoderma. *J. Am. Vet. Med. Assoc.* 222: 451–4.

41. Morris, D.O., Rook, K.A., Shofer, F.S. and Rankin, S.C. (2006). Screening of *Staphylococcus aureus*, *Staphylococcus intermedius*, and *Staphylococcus schleiferi* isolates obtained from small companion animals for antimicrobial resistance: a retrospective review of 749 isolates (2003–04). *Vet. Dermatol.* 17(5): 332–7.

42. Sasaki, T., Kikuchi, K., Tanaka, Y., *et al.* (2007). Methicillin-resistant *Staphylococcus pseudintermedius* in a veterinary teaching hospital. *J. Clin. Microbiol.* 45: 1118–25.

43. Teshager, T., Dominguez, L., Morenzo, M.A., *et al.* (2000). Isolation of an SHV-12 β-lactamase-producing *Escherichia coli* strain from a dog with recurrent urinary tract infections. *Antimicrob. Agents. Chemother.* 44: 3483–4.

44. Warren, A., Townsend, K., King, T., *et al.* (2001). Multi-drug resistant *Escherichia coli* with extended-spectrum β-lactamase activity and fluoroquinolone resistance isolated from clinical infections in dogs. *Aust. Vet. J.* 79(9): 621–3.

45. Oluoch, A.O., Kim, C.H., Weisiger, R.M., *et al.* (2001). Nonenteric *Escherichia coli* isolates from dogs: 674 cases (1990–1998). *J. Am. Vet. Med. Assoc.* 218: 381–4.

46. Cooke, C.L., Singer, R.S., Jang, S.S. *et al.* (2002). Enrofloxacin resistance in *Escherichia coli* isolated from dogs with urinary tract infections. *J. Am. Vet. Med. Assoc.* 220: 190–2.

47. Féria, C., Ferreira, E., Correia, J.D., *et al.* (2002). Patterns and mechanisms of resistance to β-lactams and β-lactamase inhibitors in uropathogenic *Escherichia coli*

11 Dogs & Cats

isolated from dogs in Portugal. *J. Antimicrob. Chemother.* 49: 77–85.

48. Ogeer-Gyles, J., Mathews, K., Weese, J.S., *et al.* (2006). Evaluation of catheter-associated urinary tract infections and multi-drug-resistant *Escherichia coli* isolates from the urine of dogs with indwelling urinary catheters. *J. Am. Vet. Med. Assoc.* 229: 1584–90.

49. Sanchez, S., Stevenson, M.A.M., Hudson, C.R., *et al.* (2002). Characterization of multidrug-resistant *Escherichia coli* isolates associated with nosocomial infections in dogs. *J. Clin. Microbiol.* 40: 3586–95.

50. Carattoli, A., Lovari, S., Franco, A., *et al.* (2005). Extended-spectrum beta-lactamases in *Escherichia coli* isolated from dogs and cats in Rome, Italy, from 2001 to 2003. *Antimicrob. Agents Chemother.* 49: 833–5.

51. Johnson, J.R., Stell, A.L., Delavari, P., *et al.* (2001). Phylogenetic and pathotypic similarities between *Escherichia coli* isolates from urinary tract infections in dogs and extraintestinal infections in humans. *J. Infect. Dis.* 183: 897–906.

52. Starcic, M., Johnson, J.R., Stell, A.L., *et al.* (2002). Haemolytic *Escherichia coli* isolated from dogs with diarrhea have characteristics of both uropathogenic and necrotoxigenic strains. *Vet. Microbiol.* 85: 361–77.

53. Williamson, N.L., Frank, L.A. and Hnilica, K.A. (2002). Effects of short-term trimethoprim-sulfamethoxazole administration on thyroid function in dogs. *J. Am. Vet. Med. Assoc.* 221: 802–6.

54. Frank, L.A., Hnilica, K.A., May, E.R., *et al.* (2005). Effects of sulfamethoxazole-trimethoprim on thyroid function in dogs. *Am. J. Vet. Res.* 66: 256–9.

55. Bidgood, T.L. and Papich, M.G. (2003). Comparison of plasma and interstitial fluid concentrations of doxycycline and meropenem following constant rate intravenous infusion in dogs. *Am. J. Vet. Res.* 64: 1040–6.

56. Bettenay, S.V., Mueller, R.S. and Dell'Osa, D. (1998). Doxycycline hydrochloride in the treatment of canine pyoderma. *Aust. Vet. Practit.* 28: 14–19.

57. Koch, H.J. and Vercelli, A. (1993). Shampoos and other topical therapies. In: *Advances in Veterinary Dermatology*, Volume 2 (eds. Ihrke, P.J., Mason, I.S. and White, S.D.). Pergamon Press, New York, pp. 409–11.

58. Cole, L.K., Papich, M.G., Kwochka, K.W., *et al.* (2005). Plasma and ear tissue concentrations of enrofloxacin and its metabolite ciprofloxacin in dogs with chronic end-stage otitis externa. In: *Proceedings of North American Veterinary Dermatology Forum* 20: 182.

59. Foster, A.P. and DeBoer, D.J. (1998). The role of *Pseudomonas* in canine ear disease. *Compendium Small Anim. Pract.* 20: 909–19.

60. Cole, L.K., Kwochka, K.W., Kowalski, J.J., *et al.* (1998). Microbial flora and antimicrobial susceptibility patterns of isolated pathogens from the horizontal ear canal and middle ear in dogs with otitis media. *J. Am. Vet. Med. Assoc.* 212: 534–8.

61. Martín Barrasa, J.L., Lupiola Gómez, P., González Lama, Z. and Tejedor Junco, M.T. (2000). Antibacterial susceptibility patterns of *Pseudomonas* strains isolated from chronic canine otitis externa. *J. Vet. Med. Ser. B* 47: 191–6.

62. Seol, B., Naglic, T., Madic, J. and Bedekovic, M. (2002). *In vitro* antimicrobial susceptibility of 183 *Pseudomonas aeruginosa* strains isolated from dogs to selected antipseudomonal agents. *J. Vet. Med. Ser. B* 49: 188–2.

63. Brothers, A.M., Gibbs, P.S. and Wooley, R.E. (2002). Development of resistant bacteria isolated from dogs with otitis externa or urinary tract infections after exposure to enrofloxacin *in vitro*. *Vet. Ther.* 3: 493–500.

64. Tejedor, M.T., Martin, J.L., Navia, M., *et al.* (2003). Mechanisms of fluoroquinolone resistance in *Pseudomonas aeruginosa* isolates from canine infections. *Vet. Microbiol.* 94: 295–301.

65. Ashworth, C.D. and Nelson, D.R. (1990). Antimicrobial potentiation of irrigation solutions containing tris-[hydroxymethyl] aminomethane-EDTA. *J. Am. Vet. Med. Assoc.* 197: 1513–4.

66. Sparks, T.A., Kemp, D.T., Wooley, R.E., *et al.* (1994). Antimicrobial effect of combinations of EDTA-tris and amikacin or neomycin on the microorganisms associated with otitis externa in dogs. *Vet. Res. Commun.* 18: 241–249.

67. Farca, A.M., Piromalli, G., Maffei, F., *et al.* (1997). Potentiating effect of EDTA-Tris on the activity of antibiotics against resistant bacteria associated with otitis, dermatitis and cystitis. *J. Small Anim. Pract.* 38: 243–5.

68. NCCLS (1998). Performance standards for antimicrobial disk and dilution susceptibility tests for bacteria isolated from animals. Proposed standard. NCCLS document M31-A. Villanova, PA: National Committee for Clinical Laboratory Standards.

69. Frimodt-Møller, N. (2002). Correlation between pharmacokinetic/pharmacodynamic parameters and efficacy for antibiotics in the treatment of urinary tract infection. *Int. J. Antimicrob. Agents* 19: 546–53.

70. Hagman, R. and Greko, C. (2005). Antimicrobial resistance in *Escherichia coli* isolated from bitches with pyometra and from urine samples from other dogs. *Vet. Rec.* 157: 193–6.

71. Pedersen, K., Pedersen, K., Jensen, H., *et al.* (2007). Occurrence of antimicrobial resistance in bacteria from diagnostic samples from dogs. *J. Antimicrob. Chemother.* 60: 775–81.

72. Meares, E.M. (1982). Prostatitis: review of pharmacokinetics and therapy. *Rev. Infect. Dis.* 4: 475–83.

73. Happonen, I., Linden, J., Saari, S., *et al.* (1998). Detection and effects of helicobacters in healthy dogs and dogs with signs of gastritis. *J. Am. Vet. Med. Assoc.* 213: 1767–74.

74. Wiinberg, B., Spohr, A., Dietz, H.H., *et al.* (2005). Quantitative analysis of inflammatory and immune responses in dogs with gastritis and their relationship to *Helicobacter* spp. infection. *J. Vet. Intern. Med.* 19: 4–14.

75. Happonen, I., Linden, J. and Westermarck, E. (2000). Effect of triple therapy on eradication of canine gastric helicobacters and gastric disease. *J. Small Anim. Pract.* 41: 1–6.

76. Watson, A.D.J. and Maddison, J.E. (2001). Systemic antibacterial drug use in dogs in Australia. *Aust. Vet. J.* 79: 740–6.

11 Dogs & Cats

77. Westermarck, E., Skrzypczak, T., Harmoinen, J., *et al.* (2005). Tylosin-responsive chronic diarrhea in dogs. *J. Vet. Intern. Med.* 19: 177–186.

78. Johnston, K.L., Lamport, A.I., Ballevre, O.P. and Batt, R.M. (2000). Effects of oral administration of metronidazole on small intestinal bacteria and nutrients of cats. *Am. J. Vet. Res.* 61: 1106–12.

79. Speakman, A.J., Dawson, S., Corkill, J.E., *et al.* (2000). Antibiotic susceptibility of canine *Bordetella bronchiseptica* isolates. *Vet. Microbiol.* 71: 193–200.

80. Streppa, H.K., Singer, M.J. and Budsberg, S.C. (2001). Applications of local antimicrobial delivery systems in veterinary medicine. *J. Am. Vet. Med. Assoc.* 219: 40–8.

81. Rahal, J.J. and Simberkoff, M.S. (1979). Bactericidal and bacteriostatic action of chloramphenicol against meningeal pathogens. *Antimicrob. Agents Chemother.* 16: 13–8.

82. Greene, C.E. and Dearmin, M.G. (2006). Surgical and traumatic wound infections. In: *Infectious Diseases of the Dog and the Cat*, 3rd edn (ed. Greene, C.E.). Saunders Elsevier, St. Louis, Missouri, pp. 935–61.

83. Lloyd, D.H., Lamport, A.I. and Feeney, C. (1996). Sensitivity to antibiotics amongst cutaneous and mucosal isolates of canine pathogenic staphylococci in the UK, 1980–96. *Vet. Dermatol.* 7: 171–5.

84. Myllyniemi, A.L., Gindonis, V., Nykäsenoja, S. and Koppinen, J. (2004). FINRES-Vet 2002-2003, Finnish Veterinary Antimicrobial Resistance Monitoring and Consumption of Antimicrobial Agents. National Veterinary and Food Research Institute, Helsinki, Finland.

85. Wissing, A., Nicolet, J. and Boerlin, P. (2001). Antimicrobial resistance situation in Swiss veterinary medicine. *Schweizer Archiv für Tierheilkunde* 143: 503–10.

86. Hartmann, F.A., White, D.G., West, S.E., *et al.* (2005). Molecular characterization of *Staphylococcus intermedius* carriage by healthy dogs and comparison of antimicrobial susceptibility patterns to isolates from dogs with pyoderma. *Vet. Microbiol.* 108: 119–31.

87. Strain, G.M., Merchant, S.R., Neer, M. and Tedford, B.L. (1995). Ototoxicity assessment of a gentamicin sulfate otic preparation in dogs. *Am. J. Vet. Res.* 56: 532–8.

88. Barsanti, J.A. (2006). Genitourinary infections. In: *Infectious Diseases of the Dog and the Cat*, 3rd Edn (ed. Greene, C.E.). Saunders Elsevier, St. Louis, Missouri, pp. 935–61.

89. Papich, M.G. (2007). *Saunders Handbook of Veterinary Drugs*, 2nd Edn. Saunders/Elsevier St. Louis Missouri, USA.

11 Dogs & Cats

Chapter 12

GUIDELINES FOR ANTIMICROBIAL USE IN AQUACULTURE

Peter R. Smith, Alain Le Breton, Tor Einar Horsberg and Flavio Corsin

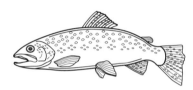

Aquaculture is a very significant and rapidly expanding industry, with a production in 2004 of 60 million tonnes with an estimated value of US$ 70.3 billion (FAO, 2006). Farmed fish now contribute approximately 50% of the world's fish food production. Food production in the aquatic environment is largely an Asian activity with over 90% of world production coming from this region. In quantity terms, China is responsible for approximately 70% of world production, Japan and the rest of the Asia-Pacific region for a further 22%. Western Europe (3.5%) and North America (1.3%) account for only a small fraction of world production (1). Approximately 40% of the global fish production, most of which derives from aquaculture, is traded internationally, with exports exceeding that of commodities such as meat, dairy, cereals, sugar and coffee (1).

Aquaculture production is divided roughly equally between marine or brackish water (57%) and freshwater (43%) and in terms of value, fish are the dominant aquaculture product (54%) followed by crustaceans (20%) and molluscs (14%). When considered by species, the world production is dominated by carp (18 million tonnes) followed by oysters and kelp (both over 4 million tonnes). Considered in value terms, however, shrimp and salmonids become more significant. In addition to the production of fish for consumption there is also a large market in non-food, ornamental fish where there is little regulation, although this is beginning to change.

12.1 Aquaculture diversity

It is impossible to overstate the diversity of activities that must be included under the term aquaculture. Although, in 2004, 25 species belonging to a number of different phyla accounted for over 80% of the world aquaculture production, the farming of a total of 442 species is reported in the FAO FISHSTAT Plus database as having occurred at any time between 1950 and 2004 or still ongoing.

The vast range of species farmed is reflected in the diversity of culture systems and environments encountered. Temperatures can vary over at least a 30°C range and salinity can vary from zero to 40 g/l. The nutrient levels in aquaculture systems also vary over a wide range. Some systems operate best with pure spring water whilst, at the other end of the spectrum, some involve the deliberate eutrophication of the

12 Aquaculture

water. Aquaculture can be conducted in freshwater, brackishwater and full strength seawater. Equally, systems vary with respect to their exposure to bacteria present in human or animal wastes.

The socio-economic environments within which aquaculture operates also vary over the full range found in the world, from small-scale systems most popular in the Asian region, to industrial-level operations, and both the scientific and technical infrastructure available to aquaculture producers and the regulatory environments within which they operate show wide variations (1).

A significant proportion of aquacultural production occurs in low-income, food-deficient countries (LIFDC). In such countries, small scale 'peasant' aquaculture plays a major role in meeting subsistence nutritional requirements and as a vital source of employment, profit and foreign exchange earnings. At the other end of the spectrum, aquaculture is often run by sophisticated, multinational companies. It would, however, be a mistake to associate the size of aquaculture operations and the extent to which they are involved in international trade with any geographical location or with any species. Small-scale and large industrial aquaculture operations coexist in most countries.

12.2 Antimicrobial use in aquaculture

Given the huge diversity characterising the aquaculture sector, it is obvious that by treating antimicrobial agent use in aquaculture as a single category only very broad generalisations can be made. Possibly the most valid is that, with few exceptions (2), we have limited data relating to aspects of antimicrobial use in world aquaculture, such as the amounts used, the range of agents employed and the rationale for their use. For most species farmed we also lack adequate knowledge of the pharmacokinetics and pharmacodynamics of administrations.

Some estimates of the amounts of antimicrobial agent use can be made for some countries. In Europe, the amounts of antimicrobial use would appear to be related to the extent to which appropriate husbandry techniques have been developed and to the availability of vaccines effective against the dominant diseases. In Norway (3), use has been estimated at 2 g per metric tonnes production. This figure is most likely also representative for other European countries where Atlantic salmon is the dominant species, whereas in other European countries (4, 5) the use has been estimated to lie in the range 10–100 g/t. In Chilean salmonid culture, where there is as yet no effective vaccine of the dominant bacterial disease, piscirickettiosis, use has been estimated at 200 g/t (6). There are very few data allowing any estimate for use in Asian aquaculture, but there are indications for a significantly higher consumption than recorded for Europe (7).

With respect to the range of agents that are employed in aquaculture there are wide variations in the quality of the available data (8). At one end of the spectrum there are countries, mainly in northern Europe and northern America, where availability is very highly regulated and where, in general, very few (two or three) agents have been granted Marketing Authorisations (MA) (9). At the other end there are countries where use is limited only by market availability and price. Despite huge country-to-country variations, the agents most frequently reported as being used belong to the tetracyclines, the potentiated sulfonamides and to the first- and second-generation quinolones.

There are few data relating to the rationale for antimicrobial use in aquaculture and we are forced to offer only a series of generalisations. The evidence suggests that the vast majority of antimicrobial use in aquaculture involves the presentation of medicated feed, is mostly metaphylactic and is only initiated in response to an overt infection in farmed animals. There are, however, consistent reports of prophylactic use in shrimp and mollusc hatchery production. Voluntary use of antimicrobials as growth promoters in any aspect of aquaculture is generally rare.

A very significant proportion of world aquaculture production occurs in LIFDC where the technical or professional support available to producers is very limited. As a consequence it is probable that the majority of antimicrobial use in world aquaculture is not associated with any classification of the target bacterium or of its susceptibility to the range of available antimicrobials. This situation can be contrasted with the conditions obtaining in the more industrialised part of the sector. Here technical support is increasingly available, but it can be argued that we still face a serious shortfall in the science that is needed to advise the advisors and in servicing the millions of producers involved in the aquaculture sector, especially in Asian countries.

12.3 Therapy of diseases encountered in aquaculture

In commercial aquaculture the diseases to which antimicrobial therapies are most commonly applied are those occurring in the production of finfish and crustaceans (shrimp and prawns). In mollusc culture systems the use of antimicrobials is almost completely confined to the very early larval stages of production, and the amounts used are therefore relatively small. Antimicrobial use in ornamental fish is largely unregulated and has rarely been quantified, but is thought to be considerable and the significance of this use is increased by the proximity of these fish to humans.

In human and land-based animal medicine, where a wide range of agents are available to health-care specialists, it is possible for them to select an appropriate therapeutic agent on the basis of records of its past performance in reducing losses to the specific infectious disease they are faced with. These conditions do not, however, apply in aquaculture. A distinguishing characteristic of this industry is the very limited number of antimicrobials that are available. In those countries that have a significant scientific infrastructure and a developed regulatory environment, the range of agents from which a choice can be made is frequently extremely limited. For example, with respect to 25 European countries, the mean number of antimicrobials licensed for use in aquaculture is currently 2 ± 1.2 and in none of these countries have more than five agents been licensed (9). In countries with a less developed scientific infrastructure, regulations tend to be limited or only weakly enforced. Thus, in these countries the range of agents used in aquaculture tends to be greater. In these countries therapeutic agents are frequently chosen by the farmers themselves with very limited input from trained health-care professionals, although things have changed significantly over the years.

The choice of therapeutic agents in aquaculture is further complicated by the general absence of standardised therapeutic regimen and by the serious lack of field data on clinical efficacy of any therapies. Scanning the published scientific literature reveals that even data on the efficacy generated in small-scale laboratory trials have been rarely reported. In practice, the choice of therapeutic agent is frequently influenced as much by considerations of agent availability, regulations and bacterial susceptibility as it is by considerations of the nature of the disease being treated.

At the present state of our knowledge it is not possible to provide a list of the antimicrobial agents that would be most effective in treating any specific disease condition. The diversities among aquaculture species and aquatic farming environments and technologies are much bigger than for terrestrial animals, making any such attempts bogus. Table 12.1 is a compilation of the licensing status for antimicrobial agents in several countries. It demonstrates a great variation in licensed products, a variation that is a result of tradition and economy rather than scientific data. The table summarises the various disease conditions that have been treated by various agents and lists the countries in which those agents have been licensed. In several countries, off-label use of antibacterials is the rule rather than the exception. It should be noted that the association in the table of a particular agent with a particular disease should not be taken to imply that there are good-quality data demonstrating efficacy. Equally, the demonstration of efficacy in one fish species in one environment cannot be taken as evidence that efficacy will be achieved in treating the same species or another species in a different environment. Many environmental conditions such as water quality parameters will interfere with the efficacy of the treatment, especially when immersion treatments are done. Table 12.1 does not include any data or recommendation as to the most appropriate treatment regimen for any agent. This omission is partly a consequence of the general lack of good empirical data. However, factors such as fish species and the salinity and temperature of the environment of the treated animals will have significant pharmacokinetic impacts.

12.4 Pharmacokinetics and pharmacodynamics

Pharmacokinetic (PK) studies address the time course of antimicrobial concentrations in the body, while pharmacodynamic (PD) studies address the relationship between those concentrations and the antimicrobial effect (10). The relationship between PK and PD parameters are discussed in great detail in Chapter 6, thus, only aspects regarding bacteria pathogenic to aquaculture species are discussed here. PK and PD studies have an important role in determining breakpoints suitable for interpreting susceptibility tests (see below). They also have a major, but with respect

12 Aquaculture

12 Aquaculture

Table 12.1 Antimicrobial agents and their applications in aquaculture

Antimicrobial		Indication		Licensed for aquatic species
Family	Drug	Species	Diseases	Country
β-Lactamas	Amoxicillin	Salmonids, sea bass, sea bream, yellowtail, catfish, eels, tilapia	Furunculosis, bacterial gill diseases, pasteurellosis, edwardsiellosis, streptococcosis	UK, Romania, Italy, Greece
Tetracyclines	Oxytetracycline and chlortetracycline	Salmonids, channel catfish, carps, marine species, ornamental fish	Vibriosis, pasteurellosis, flexibacteriosis, infections with segmented filamentous bacteria, columnaris, yersiniosis, furunculosis, cold water vibriosis, botulism, Pseudomonas infections, Aeromonas infections flavobacteriosis, streptococcosis	EU countries, most Asian countries, USA, Canada, Japan
Quinolones and fluoroquinolones	Nalidixic acid	Salmonids, eels, carps, goldfish ornamental fish	Furunculosis, vibriosis, Pseudomonas infections	Japan
	Oxolinic acid	Eels, carps, goldfish, salmonids, turbot	Pseudomonas infections, Serratia infections, edwardsiellosis, vibriosis, cold water vibriosis, furunculosis	Denmark, Greece, France, Norway, Iceland, Bulgaria
	Flumequine	Salmonids, marine species, ornamental fish	Pasteurellosis, vibriosis, flexibacteriosis, furunculosis, yersiniosis	Croatia, Czech Rep, France, Hungary, Italy, Latvia, Slovakia
	Enrofloxacin	Salmonids, ornamental fish	Bacterial kidney disease, vibriosis, furunculosis, streptococcosis	
	Sarafloxacin	Salmonids, channel catfish	Furunculosis, yersiniosis, edwardsiellosis	
Macrolides	Erythromycin	Yellowtail, salmonids	Streptococcosis, lactococcosis, bacterial kidney disease, piscirickettiosis, Chlamydia infections	
	Spiramycin, josamycin	Yellowtail	Streptococcosis	Japan
Amphenicols	Florfenicol	Salmonids, marine species, eels, ornamental fish	Flavobacterium psychrophilum infections, furunculosis, vibriosis, flexibacteriosis, pasteurellosis, edwardsiellosis	UK, Ireland, Latvia, Slovenia, Norway, Bulgaria, Denmark, Lithuania
Sulfonamides	Sulfamerazine Sulfadimethoxine Sulfadimidine	Fresh water salmonids Rainbow trout, Channel catfish Fresh water salmonids, carps	Furunculosis	USA
Potentiated sulfonamides	Trimetoprim + sulfadiadine or sulfamethoxazole	Salmonids, ornamental fish, catfish, marine species	Aeromonas infections, yersiniosis, edwardsiellosis, vibriosis, pasteurellosis	USA, Canada, UK, Denmark, Croatia, Norway, France, Slovenia, Italy, Greece, Germany
	Ormethoprim + sulfadimethoxine	Salmonids, channel catfish	Furunculosis, edwardsiellosis	USA

to aquaculture, largely unfulfilled, potential in the design of therapeutic regimen. In considering PK/PD approaches it is important to note that what data we have relates almost exclusively to species farmed in Europe. Studies relating to those species that contribute to the vast majority of world aquaculture production are rare to non-existent (11).

12.4.1 Pharmacodynamics properties

The minimum concentration required to inhibit *in vitro* growth (MIC) of different antimicrobial agents against fish pathogenic bacteria is a key pharmacodynamic parameter. A large number of reports of MIC values for bacteria associated with disease in aquatic organisms have been published over the years (12–18). Other parameters that measure bacterial susceptibility, such as the concentration required to kill (MBC), the concentration required to prevent mutations emerging (MPC) (19) and the minimum concentration that exerts selective pressure for resistant variants (MSC) (20) have been reported much less frequently.

When applying MIC values to PK/PD modelling, three factors must be considered:

1. The concentrations required to inhibit a bacterium in laboratory media may not be the same as the concentration required in the host.
2. Any numerical value of any *in vitro* MIC is dependent on the test protocol used to determine it.
3. In PK/PD modelling it is the MIC characterising susceptible strains that is needed.

Unfortunately, the available studies of MIC have used a variety of test protocols and this limits the extent to which the numerical values they have reported can be compared. It is only very recently that standard protocols for determining MIC values for aquatic bacteria have been published (21). Miller and Reimschuessel (18) (Table 12.2) have used these protocols to establish epidemiological cut-off values that allow the characterisation of isolates of *Aeromonas salmonicida* as wild type (WT) or non-wild type (NWT) according to the procedures recommended by the European Committee on Antimicrobial Susceptibility Testing (EUCAST) (22, 23). The cut-off values estimated for WT isolates represent the type of data that will be of most value in PK/PD modelling.

12.4.2 Pharmacokinetic properties

A number of pharmacokinetic studies in different fish species have been published over the years, and results from more than 400 papers have recently been compiled in a searchable database (11). Samuelsen (24) has recently published a valuable review of the pharmacokinetic data available for the quinolone group of agents.

Unfortunately, the quantitative data that has been generated in different studies shows very significant variation. In part, this variation is a function of the very many factors that complicate the measurement of the pharmacokinetic properties of agents in fish. Variation can be expected when different administration regimen are used and when different fish species are studied. Equally, environmental factors such

Table 12.2 Epidemiological cut-off values estimated by Miller and Reimschuessel (18) from data on 217 strains of *Aeromonas salmonicida*

Agent	Epidemiological cut-off values			
	MIC (mg/l) M49-A (CLSI, 2006b)		Disc diffusion (mm) M42-A (CLSI, 2006a)	
	WT[a]	NWT[a]	WT[a]	NWT[a]
Oxytetracycline	≤1	≤8	≤28	≤23
Florfenicol	≤4	≤8	≤31	≤30
Oxolinic acid	≤0.125	≤1	≤30	≤25
Ormetoprim- sulfadimethoxine	≤10	≤30	≤20	≤16

[a] The terms WT and NWT have been defined by EUCAST (22).

as temperature (25–28) and salinity (29) will also influence PK values.

Difficulties in estimating relevant measures for PK parameters also arise from the fact that most administrations to fish are metaphylactic treatments of large populations performed by the presentation of medicated feed. In such treatments, large inter-individual variations in plasma- and tissue concentrations of the agent are inevitable. The limited data available suggests that, with respect to florfenicol, the degree of fish-to-fish variation is greater in the field (30) than in laboratory trials where healthy fish were given a standard treatment (31). Not only do these variations in the concentration achieved in different members of the population result in a substantial risk of

sub-optimal tissue concentrations in a large proportion of the treated population, they also raise serious questions as to the appropriate statistic that should be used to characterise the concentrations achieved in a population (32, 33). The inappetance of infected fish also raises problems for estimation of PK values for oral administrations. In a number of studies of treatments on commercial farms, agent concentrations were below the limit of detection in all moribund fish examined at the end of a period of therapy.

Thus, there are major theoretical and practical problems associated with the collection of PK values relevant to commercial treatments. The data in Table 12.3 allows a comparison of the PK parameters

Table 12.3 Some pharmacokinetic properties of antimicrobial agents in Atlantic salmon held at 10–12°C in seawater (34)

Agent	Route and dose (mg/kg)	VD_{ss} (l kg)	CL_T (l h kg)	$t_{1/2\beta}$ (h)	AUC (µg h ml)	C_{max} (µg ml)	T_{max} (h)	F (%)
Enrofloxacin	IV (10)	6.1	0.14	34.2	72.4			
	oral (10)				40.2	1.54	6	55
Sarafloxacin	IV (10)	2.3	0.10	24.0	100.7			
	oral (10)				2.2	0.08	12	2
Difloxacin	IV (4)	4.2	0.07	46.4	59.0			
	oral (4)				33.6	0.53	6	57
Flumequine	IV (25)	3.5	0.18	22.8	140.2			
	oral (25)				62.7	1.42	6	45
Oxolinic acid	IV (25)	5.4	0.28	18.2	89.1			
	oral (25)				26.8	0.61	12	30
Oxytetracycline	IV (50)	1.3	0.02	63.9	2692.2			
	oral (50)				77.7	1.80	6	3
Doxycycline	IV (12.5)	4.0	0.05	67.2	238.4			
	oral (12.5)				<4.6	<0.1	—	<2
Florfenicol	IV (10)	1.1	0.09	12.2	116.3			
	oral (10)				112.0	4.41	12	96
Amoxicillin	IV (50)	2.1	0.23	13.4	220.6			
	oral (50)				<4.6	<0.1	—	<2
Trimethoprim	IV (5)	2.0	0.07	22.4	69,5			
	oral (5)				66.7	1.52	12	96
Sulfadiazine	IV (25)	0.7	0.02	21.5	1121.9			
	oral (25)				556.8	7.92	24	50

VD_{ss}, volume of distribution at steady state;
CL_T, total body clearance;
$t_{1/2\beta}$, elimination half-life;
AUC, area under the plasma concentration versus time curve;
C_{max}, maximum plasma concentration;
T_{max}, time to maximum plasma concentration;
F, bioavailability.

for a number of agents following their single-dose administration to Atlantic salmon (34).

12.5 Antimicrobial susceptibility testing of fish pathogens

In recent years, some progress has been made in developing standard methods for determining the *in vitro* susceptibility of bacteria associated with aquatic animal disease. Alderman and Smith (35) reported a set of susceptibility test protocols that had been developed by a group of 24 scientists from 17 countries. These protocols have been modified and importantly associated with appropriate control criteria in the Clinical and Laboratory Science Institute's (CLSI) guidelines M42-A (36) and M49-A (21). Given the extent of their development, the degree of consultation that has been involved in the production and the absence of any serious alternative, it is argued that these protocols should be adopted as the industry standard methods for determining *in vitro* susceptibility. The recent survey of current practice (37) revealed that the majority (90%) of responding laboratories employed disc diffusion protocols in susceptibility testing of clinical isolates from aquatic animals.

The practical determination of resistance or susceptibility in a bacterium in a clinical context is, however, a two-step process. After laboratory tests have been employed to obtain a measure of *in vitro* susceptibility, the essential second step is to interpret the meaning of that measure, in any specific clinical context, by applying appropriate breakpoints. At the present moment no clinically relevant breakpoints have been established for susceptibility test data generated from bacteria associated with aquatic animal disease by the application of standard minimum inhibitory concentration or disc diffusion methods. Current studies have been focused on establishing epidemiological cut-off values (22) that can be used as a first approximation for such breakpoints (23). The issue as to whether useful laboratory-independent cut-off values can be established or whether the degree of inter-laboratory variation (38, 39) will require that we establish standard protocols for generating laboratory- and species-specific values (40) has yet to be resolved. However, following a study of the distribution of data from 217 strains of *A. salmonicida*, Miller and Reimschuessel (18) have suggested laboratory-independent epidemiological cut-off values that could

be applied to disc diffusion data generated by M42-A (36) for this species. A comparison of these values (Table 12.2) with the breakpoints currently in use in laboratories surveyed by Smith (37) is disturbing. The extent to which these cut-off values are considerably larger than the majority of breakpoints in use, raises the possibility that many laboratories are reporting isolates with NWT susceptibilities as clinically susceptible. In the period before appropriate cut-off values or breakpoints can be established from empirical data there is an urgent requirement to reduce the errors associated with the interpretation of disc diffusion data.

Kronvall *et al.* (40) have suggested that epidemiological cut-off values can usefully be set by calculating the mean less 2.5 standard deviations of the zones generated for fully susceptible strains. The standard deviations of the distributions of zone sizes for nine agents against fully susceptible *A. salmonicida* and four agents against *Vibrio anguillarum* have all been shown to be within the range 3–4 mm (unpublished data). If this holds true for other species, calculating the mean zone size for susceptible species and subtracting 10 mm would represent a simple, if crude, method for generating a first approximation of a cut-off value. This work suggests that, in the period before consensus breakpoints become available, a recommendation not to proceed with a treatment should be given by a laboratory every time the isolated bacterium generated a zone that was 10 mm smaller that the mean normally recorded, in that laboratory, for fully susceptible isolates of the same species.

12.6 Negative impacts of antimicrobial use in aquaculture

12.6.1 Negative aspects associated with resistance

Antimicrobial use in aquaculture will and does provide the conditions for the emergence of bacteria that are resistant to antimicrobials. The bacteria in which such resistant variants are most likely to occur are those associated with fish diseases (41). Thus, there is a negative feedback loop in aquacultural use. The more antimicrobials are used, the more likely they are to be rendered useless. This negative feedback provides the most compelling reasons for prudence in the use of antimicrobials in aquaculture. Irrational or excessive use of any agent will have a direct impact on the future therapeutic value of any agent. In many countries there is an extremely limited number of agents licensed for use and this exacerbates the problem.

The possibility that antimicrobial use in aquaculture might also have an impact on the treatment of infections in human and other land-based animals was first raised close to 40 years ago (42), but in the intervening years we have failed to characterise, either qualitatively or quantitatively, the extent of this risk. Smith (43) has presented mathematical models suggesting that the significance of selection of bacteria with transferable resistances as a result of the non-human use of antimicrobials, is only likely to impact on human therapy in situations where the frequency of those resistances in human pathogens is low.

The potential risks presented by aquacultural use are significantly different from those presented by use in land-based animals. With respect to agricultural use of antimicrobials, the major risks are associated with the selection, in treated animals, of resistant variants of bacteria capable of infecting humans (44). With aquacultural use this exposure pathway is generally considered to be less significant, and the major risks are those associated with selection of bacteria containing resistance genes that could be transferred to human pathogens. There are ample data (45) that the genes encoding resistance in human pathogens and in bacteria associated with aquaculture are highly related indicating that, in nature, these genes are capable of transfer between the two groups of bacteria. There are, however, much less data demonstrating the dominant direction of this gene flow or the consequence of increased frequencies of these genes in aquaculture on their frequencies in human pathogens.

The recent WHO/FAO/OIE Expert Group (46) identified the major risks to human health associated with aquacultural use of antimicrobials as being those arising from the emergence of transferable resistances in the bacteria associated with fish disease and in those present in the aquacultural environment. They recommended that the emergence of such transferable resistances should be regularly monitored. However, any calls for such monitoring and surveillance will be of little value until validated and standardised laboratory methods that would be capable of generating relevant data have been developed.

12.6.2 Negative impacts associated with residues

Although arguably the most significant adverse effects resulting from aquacultural use of antimicrobials may be those associated with the emergence of resistant bacteria (41), it is probable that on a global scale considerations of drug residues have had a greater impact on antimicrobial agent use, in addition to significant economic consequences for several exporting countries. There are few, if any, reports of adverse reactions in humans to drug residues in aquaculture products. There are significant regulations governing the presence of such residues (1). These regulations, particularly those that govern international trade, have stimulated rapid improvements in the ability of many countries to detect and monitor such residues, although in view of the paucity of aquaculture commodities covered by the Codex Alimentarius, the requirements imposed by countries to a great extent still lack harmonisation. The introduction of residue testing by large retailers has also had a major impact on antimicrobial agent use.

12.7 Towards improvements of antimicrobial use in aquaculture

Improvements in the use of antimicrobials in aquaculture would require the design of administration regimen that optimise clinical efficacy whilst minimising the development of resistance, the environmental impact and the presence of residues in food products. The lack of fundamental data presents major difficulties for the task of generating specific guidelines for the rational, evidence-based use of antimicrobial agents in aquaculture. Although for some fish species such as salmonids, progress has been made in collecting the PK/PD data that this task would require, for others, and notably those that make the largest contribution to world production, data collection has hardly begun (11).

The example of northern European salmonid culture in general and that of Norwegian in particular (3, 47), demonstrates that economically successful aquaculture can be achieved without extensive use of antimicrobials. Equally, some National Federations of Producers, such as the French, strongly promote this approach and have published a handbook of

Good Health Management Practices in Aquaculture (48). Several examples from the shrimp farming sector have also indicated that the application of Better Management Practice protocols can lead to successful production without reliance on antimicrobials. Corsin *et al.* (49) and Padiyar *et al.* (50) have demonstrated that the application of these production management approaches is gradually expanding in scope.

The wide variety of situations where antimicrobials are used in aquaculture also presents difficulties in making specific recommendation as to how the use of these agents can be improved. However, a number of general considerations can be identified.

12.7.1 Disease prevention

Well-fed animals that are living in an environment that is compatible with their physiological needs are less likely to be infected by pathogenic bacteria. As a consequence, optimising husbandry practices must always be first line of defence against infectious disease. In this context it is worth noting that adverse living conditions frequently arise as a function of overstocking. The specific stocking densities appropriate for any environment are determined by the innate quality of that environment, but overstocking will always lead to an increased disease risk. Here the appropriate long-term response is not to continue to rely on antimicrobials to control the losses to disease, but to reduce the stocking densities to a more appropriate level.

Many aquaculture enterprises require that animals be imported into the farm. Monitoring the health status of these animals and particularly their examination for sub-clinical or covert infection, is an essential step in reducing subsequent disease and, therefore, in avoiding the need for antimicrobials.

Vaccines have been developed for some diseases of fin-fish. The use of some of these vaccines has been demonstrated to have a major role in reducing infection and therefore the need for therapy. However, crustaceans lack an adaptive immune system and, therefore, vaccines cannot provide a method of reducing antimicrobial use in shrimp aquaculture.

12.7.2 Appropriate diagnosis

Antimicrobial therapy can only function by reducing the impact of a bacterium on the health of the host. Beneficial consequences for the hosts can, therefore, be expected only when the bacterial infection is a major factor in the morbidity or mortality of a population. The aim of any diagnosis must not only be the detection of a particular bacterium but also, and critically, an assessment of its role in the disease process.

The isolation of a particular bacterium from a moribund host cannot be taken as evidence that the infection is the cause of the morbidity. Many bacterial infections detected in aquatic animals are secondary or opportunistic and the underlying cause may be environmental, infection by viruses or infestation by parasites. In such situations antimicrobial therapy would frequently be inappropriate.

'Diagnosis from a distance' must always be treated with some caution. The examination in a laboratory of a diseased animal will always tend to lead to an exaggeration of the role of the isolated pathogen. Whenever possible laboratory studies must be associated with field observation and interpreted within the context of the total clinical picture.

12.7.3 Appropriate therapy

In any situation, the success of any antimicrobial therapy will be a function of the choice of the most appropriate agent. Ideally, a recommendation could be made that the selection of agent should be made by a trained fish health professional from those licensed for the application. The selection of an agent that had been granted an MA for a particular application would go a long way to reducing inappropriate choices. However, in many countries, there is not only a lack of trained fish health professionals, but there is also a complete absence of agents licensed for use in aquaculture. Even in countries that have issued MAs for aquaculture, the number of agents that have been licensed is normally so small that the degree of choice is very limited.

The administration of antimicrobials to treat infections associated with bacteria that are clinically resistant cannot benefit the infected animal and can have only negative impacts. Antimicrobial use should, therefore, always be informed by data from susceptibility testing of the target bacterium. The current lack of validated breakpoints for the correct interpretation of these data does not mean that such data has no value. The reduction in susceptibility that arises from the acquisition by a bacterium of a gene encoding a specific, positive-function resistance is normally so significant that it is relatively easy for anybody with a

12 Aquaculture

little experience to detect. It should be noted that this type of mechanism is involved in the majority of cases of clinical resistance (45). Problems with the interpretation of disc diffusion data arise only when resistance is mediated by chromosomal mutations in the target bacterium or by other mechanisms that result in low, but clinically significant, reductions in susceptibility.

The success of antimicrobial therapy is a function of its efficacious administration to the infected population. In the majority of cases antimicrobials are administered in medicated feed. When this is the case, care should be taken to ensure that the target population is feeding at an adequate level to ensure that therapeutic concentrations of the agent can be achieved.

12.8   The way forward

Prudent use of antimicrobials has the overall aim of reducing antimicrobial use and the example of the Norwegian salmon farming industry illustrates that this is an achievable goal. It has been argued that, in this industry, a combination of improved husbandry (51) and the availability of vaccines that provided efficacious protection against the dominant diseases (47), made a major contribution to the dramatic decline in antimicrobial use. However, it also important to note that this industry was farming a high value product in a country with a highly developed scientific infrastructure; and that there were a significant number of trained professionals involved in providing a fish health service to a relatively small number of producers. It is also important to note the care and research that contributed to the design of the regulatory environment constructed for this industry.

It has to be recognised that, at least in the short-term, the replication of these conditions would be difficult in many countries. This is particularly true of those LIFDC that are involved in a significant proportion of world production. In these countries, the underdeveloped state of the scientific and technical infrastructure and the difficulties faced in addressing the needs of millions of producers have the consequence that antimicrobial therapies are frequently initiated without the involvement of health-care professionals or the performance of any susceptibility testing or even the identification of a specific disease condition. Prudent use is difficult to achieve in such contexts.

It is highly unlikely that progress towards prudent use could be made simply by formulating further regulations if developmental and educational programmes are not initiated at the same time. If prudent antimicrobial use is to be achieved in global aquaculture the primary focus must be on the development of scientific infrastructures and the education of fish health workers and fish farmers. Several efforts are now ongoing towards the introduction of better management of farms to prevent health problems. The implementation of Better Management Practices (BMP) especially in shrimp farming have proven particularly successful in countries like India and Vietnam and successfully led to the prudent use of antimicrobials by farming communities (52). These approaches are generally strengthened through the establishment of farmer groups which, among other benefits, improves access to extension services and reduces the risks of experiencing animal health problems (49).

Regulation and education, if they are to be effective, will have to be based on the product of research. This chapter has clearly identified the need for more research, but we must be careful to identify the questions that we require to be investigated. There is an urgent need for veterinarians and other health care workers to identify the types of information they require and to communicate these requirements both to research scientists and those that fund their work.

References

1. FAO. State of the world aquaculture (2006). Inland Water Resources and Aquaculture Service, Fishery Resources Division, Fisheries Department, FAO Fisheries Technical Paper No. 500. Rome, FAO, p. 134.
2. Subasinghe, R.P., Barg, U. and Tacon, A. (2000). Chemicals in Asian aquaculture: need, usage, issues and challenges. In: *Proceedings of the Meeting on the Use of Chemicals in Aquaculture in Asia Arthur* (eds. J.R., Lavilla-Pitogo, C.R. and Subasinghe, P.R.), 20–22 May 1996, Tigbauan, Iloilo, Philippines, p. 235.
3. Lillehaug, A., Lunestad, B.T. and Grave, K. (2003). Epidemiological description of bacterial diseases in Norwegian aquaculture – a description based on antibiotic prescription data for the ten-year period 1991 to 2000. *Dis. Aquat. Org.* 53: 115–25.
4. Moulin, G. and Roux, S. (2006). Suivi des ventes de médicaments vétérinaires contenant des antibiotiques en France en 2004. Rapport de l'AFSSA-ANMV, 2006. 38 p. Available at: http://www.anmv.afssa.fr. Accessed on: 13 November 2007.

5. Rigos, G., Nengas, I., Alexis, M. and Trosi, G.M. (2004). Potential drug (oxytetracycline and oxolinic acid) pollution from Mediterranean sparid farms. *Aquat. Toxicol.* 69: 281–8.

6. Bravo, S., Dolz, H., Silva, M.T., Lagos, C., Millanao, A. and Urbina, M. (2005). Informe final. Diagnostico del uso de fármacos y otros productos químicos en la acuicultura. Universidad Austral de Chile. Facultad de Pesquerias y Oceanografia, Instituto de Acuicultura. Casilla 1327. Puerto Montt, Chile. Proyecto No. 2003–28.

7. Van, P.T. (2005). Current status of aquatic veterinary drugs usage for usage in Aquaculture in Vietnam. In: *Antibiotic Resistance in Asian Aquaculture Environment,* Proceedings of the international workshop held in Chiang Mai, Thailand, February 2005.

8. Schnick, R.A., Alderman, D.J., Armstrong, R., *et al.* (1997). Worldwide aquaculture drug and vaccine registration progress. *Bull. Eur. Assoc. Fish Pat.* 17: 251–60.

9. Guichard, B. and Licek, E. (2006). A comparative study of antibiotics registered for use in farmed fish in European countries. Poster presented at the First OIE Global Conference on Aquatic Animal Health, 10 October 2006, Bergen, Norway.

10. Gunderson, B.W., Ross, G.H., Ibrahim, K.H., Rotschafer, J.C. (2001). What do we really know about antibiotic pharmacodynamics? *Pharmacotherapy* 21: 302–18.

11. Reimschuessel, R., Stewart, L., Squibb, E., *et al.* (2005). Fish drug analysis – Phish-Pharm: a searchable database of pharmacokinetics data in fish. *AAPS J.* 07: E288–E327.

12. Nusbaum, K.E. and Shotts, E.B. (1981). Action of selected antibiotics on four common bacteria associated with diseases of fish. *J. Fish Dis.* 4: 397–404.

13. Inglis, V. and Richards, R.H. (1991). The *in vitro* susceptibility of *Aeromonas salmonicida* and other fish pathogenic bacteria to 29 antimicrobial agents. *J. Fish Dis.* 14: 641–50.

14. Bruun, M.S., Schmidt, A.S., Madsen, L. and Dalsgaard, I. (2000). Antimicrobial resistance patterns in Danish isolates of *Flavobacterium psychrophilum. Aquaculture* 187: 201–212.

15. Michel, C. and Blanc, G. (2001). Minimal inhibitory concentration methodology in aquaculture: the temperature effect. *Aquaculture* 196: 311–8.

16. Uhland, F.C. and Higgins, R. (2006). Evaluation of the susceptibility of *Aeromonas salmonicida* to oxytetracycline and tetracycline using antimicrobial disk diffusion and dilution susceptibility tests. *Aquaculture* 257: 111–7.

17. Smith, P. and Hiney, M. (2005). Towards setting breakpoints for oxolinic acid susceptibility of *Aeromonas salmonicida* using distribution of data generated by standard test protocols. *Aquaculture* 250: 22–6.

18. Miller, R. and Reimschuessel, R. (2006). Epidemiological cutoff values for antimicrobial agents against *Aeromonas salmonicida* isolates determined by frequency distributions of minimal inhibitory concentration and diameter of zone of inhibition data. *Am. J. Vet. Res.* 67: 1837–43.

19. Rybak, M.J. (2006). Pharmacodynamics: relation to antimicrobial resistance. *Am. J. Infect. Control* 34: 38–45.

20. O'Reilly, A. and Smith, P. (1999). Development of methods for predicting the minimum concentrations of oxytetracycline capable of exerting a selection for resistance to this agent. *Aquaculture* 180: 1–11.

21. Clinical and Laboratory Standards Institute. (2006). Methods for broth dilution susceptibility testing of bacteria isolated from aquatic animals. Approved guideline M49-A. Clinical and Laboratory Standards Institute, Wayne, Pennsylvania.

22. EUCAST (2000). Terminology relating to methods for the determination of susceptibility of bacteria to antimicrobial agents. EUCAST Definitive document E. Def 1.2 May 2000. Available at: http://www.srga.org/Eucastwt/eucast-definitions.htm Accessed on: 17 November 2007.

23. Kahlmeter, G., Brown, D.F.J., Goldstein, F.W., *et al.* (2003). European harmonization of MIC breakpoints for antimicrobial susceptibility testing of bacteria. *J. Antimicrob. Chemother.* 52: 145–8.

24. Samuelsen, O.B. (2006). Pharmacokinetics of quinolones in fish: a review. *Aquaculture* 255: 55–75.

25. Björklund, H. and Bylund, G. (1990). Temperature-related absorption and excretion of oxytetracycline in rainbow trout (*Salmo gairdneri* R.). *Aquaculture* 84: 363–72.

26. Kleinow, K.M., Jarboe, H.H. and Shoemaker, K.E. (1994). Comparative pharmacokinetics and bioavailability of oxolinic acid in channel catfish (*Ictalurus punctatus*) and rainbow trout (*Oncorhynchus mykiss*). *Can. J. Fish Aquat. Sci.* 51: 1205–11.

27. Sohlberg, S., Aulie, A. and Söli, N.E. (1994). Temperature-dependent absorption and elimination of flumequine in rainbow trout (*Oncorhynchus mykiss* Waldbaum) in freshwater. *Aquaculture* 119: 1–10.

28. Samuelsen, O.B. (2006). Multiple dose pharmacokinetic study of oxolinic acid in cod, *Gadus morhua* L. *Aquacult. Int.* 14: 443–50.

29. Sohlberg, S., Ingebrigtsen, K., Hansen, M.K., Hayton, W.L. and Horsberg, T.E. (2002). Flumequine in Atlantic salmon *Salmo salar*: disposition in fish held in sea water versus fresh water. *Dis. Aquat. Org.* 49: 39–44.

30. Coyne, R., Smith, P., Dalsgaard, I., *et al.* (2006). Winter ulcer disease of post-smolt Atlantic salmon: an unsuitable case for treatment? *Aquaculture* 253: 171–78.

31. Horsberg, T.E., Hoff, K.A. and Nordmo, R. (1996). Pharmacokinetics of florfenicol and its metabolite florfenicol amine in Atlantic salmon. *J. Aquat. Anim. Health* 8: 292–301.

32. Coyne, R., Bergh, Ø., Samuelsen, O., *et al.* (2004). Attempt to validate breakpoint MIC values estimated from pharmacokinetic data obtained during oxolinic acid therapy of winter ulcer disease in Atlantic salmon (*Salmo salar*). *Aquaculture* 238: 51–66.

33. Coyne, R., Samuelsen, O., Bergh, Ø., *et al.* (2004). On the validity of setting breakpoint minimum inhibition concentrations at one quarter of the plasma concentration achieved following oral administration of oxytetracycline. *Aquaculture* 239: 23–35.

12 Aquaculture

34. Horsberg, T.E. (2003). Aquatic animal medicine. *J. Vet. Pharmacol. Ther.* 26 (Suppl 1): 39–42.

35. Alderman, D. and Smith, P. (2001). Development of draft protocols of standard reference methods for antimicrobial agent susceptibility testing of bacteria associated with fish disease. *Aquaculture* 196: 211–43.

36. Clinical and Laboratory Standards Institute. (2006). Methods for antimicrobial disk susceptibility testing of bacteria isolated from aquatic animals. Approved guideline M42-A. Clinical and Laboratory Standards Institute, Wayne, Pennsylvania.

37. Smith, P. (2006). Breakpoints for disc diffusion susceptibility testing of bacteria associated with fish diseases: a review of current practice. *Aquaculture* 261: 1113–21.

38. NicGabhainn, S., Amedeo, M., Bergh, Ø., *et al.* (2003). The precision and robustness of published protocols for disc diffusion assays of antimicrobial agent susceptibility: an inter-laboratory study. *Aquaculture* 240: 1–18.

39. Huys, G., Cnockaert, M., Bartie, K., *et al.* (2005). Intra- and inter-laboratory performance of antibiotic disk-diffusion-susceptibility testing of bacterial control strains of relevance for monitoring aquaculture environments. *Dis. Aquat. Organ.* 66: 197–204.

40. Kronvall, G., Kahlmeter, G., Myhre, E. and Galas, M.F. (2003). A new method for normalized interpretation of antimicrobial resistance from disk test results for comparative purposes. *Clin. Microbiol. Infect.* 9: 120–32.

41. Smith, P., Hiney, M.P. and Samuelsen, O.B. (1994). Bacterial resistance to antimicrobial agents used in fish farming: a critical evaluation of method and meaning. *Annu. Rev. Fish Dis.* 4: 273–313.

42. Watanabe, T., Aoki, T., Ogata, Y. and Egusa, S.R. (1971). Factors related to fish culture. *Ann. N. Y. Acad. Sci.* 182: 383–410.

43. Smith, D.L., Harris, A.D., Johnson, J.A., Silbergeld, E.K. and Morris, G.J. (2002). Animal antibiotic use has an early but important impact on the emergence of antibiotic resistance in human commensal bacteria. *Proc. Natl. Acad. Sci. USA* 99: 6434–9.

44. Wassenaar, T.M. (2005). Use of antimicrobial agents in veterinary medicine and implications for human health. *Crit. Rev. Microbiol.* 31: 155–69.

45. Sørum, H. (2006). Antimicrobial drug resistance in fish pathogens. In: *Antimicrobial Resistance in Bacteria of Animal Origin* (ed. Aarestrup, F.M.). Washington, DC, USA: American Society for Microbiology Press, pp. 213–38.

46. WHO/FAO/OIE. (2007). Report of a Joint FAO/OIE/WHO Expert Consultation on Antimicrobial Use in Aquaculture and Antimicrobial Resistance, Seoul, Republic of Korea, 13–16 June 2006. World Health Organization, Geneva, p. 97.

47. Grave, K., Markestad, A. and Bangen, M. (1996). Comparison in prescribing patterns of antibacterial drugs in salmonid farming in Norway during the periods 1980–1988 and 1989–1994. *J. Vet. Pharmacol. Ther.* 19: 184–91.

48. Le Breton, A. and Lautraite, A. (2004). Guide de Bonnes Pratiques Sanitaires en Elevages Piscicoles. Comité Interprofessionnel des produits de l'Aquaculture (Eds.). Paris, 285 p.

49. Corsin, F., Mohan, C.V., Padiyar, A., Yamamoto, K., Chanratchakool, P. and Phillips, M.J. Codes of practice and better management: a solution for shrimp health management? In: *Diseases in Asian Aquaculture VI* (eds. Reantaso, M.B., Mohan, C.V., Crumlish, M. and Subasinghe, R.). Fish Health Section, Asian Fisheries Society. (in press).

50. Padiyar, P.A., Phillips, M.J., Bhat, B.V., *et al.* (2005). Cluster level adoption of better management practices in shrimp (*P. monodon*) farming: an experience from Andhra Pradesh, India. In: *Diseases in Asian Aquaculture VI* (eds. Reantaso, M.B., Mohan, C.V., Crumlish, M. and Subasinghe, R.). Fish Health Section, Asian Fisheries Society. (in press).

51. Smith, P. and Hiney, M. (2000). Oil-adjuvanted furunculosis vaccines in commercial fish farms: a preliminary epizootiological investigation. *Aquaculture* 190: 1–9.

52. Annon (1999). Food safety issues associated with products from Aquaculture. Report of a joint FAO/NACA/WHO Study Group. WHO Technical Report Series 883. World Health Organization, Geneva, p. 68.

12 Aquaculture

INDEX